GLENCOE

Administering Medications

Pharmacology for Health Careers

Fourth Edition

Donna F. Gauwitz, R.N., M.S.

Assistant Professor, College of Nursing

Broward Community College, Pembroke Pines, Florida

Phyllis Theiss Bayt, R.N., B.S., C.M.A.

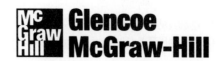

New York, New York   Columbus, Ohio   Woodland Hills, California   Peoria, Illinois

Library of Congress Cataloging-in-Publication Data

Bayt, Phyllis Theiss, 1936–
    Administering medications : pharmacology for health careers /
Phyllis Theiss Bayt, Donna Gauwitz. — 4th ed.
        p.   cm.
    Includes bibliographical references and index.
    ISBN 0-02-804876-8
    1. Drugs—Administration.   2. Pharmacology.   I. Gauwitz, Donna.
II. Title.
    [DNLM: 1. Pharmaceutical Preparations—administration & dosage
Programmed Instruction.   QV 18.2 B361a 2000]
RM147.B39   2000
615'.6—dc21
DNLM/DLC
for Library of Congress   99–15303
                                                                    CIP

While the information, recommendations, and suggestions contained herein are accurate to the best of the authors' knowledge, health care, pharmacology, and drug use are rapidly changing areas. The reader should consult the manufacturer's package insert for current drug product information before administering any drug.

Glencoe/McGraw-Hill
A Division of The **McGraw·Hill** Companies

Administering Medications: Pharmacology for Health Careers, Fourth Edition
Student Text

Send all inquiries to:
Glencoe/McGraw-Hill
8787 Orion Place
Columbus, OH 43240

ISBN 0-02-804876-8 (Student Text)
ISBN 0-02-804877-6 (Instructor's Manual)

Printed in the United States of America

5 6 7 8 9 10   066   06 05 04 03 02

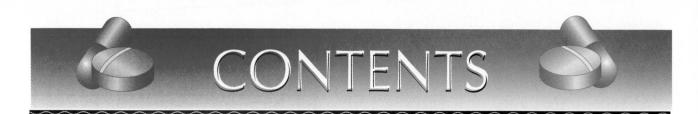

CONTENTS

Administering Medications: Pharmacology for Health Careers is designed to teach the safe administration of medications to health care students entering the nursing, medical assisting, and other allied health care professions. This textbook speaks directly to students and encourages students to identify and apply the concepts learned.

This textbook contains 20 completely revised chapters with one new chapter called "Vitamins, Minerals, and Herbs." Several chapters have been separated into two chapters in order to help students learn and retain fundamental information. "Antibiotics and Antifungals" has been pulled from the former "Drugs for Infection and Cancer" chapter and now makes up the new Chapter 6. "Drugs for the Eye and Ear" has been pulled from the old "Drugs for the Nervous and Sensory Systems" chapter and now makes up the new Chapter 7. "Drugs for the Nervous and Sensory System" is now Chapter 16. The organization of the chapters allows students and instructors to build a knowledge base starting with the fundamentals of medication administration and progressing through the drugs frequently used to treat the most common diseases. Each chapter is organized around a body system to help students fully understand drug actions.

The Chapter Review section contains new knowledge questions on terminology and chapter content. The Case Studies for Critical Thinking section gives students the opportunity to apply what they learned to real life situations. The Application section allows students the chance to familiarize themselves with drug references such as the *PDR*©. Every chapter concludes with an activity using the Internet to expose the student to research and background information that can be found on the World Wide Web.

Also new to this edition is the Patient Education feature. These sidebars contain important patient information for the health care professional to communicate to the patient. This feature also includes cultural diversity and pediatric and geriatric implications where appropriate.

Each chapter has newly revised or added procedures that reflect current practice. These procedures allow students to practice in a step-by-step manner and serve as a tool to facilitate the learning of safe and accurate administration of medication. These procedures are to be practiced under the supervision of an instructor or the nurse in charge. They may be carried out in either a teaching laboratory or on the job. The representative drug tables in Chapters 5–20 have been completely revised with common and frequently prescribed medications.

The Instructor's Manual has similarly been revised to reflect the latest practice and correlate with the textbook. All of the chapter tests have been revised and lengthened to include 60 questions per chapter. The questions are a combination of multiple choice, true or false, completion, and matching. The answers to the chapter review questions formerly found in the textbook are now included in the Instructor's Manual.

New to this edition of the Instructor's Manual are the critical thinking activities which provide students opportunities to practice their critical thinking skills. Also new are the computerized test bank and the instructor's PowerPoint presentation. This presentation allows the instructor to illustrate key points from each chapter. The presentation also includes additional critical thinking questions and questions to prompt classroom discussion. The computerized test bank allows instructors to create their own tests and measure students' knowledge of the chapter content. Correlation Charts for AAMA, AMT, SCANS, and the National Health Care Skills Standards are also included.

Together, the textbook and Instructor's Manual form a complete teaching and learning package. *Administering Medications: Pharmacology for Health Careers* will prepare students to enter the health care field with the knowledge and skills to become a resourceful and safe practitioner and a valuable asset to employers.

ACKNOWLEDGMENTS

I wish to express a heartfelt thank you to the following individuals for their assistance in this fourth edition.

Susan Cole, Executive Editor, for her guidance through this whole worthwhile project.

Sue Diehm, Production Editor, for her assistance throughout the editing phase.

William J. Gauwitz, Jr., my husband and best friend, for his expertise in typing.

I also wish to thank the following reviewers for their valuable critiques and suggestions:

Cindy A. Abel
Ivy Tech State College
Lafayette, Indiana

Sally Christiansen
Waukesha County Technical College
Pewaukee, Wisconsin

Kathleen Hess
Antonelli Medical and Professional Institute
Pottstown, Pennsylvania

Betty Jones
Gaston College
Dallas, North Carolina

Barbara Jorenby
Dakota County Technical College
Rosemount, Minnesota

Linda Oldenburg
Crestview Post-Acute Rehabilitation Services
Portland, Oregon

Kim Parks
Bradford School
Pittsburgh, Pennsylvania

Pat Schrull
Lorain County Community College
Elyria, Ohio

Brendia Winters
Houston Community College
Houston, Texas

Orientation to Medications

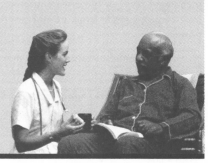

In this chapter you will learn where drugs come from, how they are standardized, and how their use is governed by law. You will also learn how to use drug references and drug cards to gather information about medications.

OBJECTIVES

After studying this chapter, you should be able to

- define *pharmacology, pharmacodynamics, pharmacy, anatomy, physiology,* and *pathology.*
- list the major sources of drugs and give examples of each.
- list the six uses of drugs.
- define drug standards and tell how they are determined.
- explain why drug standards are necessary.
- list and describe four types of names by which drugs are known.
- name three drug references and show how to use at least one.
- use drug references to prepare a drug card.
- name three major drug laws and list their main features.
- name the federal agencies that enforce the drug laws.
- explain why health workers must be familiar with drug laws.

KEY TERMS

action: a drug's chemical effects on body cells

administration: how a drug is given

adverse reaction: an unintended and undesirable effect of a drug

anatomy: the study of the structure of body parts

chemical name: describes the chemical structure of a compound

contraceptives: drugs used to control fertility and prevent pregnancy

contraindications: conditions in which the use of a certain drug is dangerous or ill-advised

controlled substances: potentially dangerous or habit-forming drugs whose sale and use are strictly regulated by law

Controlled Substances Act of 1970: regulates manufacturing and distribu-

tion of controlled substances; also known as Comprehensive Drug Abuse Prevention and Control Act

diagnostic drugs: drugs used to diagnose disease

drug: chemical substance used in the diagnosis, treatment, cure, or prevention of a disease; also called medication

drug card: index card on which you write drug information for your own reference

Drug Enforcement Administration (DEA): since 1973, the only legal U.S. drug enforcement agency

Food, Drug, and Cosmetic Act (FDCA) of 1938: mandates that drug manufacturers test all drugs for potentially harmful effects and that drug labels must be complete

Food and Drug Administration (FDA): enforcement agency for the FDCA

generic name: official nonproprietary name assigned to a drug by the manufacturer, with the approval of the United States Adopted Names Council

health maintenance: developing a healthy lifestyle; keeping existing diseases under control, and getting regular checkups

indications: diseases and disorders for which a certain drug may be used

legend drugs: prescription drugs

nonproprietary name: generic name of a drug

official name: generally, the same as the generic name of a drug; name of drug as it appears in the official reference, the *United States Pharmacopeia/National Formulary (USP/NF)*

over-the-counter (OTC) drugs: drugs available without a prescription

package insert: printed information about a pharmaceutical product

pathology: study of the disease process, including changes in structure and function of the body

pharmacodynamics: study of the body's response to a drug

pharmacokinetics: the absorption, distribution, metabolism, and excretion of drugs

pharmacology: study of drugs (uses, preparation, routes, laws, etc.)

Physicians' Desk Reference (PDR®): a widely used drug reference book that gives information about the drug products of major pharmaceutical companies

physiology: the science that deals with the functions of cells, tissues, and organs of living organisms

precautions: warnings to use care when giving drugs under certain conditions

prescription drugs: drugs that can be dispensed only with a physician's order

proprietary name: brand name of a drug

psychology: study of the normal and abnormal processes of the mind

side effects: desirable or undesirable effects of a drug apart from the primary purpose for giving the drug

standards: rules ensuring uniform quality and purity

synthetic drugs: drugs created in the laboratory from various chemicals

therapeutic effect: desired or predicted physiological response caused by a drug

trade name: licensed name under which a drug prepared by a specific manufacturer is sold; proprietary or brand name

United States Adopted Names (USAN) Council: organization that adopts the generic name of a drug

United States Pharmacopeia Dispensing Information (USPDI): official reference for pharmacists or persons administering medications

United States Pharmacopeia/National Formulary (USP/NF): official book listing standardized drugs

Not long ago, only doctors and nurses were allowed to administer medications. But times are changing; many other members of the health occupations are now asked to give or know about medications. They are also expected to observe how patients react after taking medications. These are important new responsibilities. They demand that you, a member of the health care team working with medications, also have knowledge of many health-related topics. You must know the basic principles of **pharmacology,** which is the study of drugs and their uses. You must understand how the body responds to drugs, or **pharmacodynamics.** You must also understand **pharmacokinetics,** the absorption, distribution, metabolism, and excretion of drugs. These areas require some knowledge of human **anatomy,** the study of body parts, and of **physiology,** the science that deals with the functions of cells, tissues, and organs of living organisms. You must understand the study of disease processes, including changes in the structure and function of the body, or **pathology,** and how drugs change the course of disease. You must also give attention to **psychology,** the study of the normal and abnormal processes of the mind, because a patient's mental state influences how the body reacts to drugs.

This textbook will teach you, step by step, the basics of pharmacology, pharmacodynamics, pharmacokinetics, anatomy, physiology, and pathology. You will also find suggestions for responding to patients' psychological needs, along with information you should tell patients about medications they may be taking. The uses of specific drugs for treatment of disease are discussed in connection with the body systems on which they act. As you learn general principles, most of you will also carry out practice tasks to give you experience in giving medications.

PHARMACOLOGY

A **drug** is a chemical substance used in the diagnosis, treatment, cure, or prevention of a disease. Pharmacology is the study of drugs: their uses, preparation, routes, and laws. Pharmacology includes the study of how drugs affect the human body. In medicine, we are particularly interested in the desired or predicted physiological response that a drug causes. This is the drug's **therapeutic effect.**

Pharmacology attempts to describe a drug's desirable or undesirable effects apart from the primary reason for giving the drug. These are called

side effects. Pharmacology also focuses on the proper amounts of drugs to give and how to give them. Knowledge of the laws and responsibilities surrounding drug use, along with practical experience in giving medications, will prepare you to play a vital role on the health care team.

DRUG SOURCES

Drugs come from four sources: plants, animals, minerals, and from chemicals **(synthetic drugs)** by means of biotechnology or genetic engineering.

Our ancestors long ago discovered that the roots, leaves, and seeds of certain plants had the power to cure illnesses, ease pain, and affect the mind. Today many drugs are still extracted from parts of plants. An example is digitalis, a cardiac glycoside used to treat congestive heart failure. Digitalis is made from a wildflower, purple foxglove. Drugs from the poppy plant are morphine and codeine, which are potent analgesics. Other drugs of plant origin are gums and oils. An example of a gum is psyllium seed, which is a bulk-forming laxative. Castor oil from the castor bean acts as a stimulant laxative.

Drugs of animal origin are prepared by extracting natural substances, such as hormones, from animal tissues and organs. Insulin, for example, is extracted from the pancreas of cattle and pigs. Insulin is a valuable drug used to treat diabetes mellitus by lowering the blood glucose level. Heparin, used to reduce the formation of blood clots, is taken from the intestinal linings of cattle and pigs.

Iron, iodine, calcium, sodium chloride (salt), magnesium hydrochloride (milk of magnesia), and magnesium sulfate (Epsom salts) are examples of minerals used in drug therapy. They are derived from rocks and crystals.

Many drugs are made, or synthesized, in the laboratory through chemical processes. Sulfonamide drugs such as Bactrim and Septra, for example, are frequently used in the treatment of urinary tract infections. An advantage of synthetic drugs is that they are generally less expensive than nonsynthetic drugs because they are produced in mass volume. Biotechnology and genetic engineering patch together DNA material from different organisms, making new drugs and drug products available. Insulin and vaccines can be produced this way. Humulin® insulin is a genetically engineered drug used in the treatment of diabetes mellitus.

DRUG USES

The study of drug uses will give you an understanding of one phase of health care, drug therapy. The four most familiar uses of drugs relate to disease: prevention, treatment, diagnosis, and cure. Two other types of drugs are **contraceptives,** used for the prevention of pregnancy, and drugs to promote **health maintenance.**

Disease prevention involves the administration of drugs, such as vaccines, that inoculate the body against disease microorganisms. Health maintenance helps patients maintain or enhance their current levels of health. Drugs such as vitamins and minerals are given to help keep the body healthy and strong or to keep the body systems functioning normally.

Treating disease means relieving the symptoms while the body's natural disease-fighting mechanisms do their work. Aspirin and antihistamines are examples of drugs used to treat disease symptoms. An antihistamine such as *Benadryl* is an example of a drug used to treat allergy symptoms or motion sickness. Aspirin is used to treat fever and pain. Curing disease often means eliminating disease-causing microorganisms. Antibiotics such as erythromycin and penicillin are drugs given to cure a disease such as pneumonia.

Diagnostic drugs are considered drugs because they are chemical substances used to diagnose or monitor a patient's condition. A diagnostic drug may have side effects and adverse reactions just like any other drug. For example, radiopaque dye (a contrast medium that shows up on fluoroscopes or X rays) is administered to detect gallbladder malfunctions. A radiopaque dye such as iodine may cause anaphylaxis, an immediate, severe, and frequently fatal reaction in a patient previously sensitized to the chemical (iodine). It is therefore important to ask patients if they have a shellfish allergy, which indicates a predisposition to an iodine allergy.

The prevention of pregnancy is possible with the use of contraceptives, drugs that control fertility.

Drugs often have more than one use. The drug promethazine hydrochloride (*Phenergan*), for example, is used in a variety of ways. It can control allergic reactions, treat motion sickness, induce sleep, and prevent vomiting after surgery. Some drugs have the ability to prevent as well as cure or treat disease.

DRUG STANDARDS

Drugs differ widely in strength, quality, and purity, depending on how they are manufactured. To control these differences, certain rules or **standards** have been set up that products must meet. Drug standards are required by law. The law says that all preparations called by the same drug name must be of a uniform strength, quality, and purity. A drug prepared in Indiana must meet the same standards for strength, quality, and purity as the same drug prepared in California or New Jersey. Because of drug standards, physicians who order penicillin, for example, can be sure that patients anywhere in the country will get the same basic substance from the pharmacist. Drug standards also help doctors prescribe accurate dosages and predict the results.

Drugs for which standards have been developed are listed in a special reference book called the **United States Pharmacopeia/National Formulary (USP/NF)**. The *USP/NF* is recognized by the U.S. government as the official list of drug standards, which are enforceable by the U.S. Food and Drug Administration.

Since 1975, USP has engaged in a program to include all drug substances and, to the extent possible, all drug products in the United States. The book is updated regularly, and a new edition is published every five years to keep the information up to date.

DRUG NAMES

All drugs have more than one name. In fact, most have four: a chemical name, a generic name, an official name, and one or more trade names.

The **chemical name** describes the chemical composition and molecular structure of the drug. Acetylsalicylic acid is an example of a chemical name.

The **generic name** is the official **nonproprietary name** assigned by the manufacturer with the approval of the **United States Adopted Names (USAN) Council**. The generic name is simpler than the chemical name. For example, aspirin is the generic name for acetylsalicylic acid.

The **official name** is usually the same as the generic name.

Also known as the brand, product, or **proprietary name,** the **trade name** is the name under which the drug is sold by a specific manufacturer. The name is owned by the drug company, and no other company may use it. The symbol ® to the right of the name shows that its use is restricted. A drug that is manufactured by several companies may be known by several different trade names. For example, the drug with the generic name nitroglycerin is sold by several manufacturers under such trade names as *Nitro-Bid, Nitrong,* and *Nitrostat. Bufferin* is an example of a trade, proprietary, or brand name for aspirin.

PRODUCT NAME DRUGS VERSUS GENERICS

Most drugs are known to the general public by their trade names. *Procardia* and *Adalat* are much more familiar sounding to someone who is not in the profession than is the name nifedipine. But you and your fellow health workers must be familiar with both the trade and generic names of many drugs. First, a physician may prescribe a drug by a generic name or a trade name. Because several brand names may exist for the same ingredient, such as acetaminophen, physicians are encouraged to order drugs by their generic names. In fact, state and federal governments now permit, encourage, and, in some cases, mandate that the consumer be given the generic form when buying prescription drugs. Another reason for using generic names is that it avoids confusion among similar trade names. A prescription written for a generic product allows the pharmacist to choose among nonbranded drugs available from several companies. Generic drugs are therapeutically equivalent to and much cheaper than trade name drugs.

Another reason for knowing the generic name is that drugs often have several trade names but only one generic name. If you learn the generic names, you can organize information about several trade name drugs in your mind. Of course, it is not possible to memorize all the generic and trade names for medications, but you should try to become familiar with both names of the drugs you handle daily in your work.

Where we mention specific drugs, generic names are given first and are not capitalized. Trade names are capitalized and shown in parentheses following the generic names. Only one or two common trade names are given in each case. Keep in mind that many other trade name products may be available.

DRUG REFERENCES

Several reference books provide useful information about drugs on the market. Doctors, nurses, and others in the health occupations often refer to them when planning and administering drug therapy. Drug references can help you understand why and how a particular drug is administered. For each drug, they usually include the following information:

- **description**—what the drug is made of
- **action**—how the drug works
- **indications**—what conditions the drug is used for
- **interactions**—undesirable effects produced when drugs are taken with food or with other drugs
- **contraindications**—conditions under which the drug should not be used
- **precautions**—specific warnings to consider when administering drugs to patients with specific conditions or diseases
- **adverse reactions**—unintended and undesirable effects
- **dosage and administration**—correct dose for each possible route of administration
- **how supplied**—how the drug is packaged and stored

Learning how to use the drug references will help you meet the new responsibilities of health workers in administering medications.

A common reference book is the *Physicians' Desk Reference (PDR®)*, which is available in most health facilities. The *PDR®* gives information about the drug products of major pharmaceutical companies. It is useful for checking clinical pharmacology, mechanism of action, indications, contraindications, warnings, precautions, adverse reactions, overdosage, dosage and administration, and how the product is supplied. It lists drugs by their product, generic, and chemical names and manufacturers. Color photographs in a "Product Identification" section help you identify some drugs.

The **United States Pharmacopeia Dispensing Information (USPDI)** is another drug reference, first published in 1980 in three volumes. It provides pharmacists and other health care workers with easy-to-follow information about official drugs and products. You will find Volume II useful, as this volume is written in nontechnical language that is easy for patients to understand. It is called *Advice for the Patient*. Volume III is the "Orange Book," *Approved Drug Products and Legal Requirements*. This volume includes state and federal requirements for prescribing and dispensing drugs. These volumes are updated each month in the *USPDI Update*.

Another valuable reference is the *Handbook of Nonprescription Drugs*, published by the American Pharmaceutical Association. It deals with over-the-counter information in general categories. Pharmacology textbooks and articles in nursing and other professional journals are also helpful sources of information. Some health care facilities keep their own reference lists of the drugs they use most often.

Another reference is the *American Hospital Formulary Service (AHFS) Information Book*. It contains an objective overview, in outline form, of almost every drug available in the United States. This book is updated yearly, and information is easily located with just one index at the back of the book.

COPING WITH TECHNICAL LANGUAGE

A problem with many drug references is that they are written in complex language. They use medical terms that may be unfamiliar, especially to new students. The descriptions of drugs assume that the reader has a background in anatomy, physiology, diseases, and pharmacology.

An important aim of this book is to help you learn enough about anatomy, physiology, diseases, and pharmacology to understand what you find in different drug references. You will learn important technical terms, basic principles to help you understand how drugs work, and basic information about various diseases to understand why a particular drug is prescribed.

COPING WITH CHANGING INFORMATION

Information about drugs is constantly changing. New drugs appear all the time, and old drugs are taken off the market. Drug research turns up better ways of using drugs and administering them. This means that drug references can become quickly outdated. Some reference publishers send out regular supplements with information updates. These should be checked along with the drug reference. Another place to look for current information on drug administration is **package inserts.** These are printed sheets of information inside the boxes in which drugs are packaged. This is the same information provided in the *PDR*®.

This text will help you cope with changing information on drugs. After studying the various chapters, you will know general principles about groups or classifications of drugs. Any new information that becomes available should then fit easily into your general understanding of drugs.

PREPARING YOUR OWN DRUG CARDS

Because there are so many drugs and so much information about them, no one can expect to keep all of the important facts constantly in mind. Many health workers find it useful to prepare 5 × 7 index cards containing information about the drugs they most often use in their work. This saves time, because they can find the information more quickly in their card files than in a huge drug reference. Of course, the information on the cards must be updated regularly to remain current. **Drug cards** can be designed according to your own needs. They should include this information:

- Drug name, both generic and trade.
- Drug classification, or the group a drug belongs to, such as analgesics (pain relievers), antipyretics (fever reducers), antacids, laxatives, and so on (you will learn the basic drug classifications in later chapters).
- Forms in which the drug is available (tablets, capsules, etc.).
- Action, or how the drug interacts with the organs or systems that it is supposed to affect.
- Uses of the drug.
- Side effects and adverse reactions.
- Signs of drug poisoning (toxicity).
- Route of administration.
- Dosage range and usual adult dose.
- Special instructions for giving the medication, including nursing care required (for example, what to tell the patient about expected side effects and precautions, and so on).
- A note on where you got your information (specific drug reference, package insert, etc.).

A sample drug card is shown in Figure 1.1. Beginning with Chapter 6, you will find tables at the ends of chapters listing representative drugs in the major drug categories. These tables can serve as a guide for what to include on your drug cards. As you study the drugs in Chapters 6 through 20, make a habit of preparing drug cards for the medications you expect to be giving in your health facility.

Drug
Acetaminophen (*Tylenol*)

Action
Blockade of prostaglandin stimulation of the central nervous system.
Increases peripheral blood flow and sweating.

Uses
Fever reduction, temporary relief of mild or moderate pain.

Doses
Adults and teenagers 325-500 mg every 3-4 hours, 650 mg every
4-6 hours, 1000 mg every 6 hours as needed.

Side Effects
Yellow eyes or skin (rare), bloody or black stools, pain in side and lower back, skin rash, hives, or itching; sores, ulcers or white spots on the lips or mouth, sore throat, sudden decrease in the amount of urine;
unusual bleeding or bruising; unusual tiredness or weakness.

Figure 1.1
Sample drug card.

DRUG LEGISLATION

The U.S. government regulates the composition, uses, names, labeling, and testing of drugs. Since the early 1900s, many laws have been passed to enforce the official drug standards and to protect the public from unreliable and unsafe drugs. Federal agencies have been set up to see that these laws are followed. Table 1.1 lists the major drug laws and their enforcing agencies.

TABLE 1.1: Major Drug Laws

LEGISLATIVE ACT	ENFORCEMENT AGENCY
Pure Food and Drug Act of 1906 Approves *USP/NF* and requires that drugs meet official standards Requires labeling of medicines containing morphine and other narcotics Amendment of 1912 prohibits making false claims about health benefits of a drug	None
Food, Drug, and Cosmetic Act (FDCA) of 1938 (replaced the 1906 act) Regulates content and sale of drugs and cosmetics Requires accurate labeling and warnings against unsafe use Requires government review of safety studies before selling new drugs Amendment of 1952 allows certain drugs to be dispensed by prescription only and refilled only on a doctor's order; also recognizes OTC drugs as drugs that do not require a prescription Amendment of 1962 requires proof of effectiveness and safety before marketing new drugs and full information on advantages, side effects, contraindications Certain drugs must carry Warning label indicating a side effect or if drug may be habit-forming Certain drugs must carry label "Caution: Federal law prohibits dispensing without a prescription"	**Food and Drug Administration (FDA)** Under Department of Health and Human Services Can investigate manufacturers, withdraw approval of drugs, control shipment, and testing Enforces FDCA by prosecuting offending firms and seizing goods Drug manufacturers must register with FDA and report to FDA all adverse reactions resulting from use of their products Reviews studies of safety and effectiveness of new drugs
Controlled Substances Act of 1970 Identifies and regulates manufacture and sale of narcotics and dangerous drugs Provides research into drug abuse, prevention, and dependence Provides funding for education on drug abuse, rehabilitation, and law enforcement Classifies drugs into Schedules I–V according to medical usefulness and possible abuse (Table 1.2)	**Drug Enforcement Administration (DEA)** Under Department of Justice May punish violators by fines, imprisonment, or both
Drug Regulation and Reform Act of 1978 Permits briefer investigation of new drugs, allowing consumers earlier access	FDA
Orphan Drug Act of 1983 Speeds up drugs' availability for patients with rare diseases	FDA
Drug Price Competition and Patent Term Restoration Act of 1984 Permits generic drug companies to prove bioequivalence without duplicating costly clinical trials done by original drug manufacturer Gives longer patent protection for new drugs	FDA

The first law, the Pure Food and Drug Act, was passed in 1906. This law states that only drugs listed in the *USP/NF* may be prescribed and sold, because these drugs meet the required standards. Various amendments to this act regulate prescriptions, require testing of new drugs, and call for complete information about drug effects and dangers. The **Food, Drug, and Cosmetic Act (FDCA) of 1938,** which replaced the 1906 act, spells out additional regulations concerning purity, strength, effectiveness, safety, labeling, and packaging of drugs. It also states that the federal government must review safety studies on new drugs before they can be put on the market. This provision was added after more than 100 deaths resulted from a poorly tested and mislabeled sulfanilamide product. This solution had been marketed as an "elixir" without investigating its toxicity. The FDCA is enforced by the **Food and Drug Administration (FDA).** Since 1962, the FDA has required proof that new drugs are effective as well as safe.

Another important law is the **Controlled Substances Act of 1970,** also known as the Comprehensive Drug Abuse Prevention and Control Act. It identifies the drugs that are dangerous or subject to abuse, such as narcotics, depressants, and stimulants. This law strictly regulates the manufacturing and distribution of controlled substances. It clearly stipulates that possession of a controlled substance is unlawful without a prescription. This law provides research into preventing drug abuse and drug dependence. It also provides for treatment and rehabilitation of drug abusers. It further improves the administration and regulation of the manufacture, distribution, and dispensing of controlled substances.

Controlled substances are grouped into five categories, or schedules, each with its particular restrictions, as shown in Table 1.2. Drugs with the highest abuse potential are placed in Schedule I. They have no accepted medical use in the United States. Drugs with the lowest abuse potential are placed in Schedule V. You need to be aware that these classifications are flexible. Occasionally, drugs may be added to a schedule or changed from one schedule to another

TABLE 1.2: Drug Classifications Under the Controlled Substances Act of 1970[a]

DRUGS	CHARACTERISTICS	EXAMPLES
Schedule I Drugs	High potential for abuse, severe physical and psychological dependence No accepted medical use To be used for research only Not to be prescribed: unsafe in treatment	Alfentanil, fenethylline, hashish, heroin, lysergic acid diethylamide (LSD), marijuana, methaqualone (*Quaalude*), peyote, psilocybin
Schedule II Drugs	High potential for abuse, severe physical and psychological dependence Acceptable medical uses, with restrictions Dispensed by prescription only No refills without new written prescription from physician	Amphetamines, cocaine, meperidine HCl (*Demerol*), methadone, methylphenidate hydrochloride (*Ritalin*), morphine, opium, pentobarbital (*Nembutal*), anabolic steroids, hydromorphone hydrochloride (*Dilaudid*)
Schedule III Drugs	Moderate potential for abuse, high psychological dependence, low physical dependence Acceptable medical uses By prescription only; may be refilled five times in 6 months if authorized by physician	Barbiturates, butabarbital (*Butisol*), glutethimide (*Doriden*), secobarbital (*Seconal*), *Tylenol* with codeine
Schedule IV Drugs	Lower potential for abuse than Schedule III drugs; limited psychological and physical dependence Acceptable medical uses By prescription only; may be refilled five times in 6 months if authorized by physician	Chloral hydrate (*Noctec*), chlordiazepoxide (*Librium*), diazepam (*Valium*), flurazepam HCl (*Dalmane*), oxazepam (*Serax*), phenobarbital, propoxyphene HCl (*Darvon*), lorazepam (*Ativan*), meprobamate (*Equanil*), pentazocine HCl (*Talwin*), alprazolam (*Xanax*)
Schedule V Drugs	Low potential for abuse Acceptable medical uses OTC narcotic drugs, but sold only by registered pharmacists; buyer must be 18 years and show ID	Cough syrups with codeine, e.g., guaifenesin (*Naldecon DX*) and *Cheracol* with codeine, diphenoxylate HCl with atropine sulfate (*Lomotil*[b]), *Novahistine* expectorant, *Parepectolin*

[a] Source: DEA, U.S. Department of Justice. Check with your local DEA office for current regulations.
[b] Requires a prescription.

without new legislation. A record is kept of each time a controlled substance is sold and of the amount. There are restrictions on how prescriptions can be refilled. All prescriptions must be written in ink. Oral emergency orders for Schedule II substances may be filled, but the physician must provide a written prescription within 72 hours.

Pharmacists must carefully follow the rules outlined in the Controlled Substances Act. Violation of the law is punishable by fine or imprisonment or both. The agency that enforces this act is the **Drug Enforcement Administration (DEA).**

Doctors must also follow the law in prescribing controlled substances. They need a special license, from the DEA, for each office from which they practice and must renew or register their licenses each year. They are given one tax stamp and number for each license. This number, called the DEA number, must be shown on any prescription for controlled substances.

To keep a supply of controlled substances in an office or a health facility, the staff must fill out special order forms and records. These forms show how many controlled substances are being kept at the facility, as well as who received doses of the drugs and how unused doses were disposed of. A physical inventory of all controlled substances in the office must be made every two years. (You will learn about these forms in Chapter 4.)

All drugs fall into one of the following categories:

- **controlled substances**—these are drugs that have special restrictions as to who can prescribe and sell them and how often they can be prescribed
- **over-the-counter (OTC) drugs**—these can be bought and sold without a prescription
- **prescription drugs**—also called **legend drugs,** these are drugs that require a doctor's prescription (either oral or written) to be bought and sold

YOU AND THE LAW

As a member of the health care team, you are responsible for knowing the laws controlling drug use and the names of the regulatory agencies, such as the Federal Trade Commission (FTC) and the Consumer Product Safety Commission. The latter commission enforces the Poison Prevention Packaging Act (PPPA), which mandates "childproof" drug packaging. Claiming ignorance of the law will not stand up in court if you are ever accused of irresponsible handling and administration of drugs.

How can you be sure you understand the law? As a first step, study carefully Tables 1.1 and 1.2. These tables summarize a great deal of information about federal drug laws. Be aware that the specific drugs under each schedule in the Controlled Substances Act may change. Your health facility will have an up-to-date list of controlled substances from the DEA. Get copies of federal drug laws from the library or from the FDA.

As a next step, study the laws of your state. State laws regulate such things as who may give medications, what kinds of training and supervision are required, who may keep the records, and who may take prescriptions over the phone.

Your own health agency will also have regulations for you to follow. There will be special rules, for example, if your agency receives Medicaid or Medicare funds. You should also be aware of the lines of authority in your agency—in other words, who is in charge of what and who supervises whom. You will then be able to go to the right person when you have a legal question about giving a certain drug.

Knowing the law helps to protect you from errors and possible lawsuits. But there is a more important benefit—the safety of your patient. By showing your awareness of drug laws, you help to educate your patients. You also gain their cooperation in following the law. Drug laws are designed to protect the public. Members of the public depend on your example and your support.

Define each of the terms listed below.

1. Drug _____

_____

2. Pharmacology _____

_____

3. Anatomy _____

_____

4. Physiology _____

_____

5. Drug standards _____

_____

6. PDR® _____

_____

7. USP/NF _____

_____

8. Pathology _____

_____

9. Pharmacokinetics _____

_____

Answer the following questions in the spaces provided.

10. Name four sources of drugs, and give an example of a drug that comes from each source.

Source	Example
_____	_____
_____	_____
_____	_____
_____	_____

11. Name the six therapeutic uses of drugs. Give examples.

Use	Example
_____	_____
_____	_____
_____	_____
_____	_____
_____	_____
_____	_____

12. Name the three major drug laws and the agencies that enforce them.

Law and Date   Enforcing Agency

_____   _____

_____   _____

_____   _____

13. Differentiate between these legal classifications for drugs.

OTC drugs _____

_____

_____

_____

prescription drugs _____

_____

_____

_____

controlled substances _____

_____

_____

_____

From Column 2, select the term or phrase that best matches each item in Column 1.

	Column 1	Column 2
_____	14. Chemical name	a. *Bufferin*
_____	15. Generic name	b. aspirin
_____	16. Trade name	c. acetylsalicylic acid
_____	17. *PDR*®	d. contains information about drug products provided by pharmaceutical companies
_____	18. USAN	e. same as generic name
_____	19. Official name	f. system that adopts generic names

Match the drugs to their schedules or classes as spelled out in the Controlled Substances Act of 1970.

	Schedule	Drugs
_____	20. I	a. *Seconal, Doriden, Tylenol* with codeine
_____	21. II	b. opium, morphine, *Demerol*, amphetamines, *Dilaudid*
_____	22. III	c. cough syrup with codeine, *Lomotil, Novahistine* expectorant
_____	23. IV	d. *Librium, Valium*, phenobarbital, *Noctec, Dalmane, Darvon*
_____	24. V	e. heroin, hashish, LSD, peyote, alfentanil

Continued

■ CASE STUDIES FOR CRITICAL THINKING

Respond to the following situation in the space provided.

25. Janie has just been hired for a new job in a nursing home. She wants to make sure that she knows what she is and is not allowed to do with regard to giving medications. What advice would you give her?

_____

_____

_____

_____

26. Why do we have drug standards and drug laws?

_____

_____

_____

_____

■ APPLICATIONS

Obtain a current copy of the PDR® and a medical dictionary from your school, nursing unit, or clinic. Use them to answer the questions that follow.

27. You are giving Mr. Jones regular-strength *Tylenol* every few hours after surgery. You would like to know something more about the drug, so you consult the *PDR®*. *Tylenol* is a product or trade name. Find the section in the *PDR®* that lists drugs alphabetically by product names. What color are the pages?

_____

The *PDR®* is divided into seven sections:

Manufacturer's Index (white pages): Names and addresses of drug companies, along with a list of drugs manufactured by each company.

Product Name Index (pink): Drugs listed alphabetically by generic/chemical and product names.

Product Category Index (blue): Drugs grouped according to their effects (e.g., analgesics, anesthetics, decongestants).

Generic and Chemical Name Index (yellow): Product names grouped under their generic or chemical names.

Product Identification Section (glossy): Full-color photograph and page numbers of selected medications, a quick reference for routine identification or in case of overdose or accidental poisoning.

Product Information (white): Main part of the book; gives detailed information about drug products, listed alphabetically by drug company.

Diagnostic Product Information (green): Special section for drugs used to diagnose diseases.

Continued

28. Look up *Tylenol* in the section you turned to in question 27. How many different forms of *Tylenol* are listed there? _____ Is there a small diamond to the left of any *Tylenol* form? If so, that means there is a photograph of it in the "Product Identification" section. Find the photograph.

29. Using the page number given for *Tylenol* tablets, look them up in the "Product Information" section. The generic name is listed just after the word *Tylenol*. What is it? _____

 *Inter*NET CONNECTION

There are a number of Internet Web sites that provide drug information. One pertinent site belongs to the Food and Drug Administration of the United States (http://www.fda.gov). Listed are topics on foods, cosmetics, animal and human drugs, and tobacco. Click on the Human Drug heading and explore the information presented. You will see information on the latest drug news, new drug approvals, and consumer drug information.

CHAPTER 2

Principles of Drug Action

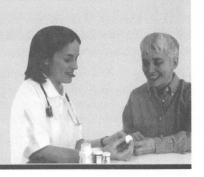

*I*n this chapter you will learn what happens to drugs when they enter the human body and how they produce their effects. You will study how drugs are affected by normal body processes, by characteristics of individual patients, and by the method and time of administration. You will also become familiar with the adverse reactions that can occur with drug administration.

OBJECTIVES

After studying this chapter, you should be able to

- state the four basic drug actions.
- name and describe the four body processes that affect drug action.
- identify at least 10 factors influencing drug action.
- differentiate between systemic and local drug effects.
- state the difference between the therapeutic effect and side effects.
- differentiate among synergism, antagonism, and potentiation.
- explain the difference between psychological and physical drug dependence.
- list five commonly abused drugs.
- state the health worker's responsibilities with regard to adverse reactions, drug dependence, and drug abuse.

KEY TERMS

absorption: passage of a substance into the bloodstream from the site of administration

action: the chemical changes in body cells and tissues caused by a drug

adverse reactions: dangerous or unexpected effects of drugs

allergy: reaction of the body cell to a foreign substance (antigen) to which it has previously developed antibodies

antagonism: the interaction of two drugs to inhibit or cancel each other's effect

antibody: a substance produced in the body that helps the body fight off foreign invaders like microorganisms and antigens

antigen: substance that stimulates production of antibodies and causes allergic reactions

biotransformation: normal body process by which substances are chemically

broken down into a water-soluble form that the body can excrete; part of the cells' work of burning fuel for growth and energy; also known as *metabolism*

capillaries: tiny blood vessels with very thin walls that let certain substances pass through them

cumulative effect: increased effects of a drug that is not completely metabolized or excreted before another dose is administered

dependence: a compulsion to continue taking a drug; can be physical and/or psychological

detoxify: eliminate substances that are toxic or poisonous to the body

distribution: transport of drugs to body cells and spaces between cells

drug abuse: taking drugs for their mood-altering effects or taking too many drugs or too much of a drug

drug misuse: overuse or careless use of any drug

dyspnea: difficult or labored breathing

effect: a physical or psychological change in a patient brought about by a drug

enzyme: a chemical that speeds up biotransformation

excretion: the removal of waste substances from the body

histamine: substance released from injured cells during an allergic reaction, responsible for allergic symptoms

idiosyncrasy: a peculiar, unusual, individual response to a drug

local: having an effect in the immediate area of administration; for example, eye-drops designed to affect only the eye

metabolism: also known as *biotransformation*

overdose: drug dose that is too large for a person's age, size, or physical condition

pharmacokinetics: study of how drugs are absorbed, distributed, metabolized, and excreted by the body

placebo: an inactive substance that has no pharmacological effect (a placebo can be a pill containing sugar or an injection of normal saline/sterile water)

potentiation: two drugs administered at the same time where one drug increases the effect of the other

reservoir: a tissue where drugs tend to collect; different drugs tend to collect in different tissues

side effects: desirable or undesirable drug effects that are not part of the treatment goal

synergism: drug interaction in which the effect of two drugs in combination is greater than the effect of each drug given separately

systemic: having an effect throughout the body

therapeutic effect: main reason for which a drug is administered

tolerance: need for increased dose of a drug to produce the same physical and/or psychological effect

toxicity: poisonous effect of prolonged exposure to high doses or too-frequent administration of a drug

withdrawal symptoms: set of physical reactions that occur when a person stops taking a drug on which he or she is physically dependent

PHARMACOKINETICS

Pharmacokinetics is the study of a drug during absorption, distribution, metabolism, and excretion. It refers to how the body handles a drug from the site of administration to the elimination of the drug. The extent to which a drug completes the processes of absorption, distribution, metabolism, and excretion depends on its ability to cross the cell membrane and the rate at which it can do so. Some drugs are free to cross the membrane, while others encounter barriers. Barriers can include either a single layer of cells or several layers of cells, such as the skin.

DRUG ACTION

Drugs are chemicals that are known to have specific effects on the body. When one of these chemicals comes in contact with body cells, it causes changes in the cell molecules. That is, the chemical combines with or alters the molecules in body cells so as to change the way the cells work. The four main drug actions are depressing, stimulating, destroying cells, and replacing substances.

Drugs do not cause cells to function in entirely new and different ways, however. Usually they either slow down or speed up the ordinary processes that the cells carry out. For example, antihistamines slow the body's natural reactions to irritation, and stimulants speed up the energy-producing functions of cells.

Some drugs destroy certain cells or parts of cells. For example, some antibiotics kill disease microorganisms, and fluorouracil (5 FU) and methotrexate kill cancer cells. Other drugs, such as potassium chloride and calcium carbonate, act to replace or supplement natural substances that the body lacks because of an organ malfunction or poor nutrition. Insulin is a drug taken, in insulin-dependent diabetes mellitus, because the pancreas is unable to produce insulin to maintain normal blood glucose levels.

Once a drug is taken, it enters into certain processes that go on in the body at all times. These processes are the body's normal means of using food and oxygen to produce energy. Energy is needed for cell growth and repair, for warmth, and for movement. Drugs are treated just like any other substance that enters the body, such as food, drink, and air. The only difference is that each drug interacts in a different way with the normal processes carried on by body cells.

These interactions are determined by many things: the size and shape of the drug molecules, their ability to dissolve in water or fat, the pH balance of drugs and cells, and the electrical charges of molecules. You should have an understanding of four basic body processes that affect drug action: absorption, distribution, metabolism/biotransformation, and excretion (Figure 2.1).

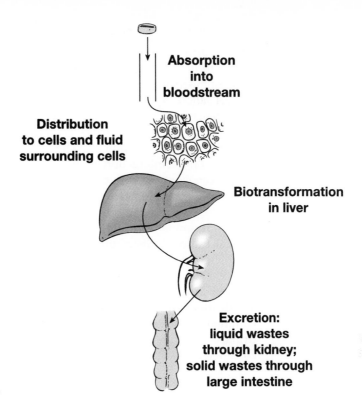

Figure 2.1
How the human
body handles drugs.

Absorption
into
bloodstream

Distribution
to cells and fluid
surrounding cells

Biotransformation
in liver

Excretion:
liquid wastes
through kidney;
solid wastes through
large intestine

ABSORPTION

The passage of a drug from the site of administration into the bloodstream is called **absorption.** How quickly a drug is absorbed is important because it determines how soon a drug becomes available to exert its action. The rate of absorption is influenced by the route of administration, the ability of the drug to dissolve, and the conditions at the site of absorption. The various routes of absorption include sublingual, oral, subcutaneous, intramuscular, intravenous, and topical. Most drugs, except topical drugs (those that are applied to the skin), must enter the bloodstream to have a therapeutic effect.

If the drug is not properly absorbed, it may not reach the organs or tissues that it is supposed to affect. The speed of absorption and the amount of absorption are important in pharmacodynamics. Drug action depends on how quickly and completely the drug is absorbed. When an exact serum level is important, blood tests can be ordered to find out how much drug is present in the bloodstream after absorption.

Sublingual drugs are placed under the tongue to dissolve and are absorbed into the bloodstream directly through the lining of the mouth. Oral drugs are swallowed and enter the bloodstream through the walls of the stomach or intestine. Subcutaneous drugs that are injected just below the skin are absorbed more slowly than intramuscular drugs, which are injected into the muscle. Intravenous drugs are administered directly into the bloodstream and have the fastest and most dependable absorption (Table 2.1).

TABLE 2.1: Drug Absorption

ROUTE OF ADMINISTRATION	ABSORPTION BEGINS	EXAMPLE
Sublingual	In the mouth	Nitroglycerin
Oral	In the stomach/intestine	Ibuprofen
IM	In the muscle	Meperidine
SUBQ, SC	Under the skin	Epinephrine, insulin
IV	In the blood stream	Antibiotics, antineoplastics

DISTRIBUTION

After a drug is absorbed, the transportation of that drug from the bloodstream to the body tissues and intended site of action is called **distribution.** Some of the drug passes out of the bloodstream through the thin walls of tiny vessels called **capillaries.** The drug then enters body cells through pores in the outer cell layers. It may also pass through cells into the fluid-filled spaces between the cells. Some drugs, such as alcohol, pass through the capillaries and enter the tissues quickly. The exact path that any given drug follows depends on the interaction between the drug and specific body tissues. Some tissues can combine with certain drugs and others cannot.

Drug distribution is affected by the chemical makeup of the drug, the amount given, the size of the patient, and the amount of protein in the blood. If distribution is slow, the effect of the drug is not felt until some time after administration. If distribution is fast, drug effects are noticed almost immediately after administration.

Some drugs tend to collect in certain organs or tissues, called drug **reservoirs.** If drugs do collect in reservoirs, they are released into the body more slowly than drugs that are evenly distributed at the start. For example, common sulfonamide drugs, such as *Bactrim* and *Septra,* often prescribed for urinary tract infections, are released slowly from tissues and are therefore considered long-lasting antibiotics.

METABOLISM/BIOTRANSFORMATION

Metabolism, or **biotransformation,** is a series of chemical reactions that inactivate a drug by converting it into a water-soluble compound so that it can be excreted by the body. This is a natural process much like the digestion of food. It is necessary so that the body can rid itself of the waste products left over after the cells make use of nutrients or drugs.

The process of metabolism occurs under the influence of **enzymes,** which are proteins. They cause chemical changes in a drug. These enzymes not only break down the drug, but also **detoxify,** or eliminate substances that are toxic to the body. Most of the metabolism and detoxification of drugs takes place in the liver. Some metabolism also takes place to some extent in the lungs, the intestines, the kidneys, and the blood.

If a person is elderly or has a decrease in liver function, there may be insufficient metabolism of the drug, and the risk for drug toxicity develops. As a member of the health care team, it is important for you to be aware of the common signs of drug toxicity.

EXCRETION

Excretion is the body's way of removing the waste products of ordinary cell processes. Drugs are excreted in the same way as other waste products. Most drugs leave the body through the kidneys and the large intestine. In the kidneys, blood is filtered and liquid waste products collect in the form of urine. In the large intestine, undigested solid wastes collect in the form of feces.

Excretion also takes place in the lungs, where gaseous wastes, such as carbon dioxide and some types of drugs, are collected from the bloodstream. These are excreted when the person exhales. Some drugs are excreted in the sweat and some even in hair. Milk glands also excrete some types of drugs. This is an important fact to know when giving medications to nursing mothers. Drugs that leave the body in a mother's milk may cause harm to the baby.

If a drug is excreted quickly, its effects are short-lived. If it is excreted slowly, its effects last longer. The rate of excretion depends on the chemical composition of the drug, the rate of metabolism, and how often the drug is administered. The condition of the excreting organs also determines how quickly and completely excretion takes place.

When a person is elderly or has kidney disease, there is an increased risk of toxicity from exposures to high doses of a drug. The dose may have to be reduced. As a member of the health care team, it is important for you to be prepared to teach patients about the excretion of drugs.

PATIENT EDUCATION

Excretion of Drugs

- Increase fluid intake to aid in excretion of drugs.
- Avoid taking laxatives, because they speed up drug excretion.
- Improper diet and lack of activity slow excretion of drugs.
- After general anesthesia, coughing and deep breathing help eliminate the anesthetic more quickly.

- Keep the skin clean to avoid irritation from drugs eliminated through the sweat glands.
- Chew gum or suck hard candy, such as lemon drops, to decrease the unpleasant effects of drugs eliminated through the saliva.
- Pregnant women should discuss all drugs, including over-the-counter drugs, with their physician to avoid possible risk to the fetus.

FACTORS AFFECTING DRUG ACTION

No two people are exactly alike, and no drug affects every human body in exactly the same way. Likewise, an individual may not react the same way to two doses of the same drug. Responses to drug action differ according to age, size, sex, genetics, physiological and pathological conditions, and psychological factors. These personal characteristics may cause slightly different drug actions in different people who receive the same drug.

Factors surrounding the administration of medications may also cause differences in people's responses to a drug. The route of administration, the time of day, the number and size of doses, diet, and environmental conditions all play a role in drug action. Physicians take these factors into account before deciding which drug to prescribe and how much to prescribe.

AGE

All drugs have standard doses that are considered safe for infants, children, and adults.

Infants' body systems are not fully developed. They lack the necessary enzymes to metabolize drugs. Growing children must not take drugs that might affect their development. The body systems of the elderly may not function as efficiently as in middle age. Older adults have decreases in kidney and liver function, which result in failure to completely metabolize or excrete drugs. For these reasons, smaller doses and different drugs are required in treating the young or the old.

SIZE

A person's size and whether he or she is fat or lean have a bearing on drug action. The goal of drug therapy is to maintain a certain concentration of a drug to achieve a desired result in the body. The proper adult dose is calculated according to a specific formula based on age and body weight. For example, the average adult dose is calculated to produce a particular effect in individuals between the ages of 15 and 65 and weighing 150 pounds.

As a result of this standard formula, drug doses for children and for elderly, very thin, and obese individuals must be calculated according to body weight. An obese individual requires a higher dose of a drug to achieve the desired result because of the high percentage of body fat. A drug works more quickly and effectively in a thin individual with a lower amount of body fat. An elderly person usually requires a smaller dose of a drug because of decreased size.

DIET

Combining certain drugs with certain foods can alter the drug's effects. For example, the effects of tetracycline (an antibiotic) are decreased when it is taken with milk and milk products. Foods rich in vitamin K, such as green leafy vegetables, decrease the effects of Coumadin on blood clotting. The absorption of the fat-soluble vitamins (A, D, E, and K) is decreased when taking mineral oil for constipation.

SEX

The sex of an individual can influence drug action. Women may react more strongly to certain drugs than men do. This is partly because of their generally smaller size and their higher proportion of body fat. Pregnant women must be extremely careful about taking any medication and must avoid taking medications without first consulting with their physician, because some drugs may harm the fetus.

GENETIC FACTORS

Each person's individual makeup causes slight differences in basic processes like metabolism and excretion, which then affect drug action. Some people are more sensitive to a drug because they lack the naturally occurring enzymes to break down drugs for excretion.

PATHOLOGICAL CONDITIONS

Diseases can strongly affect how patients respond to drugs. Disease may impair the organs necessary for metabolism and excretion. Diseases of the liver and kidneys, especially, affect the processing and elimination of drugs. Heart disease, kidney failure, diabetes, and low blood pressure are disorders known to require special care when prescribing drugs. But any disease can change the effectiveness of a drug without warning. For example, a patient who is experiencing severe cancer pain needs stronger opiates to achieve a therapeutic effect.

PSYCHOLOGICAL FACTORS

The patient's mental state is an important factor in the success or failure of drug therapy. A patient with a positive attitude is likely to respond well to medication. A patient who is in a state of depression or despair may not respond to some drugs. Strong feelings such as worry, jealousy, anger, or fear may have a noticeable effect on drug action.

Sometimes a positive drug effect occurs simply because the patient has taken something that is supposed to make him or her "feel better." A patient with a positive attitude may feel better after taking a **placebo,** an inactive substance that has no pharmacological effect. For example, a patient may report pain relief after taking a simple oral preparation of sugar.

As a member of the health care team, you can do much to create a positive attitude in the patient. One way is to review the important reasons for taking the medication. Another is to treat the patient in a cheerful and caring manner. And, finally, your own positive, confident attitude toward the drugs you administer can influence the patient's response to medication.

ROUTE OF ADMINISTRATION

Drugs are absorbed, distributed, and metabolized differently when given by different routes (see Chapter 4). The route thus affects drug action. A drug acts most quickly when injected directly into the bloodstream. Drugs injected into or under the skin or into muscles require more time to take effect. Medications administered by mouth take the longest time to show their effects.

TIME OF ADMINISTRATION

Care must always be taken to give drugs at the time of day ordered by the physician. There are many time-related factors that influence drug action. Drugs taken orally are absorbed most quickly if the gastrointestinal tract is free of food. However, certain stomach-irritating drugs are taken with meals to avoid patient discomfort. When possible, drugs that make the patient sleepy are ordered to be taken at bedtime. Drugs with stimulating effects are given at times when they will not interfere with sleep. Normal bodily functions also vary with the time of day, thus affecting drug action.

DRUG-TAKING HISTORY

Drug action depends on whether a patient has previously taken doses of the same or another drug. Some drugs tend to collect in the body producing a cumulative effect. In this case, later doses must be made smaller to avoid overmedicating the patient. Repeated doses of a drug may also make a patient less responsive to its effects. In that case, larger doses are required for the same effect.

Certain combinations of drugs can slow down or speed up effects, or they can cause unusual and sometimes dangerous reactions. This is why patients' medical histories and charts must include careful records of the drugs they have recently taken. Doctors should also check medical histories to find out whether patients are allergic to particular drugs, such as penicillin. Patients should also be questioned about food allergies, because many medications have ingredients that are found in foods. One such example is shellfish. A patient who is allergic to shellfish can have potentially fatal results if given a contrast material, often iodine, before certain hospital procedures. The chart of a patient with an allergy must be clearly marked. This is usually done on the front of the chart with a brightly colored sticker.

Drug combinations can be a problem for the elderly. They often see several doctors who may be unaware of one another and of the other drugs being prescribed. Each doctor may prescribe what is needed in a patient's particular case, unaware of the medications other doctors have prescribed. Multiple doctors and multiple drugs can lead to serious drug interactions.

ENVIRONMENTAL CONDITIONS

Extremes of weather affect the action of drugs because body functions are influenced by heat and cold. Heat relaxes the blood vessels and speeds up the circulation, so drugs act faster. Cold slows their action by constricting the blood vessels and slowing the circulation. High altitude puts the body under stress because there is less oxygen in the air. This makes some drugs ineffective.

The term drug **action** refers to the chemical changes the drug produces in cells and tissues. The drug **effect** is the combination of biological, physical, and psychological changes that take place in the body as a result of the drug action.

A drug is usually prescribed on the basis of its **therapeutic effect.** This is the desired effect, or the reason the drug is administered. However, most drugs have additional effects on the body that are not part of the goal of drug therapy. These are called **side effects.** They may be either desirable or undesirable.

A physician must always take possible side effects into account when planning drug treatment. Side effects can be harmless, mildly annoying, or dangerous. Sometimes unpleasant side effects are tolerated because of the drug's therapeutic benefit. For example, morphine is administered for its painkilling effect, but it also has the side effects of respiratory depression, constipation, and urine retention.

Many side effects can be controlled or lessened by substituting other drugs or using special procedures. For example, aspirin, taken orally, is beneficial for the treatment of arthritis, but tends to irritate the lining of the stomach. This side effect is controlled by giving the drug with milk or food. Diuretics can help ease water retention, but they may cause the body to excrete too much potassium. This situation can be corrected by giving a supplemental drug, potassium chloride, or by having the patient eat potassium-rich foods, such as bananas. Side effects are related to the actions of specific drugs. In later chapters you will learn which side effects accompany which drugs.

Drug effects are classified as either local or systemic. Some drugs affect mainly the area where they enter or are applied to the body: for example, eyedrops, sunburn creams, suppositories, and throat lozenges. These drugs are given for their **local** effects. Other drugs, such as pain medications, must travel through the bloodstream to affect cells or tissues in various parts of the body. These types of drugs are given for their **systemic** effects.

Proper administration of medications requires both knowledge of drug effects and observation of the results in the patient. The prescribed drug dosage indicates which drug and how much of the drug is needed to bring about the desired effect in a specific patient.

When you give medications, consider whether the drug is given for a local or a systemic effect. Then, while observing the patient's reaction, determine whether you are seeing the drug's therapeutic effect or a side effect. Your knowledge of drug effects is important to the work of the entire health care team—and is especially important to your patient.

ADVERSE REACTIONS

With proper administration, a drug usually has the desired effect—the patient feels better, bodily functions are restored, and side effects are under control. Occasionally, however, the body has an unexpected or dangerous response to a drug. These unexpected conditions are called **adverse reactions.** The most common adverse reactions are allergy, idiosyncrasies, tolerance, cumulative effect, overdose and toxicity, drug interactions (synergism, antagonism, and potentiation), and drug dependence. Following the discussion of adverse reactions, they are summarized, along with their causes, symptoms, and treatments, in Table 2.2. As a person giving medications, you are expected to be aware of possible reactions and notify your supervisor as soon as you notice any sign of an adverse reaction.

TABLE 2.2: Adverse Effects of Drugs

ADVERSE EFFECT	SYMPTOMS	TREATMENT	POTENTIATING DRUG
Idiosyncrasy	Opposite of expected effect	Stop medication	Genetically determined response to ordinary dose of any drug
Tolerance	Lessened effect	Increase dose or change medication	Opioid drug such as morphine or *Demerol*
Cumulation	Stronger effect	Stop medication	Alcohol (depends on patient's ability to properly excrete drug)
Toxicity	Diverse symptoms affecting multiple organs	Stop medication	Any drug given in excessive dose (e.g., central nervous system depressant)
Synergism	Stronger effect when more than one drug taken	Stop medication	Hydrochlorothiazide (*HydroDIURIL*) and enalapril (*Vaseretic*) used for hypertension
Antagonism	Weaker effect when more than one drug taken	Stop medication	Tetracycline and antacid (decreased absorption)
Potentiation	Effect of one drug increases effect of another drug	Stop medication	Acetaminophen (*Tylenol*) and codeine
Interaction	Therapeutic or adverse effect on body	If therapeutic, continue medication. If adverse effect, stop medication	Probencid and Penicillin G. Cimetidine (*Tagamet*) and theophylline; benzodiazepine antianxieties and hypnotics; warfarin and some antiarrhythmics, calcium channel blockers
Physical Dependence	Physiological need for drug	Substitute with similar drug and gradually withdraw	Opioid (e.g., as in case of cancer patient)
Psychological Dependence	Psychological craving for drug	Stop medication	Benzodiazepines, narcotics, amphetamines

DRUG ALLERGY

Drug **allergy** is an abnormal response that occurs because a person has developed **antibodies** against a particular drug. When a person takes the allergy-causing drug, called the **antigen,** the antibodies attack it. The reaction between antigen and antibodies causes damage to body tissues. The injured cells release a substance called **histamine,** which is responsible for the symptoms usually seen in allergic reactions.

Mild allergic symptoms can occur immediately after a drug is taken, or they can show up hours, days, or even weeks later. Severe allergic reactions, which can be fatal, usually begin within minutes of exposure and may require immediate emergency treatment.

The term *hypersensitivity* is often used synonymously with *allergy*. They are not the same, however, because there is not a precise definition of hypersensitivity, and it is frequently confused with other adverse reactions.

To avoid the problem of drug allergy, physicians try to find out whether patients have a history of allergies, such as hay fever, asthma, or skin rashes. They also ask whether patients have shown unusual reactions to any drugs taken in the past.

CAUTION: Drug Allergy

Mild Allergic Reaction
Symptoms: skin rash, swelling, nasal drainage, itchy eyes or skin, fever, wheezing
Treatment
Avoid reexposure to the drug; skin test to definitely diagnose the response

Severe Allergic Reaction
Symptoms: begins with irritability, extreme weakness, nausea, vomiting, and proceeds to cyanosis (bluish color to the skin), **dyspnea** (shortness of breath), severe hypotension, shock, cardiac arrest
Treatment
Notify supervisor immediately and follow instructions
Antihistamine drugs, epinephrine, bronchodilators, emergency treatment for hypotension and shock

IDIOSYNCRASY

Some people have abnormal or peculiar responses to certain drugs. These abnormal effects, or **idiosyncrasies,** are thought to be caused by an abnormal metabolism of drugs as the result of an enzyme deficiency. Individuals who have an idiosyncratic response to a drug either overreact or underreact.

TOLERANCE

Drug **tolerance** is the need for increasingly larger doses of a drug to produce the same physiological and/or psychological effects. The exact way in which tolerance develops is unknown. It can occur in some people after repeated dosages of the same or a similar drug. Drugs that frequently produce tolerance are opiates, nitrates, barbiturates, tobacco, and alcohol. For example, a cancer patient may require increasingly greater doses of morphine to relieve pain.

CUMULATIVE EFFECT

Cumulative effect occurs when the body cannot metabolize and excrete one dose of a drug completely before the next dose is given. With repeated doses, the drug starts to collect in the blood and body tissues. This can be dangerous because high concentrations of many drugs produce toxic effects. For example, cumulative toxicity occurs rapidly, as with ethyl alcohol, or slowly over time, as with lead.

OVERDOSE AND TOXICITY

Through error, poor judgment, or as a result of attempted suicide, a patient may receive a drug **overdose**—a dose that is too large for his or her age, size, and/or physical condition. This can be dangerous because any drug can act like a poison if taken in too large a dose.

Toxicity refers to the drug's ability to poison the body. Emergency measures may be needed to keep the patient alive. There may be an antidote for the poison. An antidote is a drug that has the opposite effect and can reverse the overdose symptoms.

DRUG INTERACTIONS

Sometimes two or more drugs are given to a patient as part of drug therapy, or a patient may be taking an OTC medication at home for some other ailment. Whenever a patient is taking more than one drug, the possibility of a drug interaction must be considered. Drug interaction occurs when one drug modifies the action of another drug.

Synergism. When two drugs administered together produce a more powerful response than the effect of each drug given separately, it is called **synergism.** For example, a patient may be given two drugs for hypertension. Each drug lowers blood pressure in a different way. However, the combined effect of the two drugs lowers the blood pressure more effectively than either one by itself.

Potentiation. **Potentiation** refers to the administration of two drugs at the same time wherein one drug increases the effect of the other drug. Patients who take sedatives, for example, are advised to avoid drinking alcoholic beverages. Alcohol causes sedatives to have a much stronger, possibly fatal, effect.

Antagonism. A drug interaction in which two drugs inhibit or cancel each other's effect is called **antagonism.** Drugs such as *Maalox* (an antacid) and ferrous sulfate (an iron supplement) should not be given to patients who are on oral tetracycline, an antibiotic, because the antacid and the iron supplement work against the absorption of tetracycline through the intestines.

Food can also affect drug absorption and can interact with drugs. Food-drug interactions can occur, and you should be aware of them. One example is the interaction of MAO inhibitors with tyramine-containing foods, such as alcohol, aged cheeses, beef and chicken livers, bananas, raisins, and avocados, to name a few.

There are many other ways in which drugs interact. Some of these interactions are detrimental, but not all. In fact, doctors sometimes make use of known drug interactions to control unwanted side effects or to increase the therapeutic effect of a particular drug. Probenecid is sometimes given with penicillin G. Probenecid prolongs the action of penicillin and decreases excretion of the drug. This effect results in higher blood levels or allows a smaller dose of penicillin to be given.

It is the unplanned drug interactions that are of concern in administering medications. Every member of the health care team must cooperate to observe the patient for possible drug interactions and to take appropriate action when they occur.

OTHER DRUG-RELATED DISORDERS

Some drugs, when administered over a period of time, can cause changes in body functioning or damage to certain organs. Bone marrow disease and a lower production of blood cells may result from fluorouracil therapy in cancer patients. Certain drugs may cause diseases of the liver and kidneys. Drugs can also have negative effects on behavior and emotions. Antianxiety drugs such as *Valium* have been known to disturb sleep and cause nightmares. Irritability and nervousness are common problems with many drugs.

DRUG DEPENDENCE

Drug **dependence** is a strong psychological and/or physical need to take a certain drug. This need develops when a person takes a drug over a period of time. Usually the drug was prescribed to relieve pain or to control some physical or emotional problem. Eventually, some people find they cannot seem to get along without the drug. They keep on taking it to avoid the discomfort they expect to feel if they stop.

In psychological or emotional drug dependence, a person has a drive or a craving to take a certain drug for pleasure or to relieve discomfort. There are no physical symptoms if the drug is taken away, but the person may feel anxious about not having the psychological crutch.

In physical drug dependence, the body grows so accustomed to the drug that it needs it to function. When the drug is taken away, the person develops **withdrawal symptoms** involving extreme physical discomfort. Eventually, if no further dose of the drug is administered, the body returns to normal functioning. With physical dependence, the physician may substitute another similar drug to ease the withdrawal symptoms and then gradually reduce the dosage of the substitute drug.

With both physical and psychological dependence, counseling may be needed to help the patient get along without the drug. In the case of a dying or terminal patient who is in a great deal of pain, drug dependence may be allowed to develop so that the patient can be as comfortable as possible.

DRUG DEPENDENCE OR DRUG ABUSE?

Drug dependence is a problem any health care worker may have to deal with in giving medications. The time may come when a patient asks for more pain medication, for example, and you may be worried that the patient is becoming too dependent on the drug. Is this drug abuse?

In this situation, your main responsibility is to consult the nurse in charge. The decision as to whether to medicate the patient further must be made jointly by the members of the health care team. Your own concerns may be eased, however, if you understand something about the difference between drug dependence and drug abuse.

Drug abuse refers to self-administration of a drug in chronically excessive quantities resulting in a psychological or physical dependence. Feelings of euphoria or calmness or a heightened awareness of the senses (feeling "high") are some of the reasons people take these drugs. Some experts define drug abuse as taking any drug to the point where it interferes with health and daily living patterns. The most commonly abused drugs are alcohol; nicotine; anabolic steroids; barbiturates ("downers"), sedatives or hypnotics, and depressants; marijuana (pot, dope, grass); amphetamines, and other stimulants ("uppers," "speed"); LSD and other hallucinogens; narcotics and opium; and cocaine.

Most of these commonly abused drugs are controlled substances. All of these drugs can create either physical or psychological dependence.

Drug abuse is part of a larger and more widespread problem—**drug misuse.** This is overuse or careless use of any drug, including alcohol. Drug misuse is most often a problem with people who take their own medications at home. Tranquilizers, stimulants, and pain-killing drugs are frequently misused, as are such common OTC drugs as laxatives, acetaminophen, and aspirin. Nicotine and alcohol are widely misused, and both can create serious physical as well as psychological dependence.

Both drug abuse and drug misuse endanger people's health and well-being. This includes the medical staff as well as patients. As a health care worker, you must keep medicines locked up when not in use, administer only prescribed medications, and watch for signs of drug dependence and improper use of drugs.

Complete the following statements.

1. The way a drug changes the chemistry of the body is called the drug _____ .

2. The physical changes that occur because of the drug action are called the drug _____ .

3. Absorption is _____
_____ .

4. Distribution is _____
_____ .

5. Metabolism/biotransformation is _____
_____ .

6. Excretion is _____
_____ .

7. Drug effects that result from a drug circulating through the body are called _____
_____ effects.

8. Drug effects that are confined to the area where the drug was administered are called _____
_____ effects.

9. Drugs act by _____, _____, or
_____ the work of the cells.

10. Drugs also act by _____ substances that the body fails to produce.

11. Drug action is affected by four bodily processes: _____,
_____, _____,
and _____ .

12. The organs that excrete waste are the _____,
_____, _____,
and _____ .

13. Drugs used in therapy have two kinds of effects: _____ and _____ .

14. Three symptoms of a drug allergy include _____, _____, and _____ .

15. A placebo is _____
_____ .

16. Drug abuse is _____
_____ .

17. Drug misuse is _____
_____ .

18. Idiosyncrasy is _____
_____ .

19. Five groups of drugs that are often abused are _____, _____, _____, _____, _____.

20. If you suspect drug abuse, your obligation is to _____ _____.

21. Physical drug dependence is _____ _____.

22. Psychological drug dependence is _____ _____.

Answer the following questions in the spaces provided.

23. What is the basis for treatment of drug overdose? _____ _____ _____

24. List four over-the-counter drugs that are commonly abused. _____ _____ _____

25. What two critical symptoms may occur when a patient takes an overdose of central nervous system depressants? _____ _____ _____

26. What does alcohol do for a patient who has taken an overdose? _____ _____ _____

27. What is an antidote? _____ _____ _____

28. What is an overdose? _____ _____ _____

The following is a list of patient characteristics. Place a check by those that you think might influence drug action.

_____ 29. Physical strength   _____ 34. Sex

_____ 30. Kidney disease   _____ 35. Diet

_____ 31. Deafness   _____ 36. Popularity

_____ 32. Old age   _____ 37. Infancy

_____ 33. Genes   _____ 38. Anger

Continued

_____ 39. Obesity

_____ 40. Poor circulation

_____ 41. Nervousness

_____ 42. Tallness

_____ 43. Cheerful mood

_____ 44. Political affiliation

_____ 45. Drug-taking history

_____ 46. Hair color

_____ 47. Oral hygiene

■ CASE STUDIES FOR CRITICAL THINKING

Select the term that best completes each sentence and write it in the blank.

antagonism	drug dependence	potentiation	cumulative effect	toxicity
drug allergy	drug interaction	tolerance	idiosyncrasy	

48. After taking several doses of medicine, Bill no longer seems to be affected by the drug. This may be a symptom of _____.

49. Mrs. Jones gets a stronger drug effect with each additional dose of her medication. She may be showing signs of _____.

50. Two drugs producing a greater effect than the sum of their individual effects is referred to as _____.

51. The doctor has just canceled Ms. Williams' order for a narcotic pain medication. She has been taking the pain medication regularly since her hip operation. As the usual time for her medication approaches, Ms. Williams expresses the worry that she will not be able to sleep without her medication. You see this as a possible sign of _____.

52. A drug interaction wherein two drugs inhibit or cancel the action of the other is called _____.

53. Annie Peterson is reacting in an abnormal or peculiar way to her medication. You have never seen a person react this way to the medication she is taking. Drug allergy has been ruled out. Annie's response to the drug will probably be classified as a(n) _____.

54. An adverse reaction resulting from an antibody attacking an antigen is called a(n) _____.

55. You have recently given Mr. Smith a medication ordered by his doctor. Mr. Smith is not reacting to the drug the way you expected. In talking with him, you discover that he has also been taking medication he brought with him from home. You suspect that his adverse reaction is due to a(n) _____.

56. Miss Grimes seems very sleepy and confused after receiving her medication. You check her records and discover that someone misread the doctor's order and gave Miss Grimes a dose that was much too large. You notify the supervisor immediately because you think Miss Grimes is showing signs of _____.

■ APPLICATIONS

Obtain a current copy of the PDR® from your school, nursing unit, or clinic. Use it to answer the following questions.

57. Name the form printed in the *PDR®* that the FDA and pharmaceutical manufacturers encourage health care professionals to fill out and send to the FDA's Division of Epidemiology and Surveillance.

_____

_____

Continued

58. Where do you get this form? _____

    _____

    _____

59. What does VAERS signify? _____

    _____

    _____

60. Why should the physician refer to the contraindication section of the *PDR*® or the manufacturer's package insert for each vaccine? _____

    _____

    _____

 *Inter**NET** CONNECTION*

To learn more about drug actions, go to http://www.mayohealth.org. This is the Mayo Clinic's Consumer Health Web site. Click on Medicine under the Centers listing. This will take you to the Medicine Center. Click on USP drug guide. This will take you to a listing of over 8,000 drugs. When you select a drug, you will get information on trade names, dosages, precautions, storage, and side effects.

In this chapter you will learn about three systems used in measuring medication doses. You will learn how to solve simple dosage problems and how to convert doses from one system of measurement to another. You will also review fractions to help you brush up on your math skills.

OBJECTIVES

After studying this chapter, you should be able to

- write and define the abbreviations for units of measurement in the metric, apothecary, and household systems.
- state the most common equivalents among apothecary, metric, and household measures and use a conversion table to find less common equivalents.
- convert grams to milligrams and vice versa.
- convert milliliters to teaspoons and vice versa.
- calculate the number of tablets or capsules to give when the available dose differs from the ordered dose.
- calculate doses using a procedure for converting between different units of measurement.
- calculate an adult's dose of medication.
- calculate a child's dose of medication.
- calculate drops per minute for IV therapy.

KEY TERMS

apothecary system: system of measurement in which the basic unit of volume is the minim and the basic unit of weight is the grain

Arabic numerals: 0, 1, 2, 3, 4, 5, 6, 7, 8, 9

centimeter: one-hundredth of a meter (0.01 m)

convert: to change from one unit of measurement to another

dosage range: the different amounts of a drug that will produce therapeutic effects but not serious side effects or toxicity

fraction: a way of expressing an amount that is part of a whole

grain: basic unit of weight in the apothecary system

gram: basic unit of weight in the metric system

household system: system of measurement in which the basic unit of fluid volume is the fluid ounce and the basic unit of weight is the ounce

liter: basic unit of volume in the metric system

meter: basic unit of length in the metric system

metric system: a decimal system of measurement in which the basic unit of length is the meter, the basic unit of volume is the liter, and the basic unit of weight is the gram

milliliter: one-thousandth of a liter (0.001 l); same as cubic centimeter

millimeter: one-thousandth of a meter (0.001 m)

minim: basic unit of volume in the apothecary system

Roman numerals: I, II, III, IV, V, or i, ii, iii, iv, v, and so forth

Measurement has always been an important part of prescribing and administering medications. This is so because different amounts of a drug give different effects. Some drugs are deadly poisons, but when given in tiny amounts, they can help relieve disorders. Other drugs are useless for therapy unless given in large amounts.

Most drugs have a certain **dosage range,** that is, different amounts that can produce therapeutic effects. Doctors prescribe an amount within the dosage range, depending on how strong an effect is needed and on the patient's age and physical condition. Doses below the dosage range will not produce the desired therapeutic effect. Doses above the dosage range can be harmful and possibly fatal.

To get the drug effects they want, physicians and pharmacists try to make dosages exact by measuring drugs carefully. However, they have not always used the same units of measurement. There are different measurement systems, each having its own units of weight and volume.

Three different systems of measurement are used in the medical field. You should be familiar with the units of weight and volume in each system. Dosages on a medication order may be expressed in units ranging from milliliters (or cubic centimeters) to drops, teaspoons, drams, or minims. You need to know what each of these quantities means so that you can measure out the doses properly. In addition, you may be asked to **convert** (change) from one unit or system to another in the course of your daily routine. You need to know how to use conversion tables to convert from milligrams to grams, from milliliters to teaspoons, from grains to milligrams, and so forth.

The three systems of measurement used in ordering medications are the apothecary system, the metric system, and the household system.

APOTHECARY SYSTEM

The **apothecary system** of measurement is very old and infrequently used. Only a few medications are still available in the apothecary system. It is not as precise or convenient as the metric system.

The basic unit of weight in the apothecary system is the **grain** (gr). It was originally supposed to be the weight of one grain of wheat. The basic unit of volume is the **minim** (min). A minim is the space taken up by a quantity of water that weighs the same as a grain. The fluidram, fluidounce, pint, quart, and gallon are all measurements derived from the minim. With the exception of the fluidram, the volume measurements are also considered household measurements.

Table 3.1 lists the units of weight and volume in the apothecary system. Note especially the abbreviations for these units. In the apothecary system, the abbreviation is placed before the number. You need to be able to recognize apothecary units on a medication order and write them on a medication chart.

TABLE 3.1: The Apothecary System

WEIGHT (DRY)	VOLUME (LIQUID)	EQUIVALENTS
grain (gr)	minim (min, ℳ)	A minim of liquid weighs 1 grain
dram (dr or ʒ)	fluidram (fl dr, or f ʒ)	60 grains or 60 minims = 1 dram or fluidram
ounce (oz or ℥)	fluidounce (fl oz, or f ℥)	8 drams or fluidrams = 1 ounce or fluidounce
pound (lb)	pint (pt)	
ton (t)	quart (qt)	
	gallon (gal)	

In the apothecary system, dosage quantities are written in lowercase **Roman numerals** (Table 3.2). By convention the Roman numerals are written with a bar over them after the unit of measurement; for example, ℥ ii̅ means 2 drams.

TABLE 3.2: Lowercase Roman Numerals

1	i	9	ix
2	ii	10	x
3	iii	11	xi
4	iv	12	xii
5	v	13	xiii
6	vi	14	xiv
7	vii	15	xv
8	viii		$(\overline{ss} = \frac{1}{2})$

Fractions are expressed in **Arabic numerals** rather than decimals. For example, one-quarter grain is written $\frac{1}{4}$ gr, not 0.25 gr. Arabic numerals are usually written before the unit of measurement, though some people prefer to write them after the unit to avoid confusing grains with grams in the metric system. The only exception is the quantity $\frac{1}{2}$, for which the symbol $\overline{ss}$ is used with Roman numerals after the unit.

Here are some examples:

$$f\ ℥\ \overline{vii} = 7 \text{ fluidounces}$$
$$℥\ \overline{iv} = 4 \text{ drams}$$
$$gr\ \overline{iss} = 1\frac{1}{2} \text{ grains}$$
$$5\frac{1}{4}\ dr = 5\frac{1}{4} \text{ drams}$$
$$\frac{1}{150}\ gr\ (\text{also gr}\ \tfrac{1}{150}) = \frac{1}{150} \text{ grain}$$
$$15\ gr\ (\text{also gr } 15) = 15 \text{ grains}$$
$$30\ min = 30 \text{ minims}$$

METRIC SYSTEM

The **metric system** is a decimal system that is widely used in medicine. It is a simple, logical system of measurement based on units of 10.

The basic units of metric measurements are the meter, liter, and gram. The **meter** is the unit of length; the **liter,** of volume; and the **gram,** weight.

Prefixes added to the words *meter, gram,* and *liter* indicate smaller or larger units in the system (Table 3.3). All units are a result of either multiplying or dividing by 10, 100, or 1000. The **centimeter,** for example, is 1/100th of a meter. A **millimeter** is 1/1000th of a meter. A kilometer is 1000 meters.

TABLE 3.3: Prefixes in the Metric System

deca ⟶ × 10		deci ⟶ ÷ 10	
hect ⟶ × 100		centi ⟶ ÷ 100	
kilo ⟶ × 1000		milli ⟶ ÷ 1000	
		micro ⟶ ÷ 1,000,000	

In the metric system, units of length, weight, and volume are related to each other systematically. The unit of volume most often used in preparing liquid medications is the **milliliter** (ml), which is one-thousandth of a liter. One milliliter is the liquid contents of a cube measuring 1 centimeter (cm) on a side, or 1 cubic centimeter (cc). One liter is the liquid contents of a cube measuring 10 cm on a side, or 1000 cc. One gram is equal to the weight of 1 ml (or cc) of water. One liter contains 1000 ml of water, so it weighs 1000 g (1 kilogram).

TABLE 3.4: The Metric System

WEIGHT	VOLUME	EQUIVALENTS
microgram (mcg) milligram (mg) gram (g, Gm, gm) kilogram (kg)	milliliter (ml) cubic centimeter (cc, cm^3) liter (L, l)	One milliliter (1 ml) is the same as 1 cubic centimeter (1 cc) 1000 milliliters = 1 liter = 1000 cubic centimeters 1000 micrograms = 1 milligram 1000 milligrams = 1 gram 1000 grams = 1 kilogram 100 milligrams = 0.1 gram 10 milligrams = 0.01 gram

Simple Conversions

From grams to milligrams
g × 1000 = mg
Hint: Move decimal point three places to the right
0.25 g = 250 mg

From milligrams to grams
mg ÷ 1000-g
Hint: Move decimal point three places to the left
500 mg = .500 g = 0.5 g

Metric doses are always written in Arabic numerals. Fractions of metric doses are written as decimal fractions. For example, one-half gram is 0.5 g. In reading medication orders, pay special attention to where the decimal point is placed. The differences between 0.05 g, 0.5 g, and 5.0 g are huge when it comes to doses of medicine. A mistake could prove fatal.

Table 3.4 lists the basic units of volume and weight in the metric system and their equivalents. The bottom of the table shows how to change from milligrams to grams and vice versa. Note the instructions, because these are simple conversions you will probably often make on the job. The conversions are easy if you remember the hints shown in Table 3.4.

HOUSEHOLD SYSTEM

The **household system** of measurement is familiar to most of us because we have grown up using its basic units—drops, teaspoons, tablespoons, cups, pints, quarts, and gallons.

As a result of the changing insurance industry, the average length of hospital stays has shortened and the corresponding recovery at home has lengthened. Household utensils such as teaspoons and cups vary in size and should not be used when accuracy is important. For example, the average household teaspoon can hold 4 to 5 more ml than the standard 5 ml. Therefore, the health care professional working in a doctor's office or medical clinic should encourage patients to obtain accurate measuring utensils from a pharmacy or medical supply facility.

The basic units of the household system are listed in Table 3.5. All household doses are written in Arabic numerals.

DRUGS THAT ARE HARD TO MEASURE

Certain antibiotics, anticoagulants, and insulin derived from animal sources are impossible to weigh and measure in ordinary ways. Rather than being dispensed in grams or grains, these drugs are dispensed in units (U) per cubic centimeter or milliliter, based on their strengths. Examples of these drugs are penicillin, heparin, and insulin.

TABLE 3.5: The Household System

WEIGHT (DRY)	VOLUME (LIQUID)	EQUIVALENTS
ounce (oz)	drop (gt); drops (gtt)	16 ounces = 1 pound
pound (lb)	teaspoon (t, tsp)	3 teaspoons = 1 tablespoon = ½ ounce
ton (t)	tablespoon (T, tbsp)	16 tablespoons = 1 cup = 8 fluidounces
	teacup (6 oz)	2 cups = 1 pint
	cup (c) or glass (8 oz)	2 pints = 1 quart
	pint (pt)	4 quarts = 1 gallon
	quart (qt)	
	gallon (gal)	

CONVERTING AMONG MEASUREMENT SYSTEMS

From time to time you will find it necessary to change, or convert, from one system of measurement to another. A physician may order medicine in grains, but the hospital or facility pharmacy may send up the medication in grams. Or perhaps an order written for milliliters will have to be converted into teaspoons for a patient who will be taking the medicine at home. These types of conversions are usually performed by the pharmacist or the nurse in charge. But other health workers should also know how to make simple conversions by referring to a conversion table. Table 3.6 shows the equivalents among measures in the apothecary, metric, and household systems. As you can see, the equivalents are not exact; they are only approximate. A 10 percent error usually occurs in making conversions.

TABLE 3.6: Common Measurement System Equivalents[a]

	APOTHECARY	METRIC	HOUSEHOLD
Liquid volume	1 minim (℔ or min)	0.06 ml (or cc)	1 drop
	15 minims	1 ml	15 drops (gtt)[b]
	1 fluidram (f℥)	4–5 ml	1 teaspoon (60 gtt)
	4 fluidrams	15 ml	1 tablespoon
	1 fluidounce (f℥)	30 ml	2 tablespoons (1 oz)
		180 ml	1 teacup (6 oz)
		240 ml	1 cup or glass (8 oz)
		500 ml	1 pint (16 oz)
		750 ml	1.5 pints (24 oz)
		1000 ml (1 l)	1 quart (32 oz)
Dry weight	$\frac{1}{60}$ gr	1 mg	
	1 gr	60 mg	
	$7\frac{1}{2}$ gr	500 mg (0.5 g)	
	15 gr	1000 mg (1 g)	
	60 gr (1 dram)	4 g	
	1 oz	30 g	1 oz
		500 g	1.1 lb
		1000 g (1 kg)	2.2 lb

[a]Equivalents are approximate; for example, some institutions set 1 grain equal to 64 or 65 mg for grain/milligram conversions.
[b]This figure varies; number of drops per milliliter depends on the substance being measured.

You can make most of the conversions you need if you know these basic equivalents:

$$1 \text{ mg} = \tfrac{1}{60} \text{ gr}$$
$$60 \text{ mg} = 1 \text{ gr}$$
$$1 \text{ g} = 15 \text{ gr}$$

If you can remember these, it is easy to work out other equivalents (Table 3.7). Figure 3.1 shows the relative sizes of containers you might use to measure out doses in the various systems.

TABLE 3.7: Approximate Conversions Between the Metric and Apothecary Systems

	METRIC AMOUNT	APOTHECARY AMOUNT
	2 g (2000 mg)	30 gr
	1 g (1000 mg)	15 gr
	600 mg (0.6 g)	10 gr
	100 mg (0.1 g)	$1\tfrac{1}{2}$ gr
	60 mg (0.06 g)	1 gr
	30 mg (0.03 g)	$\tfrac{1}{2}$ gr
	1 mg (0.001 g)	$\tfrac{1}{60}$ gr
	0.1 mg (0.0001 g)	$\tfrac{1}{600}$ gr
Approximation formulas	grains × 60 = milligrams milligrams ÷ 60 = grains	grams × 15 = grains grains ÷ 15 = grams

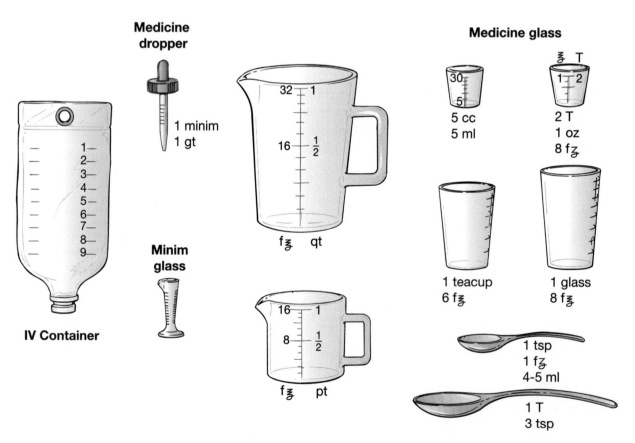

Figure 3.1
Containers for measuring doses.

Calculating dosages is much easier today than in the past. In some health facilities pharmacists now do all the calculating. They prepare drugs in unit packages that contain the correct amount of a drug for a single dose. In your facility, however, you may have to make simple dosage calculations as part of your daily routine. You need to know how to do this correctly and confidently. In medication administration, there is no room for error!

In this section, you will learn two simple procedures for calculating almost any type of dosage problem. The only math you need is multiplication and division with whole numbers and fractions. Use paper and pencil to do your calculations, and check them carefully for errors.

This chapter includes a brief review of fractions. If your arithmetic skills are weak, you will need extra practice. There are many books available in the library or bookstore to help you brush up on your basic skills.

CALCULATING THE NUMBER OF TABLETS, CAPSULES, OR MILLILITERS

This is a type of calculation you will probably encounter.

Problem 1. The doctor orders 200 mg of a drug to be given three times a day. The pharmacy sends up a bottle of 50-mg capsules. You must decide how many capsules to give for each dose.

You can use a simple formula to figure this out. The formula is:

$$\text{Desired dose (what you WANT)} \div \text{Available dose per tablet, capsule, ml (what you HAVE)} = \text{Number of tablets, capsules, ml}$$

or

$$\frac{\text{WANT}}{\text{HAVE}} = \text{Number of tablets, capsules, or ml}$$

This formula helps you set up a fraction that you can simplify using the rules for fractions. Applying the formula to Problem 1, you get:

Dose ordered (WANT): 200 mg
Available packaging (HAVE): 50-mg caps

$$\frac{\text{WANT}}{\text{HAVE}} = \frac{200 \text{ mg}}{50 \text{ mg}} = \frac{\overset{4}{\cancel{200 \text{ mg}}}}{\underset{1}{\cancel{50 \text{ mg}}}} = 4 \text{ capsules}$$

Note that the units, mg, is also crossed out above and below the divider line when simplifying. The correct dose, then, would be four capsules three times a day.

Problem 2. The doctor orders 350 mg to be given once a day. All you have on hand are 100-mg tablets. How many tablets should you give? (If the drug ordered is a liquid, ml's or cc's can be used in place of tablets or capsules.)

$$\frac{\text{WANT}}{\text{HAVE}} = \frac{350 \text{ mg}}{100 \text{ mg}} = \frac{\overset{3.5}{\cancel{350 \text{ mg}}}}{\underset{1}{\cancel{100 \text{ mg}}}} = 3\frac{1}{2} \text{ tablets}$$

Note that your answer includes a fraction of a tablet. You may administer a half or a quarter of a tablet if the tablet is scored so that it breaks easily. If it is anything other than a scored tablet, ask the nurse in charge what to do.

Dividing an unscored tablet is risky, and, of course, you should not attempt to divide capsules or enteric-coated tablets to decrease irritation to the stomach lining.

Problem 3. Now try a problem involving another unit of measurement. You are to give 20 gr of aspirin to an arthritis patient. The aspirin tablets you have are 5 gr each. How many tablets do you give?

$$\frac{\text{WANT}}{\text{HAVE}} = \frac{\overset{4}{\cancel{20 \text{ gr}}}}{\underset{1}{\cancel{5 \text{ gr}}}} = 4 \text{ tablets}$$

Note that both WANT and HAVE must be in the same unit of measurement (e.g., both milligrams or grains, etc.). This formula does not apply to a problem like this:

$$\frac{100 \text{ mg}}{5 \text{ gr}}$$

Problem 4. What if the dosage ordered is a fractional dosage? For example, let's say that the doctor orders $\frac{1}{2}$ gr and your tablets are $\frac{1}{4}$ gr. Setting up the WANT/HAVE formula, you get:

$$(\text{Remember, this line means divided by}) \longrightarrow \frac{\frac{1}{2} \text{ gr}}{\frac{1}{4} \text{ gr}}$$

To work this out, use what you know about dividing fractions. Invert the bottom fraction and turn it into a multiplication problem:

$$\frac{1}{2} \div \frac{1}{4} = \frac{1}{\underset{1}{\cancel{2}}} \times \frac{\overset{2}{\cancel{4}}}{1} = 2 \text{ tablets}$$

Problem 5. The same procedure can be applied to situations where drugs are mixed into solutions. For example, the label on a bottle of elixir says that it contains 5 gr of medication per teaspoon. The doctor has ordered 15 gr of medication.

$$\frac{\text{WANT}}{\text{HAVE}} = \frac{\overset{3}{\cancel{15 \text{ gr}}}}{\underset{1}{\cancel{5 \text{ gr}}/\text{tsp}}} = 3 \text{ tsp}$$

Problem 6. It also works for units of penicillin mixed in sterile water for injection. A vial states that it contains 100,000 units of penicillin per cubic centimeter. You are to inject 300,000 units.

$$\frac{\text{WANT}}{\text{HAVE}} = \frac{\overset{3}{\cancel{300,000 \text{ units}}}}{\underset{1}{\cancel{100,000 \text{ units}}/\text{cc}}} = 3 \text{ cc}$$

DOSAGE CALCULATIONS WITH CONVERSIONS

Suppose the doctor orders a dose in grams, but the capsules are labeled in milligrams. Perhaps the order is in grains and the tablets are labeled in milligrams. Or suppose the order is in milliliters and you want to explain to the patient how much to take at home using a teaspoon.

Dosage calculations in which you need to convert from one system or unit of measurement to another cannot be handled by the simple WANT/HAVE formula. A more complex formula is needed, but it is easy to use and can be adapted to a variety of situations. The formula is:

Dosage in ordered unit (KNOWN) × Conversion fraction (relation of UNKNOWN to KNOWN units) = Dose in desired unit (UNKNOWN)

or

KNOWN × conversion fraction = UNKNOWN

This formula is best explained in the context of some sample problems.

Problem 7. The doctor orders 0.5 g of ampicillin to be given four times a day. You want to know how many milligrams one dose would be. Your problem is:

0.5 g = ? mg (KNOWN unit is 0.5 g; UNKNOWN unit is ? mg)

To solve the problem, set up a calculation that allows you to cancel the gram unit and gives you the answer in milligrams.

$$\frac{0.5 \text{ g} \times \text{? mg}}{\text{? g}} = \text{answer in milligrams}$$

You do this by means of a conversion fraction. This fraction differs according to the particular problem. It is designed to show the equivalence between the known and unknown units of measurement. The known type of unit should be in the denominator. For this problem, the conversion fraction is:

$$\frac{\text{? mg}}{\text{? g}}$$

You must fill in the missing quantities.

First, set the quantity of either unit to 1. Then find out how many of the other units are contained in that quantity. In this case, let us set the quantity of grams at 1. One gram contains 1000 mg, so you can fill in the fraction as follows:

$$\frac{1000 \text{ mg}}{1 \text{ g}}$$

Note that this fraction is equal to 1, because the numerator and the denominator both represent the same quantity, only in different units. Remember, the denominator must be in the same unit of measurement as the KNOWN dose.

Now you can solve the problem by first canceling the gram unit and multiplying:

$$0.5 \text{ g} \times \frac{1000 \text{ mg}}{1 \text{ g}} = 0.5 \times 1000 \text{ mg} = 500 \text{ mg}$$

Problem 8. For another example, let us convert between household measures. You are to give a patient 6 tsp of milk of magnesia as necessary for constipation. How many tablespoons would that be? In other words, 6 tsp = ? T (KNOWN unit is 6 tsp, UNKNOWN is ? T).

Set up the calculation so that you can cancel out the teaspoons and get the answer in tablespoons:

$$6 \text{ tsp} \times \frac{\text{? T}}{\text{? tsp}} = \text{answer in tablespoons}$$

You know that 3 tsp = 1 T, so you can fill in the conversion fraction as 1 T/3 tsp. Proceed to solve as follows:

$$\overset{2}{\cancel{6\ \text{tsp}}} \times \frac{1\ \text{T}}{\cancel{3\ \text{tsp}}} = 2\ \text{T}$$

Problem 9. Next, we'll try a problem that involves converting from one measurement system to another. The order is Pro-Banthine gr $\overline{\text{ss}}$. The tablets are labeled in milligrams. Can you use the described procedure to find out how many milligrams equal $\frac{1}{2}$ gr?

$$\frac{1}{2}\ \text{gr} \times \frac{?\ \text{mg}}{?\ \text{gr}} = \text{answer in mg}$$

From Table 3.7, you know that 1 gr = 60 mg, so:

$$\frac{1}{\cancel{2}}\text{gr} \times \frac{\overset{30}{\cancel{60}}\ \text{mg}}{1\ \cancel{\text{gr}}} = 30\ \text{mg}$$

Now, suppose the tablets of *Pro-Banthine* are 15 mg each. How many 15-mg tablets would it take to make 30 mg? Use the WANT/HAVE formula, now that you have converted from grains to milligrams. You will give the patient two tablets.

$$\frac{\text{WANT}}{\text{HAVE}} = \frac{\overset{2}{\cancel{30}}\ \text{mg}}{\underset{1}{\cancel{15}}\ \text{mg}} = 2\ \text{tablets}$$

CHILDREN'S DOSES

As you learned in Chapter 2, children need smaller doses of medicine than adults. There are two ways to adjust dosages for children: by age and by weight. In both cases, you can use the basic KNOWN/UNKNOWN procedure. Table 3.8 shows how children and adults are defined for the purpose of calculating doses.

Adjusting Doses by Age. You should know how to check or verify pediatric doses. A 6-month-old infant is to be given tetracycline. The usual adult dose is 250 mg. Set up the problem as follows:

$$\text{Patient's age (in months)} \times \frac{\text{Usual adult dose}}{\text{Adult age (in months)}} = \text{Child's dose}$$

The adult age is always 150 months (12 $\frac{1}{2}$ years) in this method of calculating. After filling in the proper numbers for your problem, you have:

$$6\ \cancel{\text{months}} \times \frac{250\ \text{mg}}{150\ \cancel{\text{months}}} = \frac{1500\ \text{mg}}{150} = 10\ \text{mg}$$

The infant would therefore be given 10 mg of tetracycline.

TABLE 3.8: Adjusting Doses by Age and Weight

	AGE	WEIGHT
Infant	0–24 months (up to 2 years)	Less than 40 lb
Child	25–150 months (2 to 12 $\frac{1}{2}$ years)	Less than 150 lb
Adult	More than 150 months (more than 12 $\frac{1}{2}$ years)	150 lb or more

Suppose you were giving tetracycline to an 8-year-old child. Eight years is the same as 96 months (8 × 12 = 96), so your problem looks like this:

$$96 \text{ months} \times \frac{250 \text{ mg}}{150 \text{ months}} = \frac{24,000 \text{ mg}}{150} = 160 \text{ mg}$$

Adjusting Doses by Weight. You can figure out a child's dose by weight as well as by age. This formula assumes an adult weight of 150 lbs.

$$\text{Patient's weight} \times \frac{\text{Usual adult dose}}{\text{Adult weight (always 150 lbs)}} = \text{Child's dose}$$

A doctor orders *Dilantin* for a 30-lb child. The usual adult dose is 100 mg. Your calculation will look like this:

$$\overset{1}{\cancel{30 \text{ lb}}} \times \frac{100 \text{ mg}}{\underset{5}{\cancel{150 \text{ lb}}}} = \frac{100 \text{ mg}}{5} = 20 \text{ mg}$$

PARENTERAL THERAPY

Another important formula is one used with parenteral, or intravenous (IV), therapy. We will work with one simple formula, but books are available that cover this subject in detail. This formula allows you to calculate drops per minute for most physician's orders relating to this type of patient care. However, there are IV pumps and controllers that figure drip rates.

Suppose the doctor orders an infusion for a patient and specifies the amount of solution and the amount of time for it to be administered. You need to calculate the rate of flow or the number of drops per minute after you select the size of the IV tubing or drop factor. (The drop factor of the tubing for an adult is either 15 or 16 drops per 1 ml, and for a child, 60 microdrops per 1 ml.) You need the fraction 1 hour/60 minutes to complete the problem. The IV container will give you one of these drop factors.

Problem 10. The doctor orders 120 ml of 5 percent D/W (dextrose and water) to be given over 6 hours. The drop factor is 60 microdrops per 1 ml. How many microdrops would you administer in 1 minute?

$$120 \text{ ml in a 6-hour period} = \frac{120 \text{ ml}}{6 \text{ hours}}$$

Convert milliliters per hour to microdrops per minute:

$$\frac{120 \text{ ml}}{6 \text{ hour}} = \frac{? \text{ microdrops}}{? \text{ minutes}}$$

Write in one line as follows:

$$\frac{120 \text{ ml}}{6 \text{ hour}} \times \frac{60 \text{ microdrops}}{1 \text{ ml}} \times \frac{1 \text{ hour}}{60 \text{ minutes}}$$

Cancel the labels and the numbers that are equal:

$$\frac{\overset{20}{\cancel{120 \text{ ml}}}}{\underset{1}{\cancel{6 \text{ hour}}}} \times \frac{\overset{1}{\cancel{60} \text{ microdrops}}}{1 \text{ } \cancel{ml}} \times \frac{1 \text{ } \cancel{hour}}{\underset{1}{\cancel{60} \text{ minutes}}} = \frac{20 \text{ microdrops}}{1 \text{ minute}}$$

After canceling and then multiplying across terms, you will find that the order of 120 ml given over a 6-hour period would be administered at the rate of 20 microdrops per minute.

Problem 11. How many drops per minute would you administer if the doctor ordered 1000 cc of 5 percent D/W in a 12-hour period?

$$1000 \text{ ml in a } 12\text{-hour period} = \frac{1000 \text{ cc}}{12 \text{ hour}}$$

Convert milliliters per hour to microdrops per minute:

$$\frac{1000 \text{ cc}}{12 \text{ hour}} = \frac{? \text{ gtt}}{? \text{ minutes}}$$

Write in one line as follows:

$$\frac{1000 \text{ cc}}{12 \text{ hour}} \times \frac{15 \text{ gtt}}{1 \text{ cc}} \times \frac{1 \text{ hour}}{60 \text{ minutes}}$$

Cancel the labels and the numbers that are equal:

$$\frac{\overset{250}{\cancel{1000}} \cancel{\text{cc}}}{12 \cancel{\text{hour}}} \times \frac{\overset{1}{\cancel{15}} \cancel{\text{gtt}}}{1 \cancel{\text{cc}}} \times \frac{1 \cancel{\text{hour}}}{\underset{\underset{1}{4}}{\cancel{60}} \text{ minutes}} \times \frac{250}{12} = 20.8 \text{ or } \frac{21 \text{ gtt}}{1 \text{ minute}}$$

The order for 1000 cc given over a 12-hour period would be administered at the rate of 21 drops per minute.

WHEN IN DOUBT

As one who gives medications, you share in the health care team's responsibility for making sure that the patient gets the correct dose. To meet this responsibility, you must learn all you can about dosage calculation and conversions among measurement systems. If you study hard and do the practice exercises until you have mastered them, you will be prepared to handle most routine dosage questions. It is safe practice, however, to have your supervisor check all calculations.

MATH REVIEW: FRACTIONS

A **fraction** is a way of expressing an amount that is part of a whole, as shown in Figure 3.2. The more parts the whole is divided into, the smaller each part is, as you can see in Figure 3.3. The whole can be a set of anything; for example, nine squares or 100 mg. Figure 3.4 shows two sets that each make up a whole.

Figure 3.5 shows how to express a fractional amount of a whole. The top number of a fraction is the numerator. It is the number of parts you are taking of the whole. The bottom number of a fraction is the denominator. This number tells how many equal parts the whole is divided into.

Figure 3.2
A fraction indicates an amount that is part of a whole.

Figure 3.3
Dividing the whole into greater numbers of parts causes each part to become smaller.

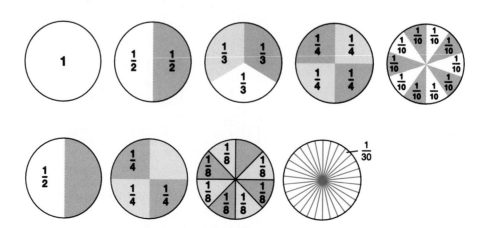

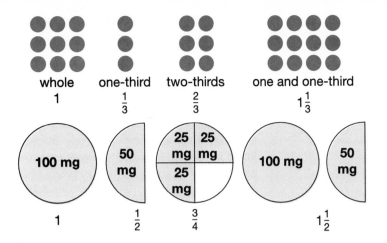

Figure 3.4
Whole sets and parts. The last item in each set is a whole plus part of another set.

whole
1

one-third
$\frac{1}{3}$

two-thirds
$\frac{2}{3}$

one and one-third
$1\frac{1}{3}$

100 mg
1

50 mg
$\frac{1}{2}$

25 mg | 25 mg | 25 mg
$\frac{3}{4}$

100 mg
$1\frac{1}{2}$

50 mg

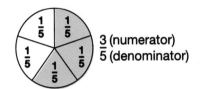

$\frac{3}{5}$ (numerator)
(denominator)

Figure 3.5
Expressing a fractional amount of a whole.

A fraction is also a way of expressing a relationship between two numbers or quantities. For example, $\frac{3}{4}$ means 3 divided by 4, which can also be expressed as

$$3 \div 4 \quad \text{or} \quad 4\overline{)3} \quad \text{or} \quad 3:4$$

A relationship expressed as 350 mg/25 mg means the same as

$$350 \text{ mg} \div 25 \text{ mg} \quad \text{or} \quad 25\text{mg}\overline{)350 \text{ mg}} \quad \text{or} \quad 350 \text{ mg} : 25 \text{ mg}$$

SIMPLIFYING FRACTIONS

To make calculations easier, fractions may be reduced to their lowest terms. To reduce a fraction to its lowest terms, divide both the numerator and the denominator by the largest number that will go into both of them evenly. If no number can be evenly divided into both the numerator and the denominator, you cannot reduce the fraction, because it is already in its lowest terms. When you reduce a fraction, the amount stays the same, but the fraction is easier to work with (Figure 3.6).

Canceling is a shortcut way of showing that you have divided the top and bottom numbers of the fraction by the same number. For example, if you want to reduce $\frac{3}{15}$ to its lowest terms, you divide the top and bottom numbers by the largest number that will go into them evenly; in this case, 3. Three goes into 3 once, so you cancel out the 3 and write 1. Three goes into 15 five times, so you cancel out the 15 and write 5. Thus, after reducing to lowest terms, the fraction is $\frac{1}{5}$.

$$\frac{3}{15} \quad \frac{\overset{1}{\cancel{3}}}{\underset{5}{\cancel{15}}} \quad \frac{1}{5}$$

Figure 3.6
Reducing fractions to lowest terms.

$\frac{4}{8}$

$\frac{1}{2}$

$$\frac{4}{8} = \frac{4 \div 4}{8 \div 4} = \frac{1}{2}$$

$$\frac{6}{9} = \frac{6 \div 3}{9 \div 3} = \frac{2}{3}$$

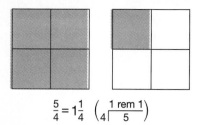

$$\frac{5}{4} = 1\frac{1}{4} \quad \left(4\overline{)\frac{1 \text{ rem } 1}{5}}\right)$$

Figure 3.7
Changing an improper fraction to a mixed number.

You can also cancel units of measurement, as long as the same type of unit appears in both the numerator and the denominator.

$$\frac{18 \text{ mg}}{25 \text{ mg}} \quad \text{or} \quad \frac{3 \text{ gr}}{5 \text{ gr}} \quad \text{but not} \quad \frac{3 \text{ gr}}{50 \text{ mg}}$$

To simplify an improper fraction (or top-heavy fraction) where the numerator is larger than the denominator, turn it into a mixed number (whole number and fraction). Improper fractions are changed to mixed numbers only in giving the final answer to a problem. During calculations, mixed numbers are awkward to work with and must be changed to improper fractions. Divide the numerator by the denominator. Express the remainder as a fraction with the same denominator (Figure 3.7).

MULTIPLYING FRACTIONS

To multiply a fraction by another fraction, multiply numerator by numerator and denominator by denominator.

$$\frac{3}{10} \times \frac{1}{10} = \frac{3 \times 1}{10 \times 10} = \frac{3}{100}$$

$$\frac{5}{8} \times \frac{2}{3} = \frac{5 \times 2}{8 \times 3} = \frac{10}{24}$$

Remember to reduce the answer to lowest terms.

$$\frac{\overset{5}{\cancel{10}}}{\underset{12}{\cancel{24}}} = \frac{5}{12} \text{ (top and bottom divided by 2)}$$

To multiply a fraction by a whole number, multiply the whole number by the numerator of the fraction. Express the whole number as a fraction by giving it the denominator 1. Then place the product over the denominator and simplify.

$$\frac{7}{9} \times 2 = \frac{7}{9} \times \frac{2}{1} = \frac{14}{9} = 1\frac{5}{9}$$

In multiplying fractions, you are allowed to cancel across the times sign.

$$\frac{3}{\underset{1}{\cancel{4}}} \times \frac{\overset{1}{\cancel{4}}}{5} = \frac{3 \times 1}{1 \times 5} = \frac{3}{5}$$

$$\frac{\overset{4}{\cancel{8}}}{9} \times \frac{5}{\underset{7}{\cancel{14}}} = \frac{4 \times 5}{9 \times 7} = \frac{20}{63}$$

When you cancel, you divide the denominator of one fraction and the numerator of the opposite fraction by the same number. This makes it easier to work the problem because you are dealing with smaller numbers. In the same way, you can cancel identical units of measurement across the times sign. This is an important step for certain formulas in dosage calculation.

$$2 \text{ tsp} \times \frac{5 \text{ ml}}{1 \text{ tsp}} = 10 \text{ ml}$$

$$\overset{.5}{\cancel{7.5}} \text{ gr} \times \frac{1 \text{ g}}{\underset{1}{\cancel{15}} \text{ gr}} = 0.5 \text{ g}$$

DIVIDING FRACTIONS

To divide fractions, invert (flip over) the divisor, then multiply the two fractions.

$$\frac{1}{2} \div \frac{2}{3} = \frac{1}{2} \times \frac{3}{2} = \frac{3}{4}$$

$$\frac{5}{8} \div \frac{5}{9} = \frac{\cancel{5}^{1}}{8} \times \frac{9}{\cancel{5}_{1}} = \frac{9}{8}$$

$$\frac{4}{5} \div 3 = \frac{4}{5} \times \frac{1}{3} = \frac{4}{15}$$

DECIMAL FRACTIONS

When working with metric measures, fractions are expressed as decimals. The placement of numbers in relation to the decimal point shows that their values are multiples of 10 (Figure 3.8). Here are some examples of various whole numbers and fractions expressed as decimals.

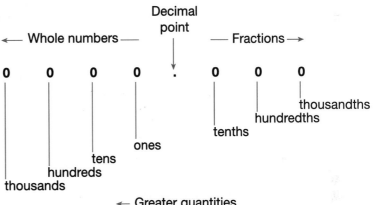

Figure 3.8
Number values in decimal fractions.

$$1.0 = 1\frac{0}{10} = 1$$

$$0.75 = \frac{75}{100} = \frac{3}{4}$$

$$0.66 = \frac{66}{100} = \frac{2}{3}$$

$$0.5 = \frac{5}{10} = \frac{1}{2}$$

$$0.33 = \frac{33}{100} = \frac{1}{3}$$

$$0.25 = \frac{25}{100} = \frac{1}{4}$$

$$0.125 = \frac{125}{1000} = \frac{1}{8}$$

Any decimal fraction can be expressed as a regular or common fraction. In these examples, note the position of the final digit relative to the decimal point.

$$0.48 = \frac{48}{100} = \frac{\cancel{48}^{12}}{\cancel{100}_{25}} = \frac{12}{25}$$
$$\underset{\text{hundredths}}{\uparrow}$$

$$1.6 = 1\frac{6}{10} = 1\frac{\cancel{6}^{\,\cancel{3}}}{\cancel{10}_{\,5}} = 1\frac{3}{5}$$

tenths

Any common fraction can be changed to a decimal fraction by dividing the numerator by the denominator.

$$\frac{1}{3} = 3\overline{)1.00}^{\;0.333...} = 0.33$$
$$\frac{9}{10}$$
$$\frac{9}{1}$$

To multiply decimal fractions, such as 1.5×0.35, set up the multiplication like a normal multiplication problem.

$$
\begin{array}{r}
1.5 \\
\times\ 0.35 \\
\hline
75 \\
45\ \ \\
\hline
0.525
\end{array}
$$

To decide where the decimal goes, look at the original problem, and count the total number of places shown to the right of the decimal points in the two numbers; in this case, 3.

$$1.5 \times 0.35 = 0.525$$
$$1 \qquad 2\,3 \qquad 3\,2\,1$$

Then, starting from the last digit of the answer, count that many places to the left, and place the decimal directly after that digit. Placing the decimal point correctly is extremely important when calculating medications, because a misplaced decimal means a huge error in the dose.

To divide a decimal fraction, such as $30 \div 1.5$, arrange the numbers as in a regular division problem. If there is a decimal fraction in the divisor, move it to the right of the rightmost digit. Count the number of places you move it. Then move the decimal point in the dividend the same number of places to the right. Place the decimal point in the answer (quotient) directly above the decimal point in the dividend.

$$\text{divisor} \rightarrow 1.5\overline{)30.0}^{\;20.} \leftarrow \text{quotient} \;\;\leftarrow \text{dividend}$$

If the divisor is not a decimal fraction, the decimal point in the quotient is directly above the one in the dividend.

$$15\overline{)30.0}^{\;2.0}$$

Define each of the terms listed below.

1. Dosage range _____
   _____
   _____

2. Grain _____
   _____
   _____

3. Metric system _____
   _____
   _____

4. Minim _____
   _____
   _____

5. Liter _____
   _____
   _____

6. Meter _____
   _____
   _____

7. Fraction _____
   _____
   _____

8. Centimeter _____
   _____
   _____

9. Milliliter _____
   _____
   _____

Write abbreviations for these units of measurement.

10. Minim _____   15. Drop _____

11. Grain _____   16. Pint _____

12. Dram _____   17. Tablespoon _____

13. Fluidram _____   18. Pound _____

14. Ounce _____   19. Milligram _____

Continued

20. Milliliter _____
21. Cubic centimeter _____
22. Liter _____
23. Gram _____

Practice decoding abbreviations. The following dosage orders are given using Roman numerals and abbreviations for the apothecary system of measurement. Write them out in full, using Arabic numerals.

24. ℥ $\overline{\text{iv}}$ _____
25. gr $\overline{\text{iss}}$ _____
26. m $\overline{\text{ii}}$ _____
27. f ℥ $\overline{\text{ix}}$ _____

Fill in the blanks. Refer to Tables 3.4, 3.6, and 3.7 if necessary.

28. A grain weighs the same as _____ minim(s) of liquid.
29. One minim is the same as _____ drop(s).
30. One milliliter is approximately equivalent to _____ drop(s).
31. Fifteen grains is about _____ gram(s).
32. One grain is about _____ milligram(s).
33. One gram is equal to _____ milligrams.
34. One milliliter is the same as _____ cubic centimeter(s).
35. One-half of a gram equals _____ milligram(s).
36. One liter (1000 cc) is about _____ quart(s).

Reduce these fractions to the lowest terms.

37. $\frac{4}{8}$ = _____
38. $\frac{3}{9}$ = _____
39. $\frac{24}{32}$ = _____
40. $\frac{21}{28}$ = _____
41. $\frac{250}{1000}$ = _____
42. $\frac{25}{45}$ = _____

Change these improper fractions to mixed numbers.

43. $\frac{8}{3}$ = _____
44. $\frac{5}{2}$ = _____
45. $\frac{17}{12}$ = _____
46. $\frac{55}{20}$ = _____
47. $\frac{18}{4}$ = _____
48. $\frac{68}{3}$ = _____
49. $\frac{350}{100}$ = _____
50. $\frac{27}{5}$ = _____

Multiply these fractions and reduce them to the lowest terms.

51. $\frac{3}{10} \times \frac{1}{10}$ = _____
52. $2 \times \frac{5}{8}$ = _____
53. 250 mg $\times$ 1 gr/60 mg = _____
54. $\frac{5}{8} \times \frac{2}{3}$ = _____
55. $\frac{5}{4} \times \frac{7}{6}$ = _____
56. 3 gr $\times$ 60 mg/1 gr = _____

Divide these fractions and reduce them to the lowest terms.

57. $\frac{1}{2} \div \frac{2}{3}$ = _____
58. $\frac{1}{60} \div 3$ = _____
59. $\frac{5}{8} \div \frac{5}{9}$ = _____
60. $1 \div \frac{1}{600}$ = _____

Continued

Write these fractions as decimals.

61. $\frac{1}{2}$ = _____   66. $\frac{1}{3}$ = _____

62. $\frac{1}{4}$ = _____   67. $\frac{2}{3}$ = _____

63. $\frac{3}{4}$ = _____   68. $\frac{6}{10}$ = _____

64. $\frac{25}{100}$ = _____   69. $\frac{89}{100}$ = _____

65. $\frac{23}{1000}$ = _____   70. $3\frac{3}{4}$ = _____

Change these decimals to fractions and reduce them to the lowest terms.

71. 0.75 = _____   74. 0.2 = _____

72. 1.5 = _____   75. 5.66 = _____

73. 0.005 = _____   76. 0.375 = _____

Multiply or divide these decimals as directed.

77. 1.5 × 3 = _____   80. 1.5 × 0.3 = _____

78. 1.5 × 0.03 = _____   81. 2.75 × 0.1 = _____

79. 7.5 ÷ 25 = _____   82. 7.5 ÷ 2.5 = _____

Convert from grams to milligrams or from milligrams to grams as directed.

83. 0.1 g = _____ mg   87. 2.5 g = _____ mg

84. 0.03 g = _____ mg   88. 0.125 g = _____ mg

85. 325 mg = _____ g   89. 1200 mg = _____ g

86. 3000 mg = _____ g   90. 5 mg = _____ g

■ CASE STUDIES FOR CRITICAL THINKING

Solve the following problems.

91. 0.1 mg = _____ gr   95. 150 mg = _____ gr

92. 0.5 mg = _____ gr   96. _____ mg = 5 gr

93. _____ mg = $\frac{1}{60}$ gr   97. 1 g = _____ gr

94. 4 mg = _____ gr   98. _____ g = $7\frac{1}{2}$ gr

Use the WANT/HAVE formula to solve these dosage problems.

99. The doctor orders 250 mg of a drug. You have 100-mg scored tablets on hand. You will give the patient _____ tablets.

100. The medication order calls for a dose of $1\frac{1}{4}$ gr aspirin. Aspirin comes in scored tablets of 5 gr each. You will give the patient _____ tablet.

101. The physician orders 75 mg of a drug. You have capsules of 25 mg each. You give the patient _____ capsules.

102. An injectable antibiotic is packaged 100,000 units/cc. The doctor orders 400,000 units. A nurse will administer _____ to the patient parenterally.

Continued

103. A solution contains 25 mg of a drug per teaspoon. The doctor orders 50 mg. You give _____ tsp.

104. You have $\frac{1}{2}$-gr tablets. You want to give $\frac{1}{4}$ gr. You administer _____ tablet(s).

105. The doctor's order is to give gr $\overline{xv}$. The medicine bottle shows that each 5-ml teaspoon contains $7\frac{1}{2}$ gr. You give _____ tsp. (Hint: $7\frac{1}{2}$ gr $= \frac{15}{2}$ gr.)

Solve these dosage problems using Table 3.7 as a resource.

106. The doctor orders 600 mg. The dosage form on hand is gr $\overline{x}$ tablets. You give _____ tablet(s). (Hint: Find 600 mg = ? gr; then use the WANT/HAVE formula.)

107. You have $\frac{1}{4}$-gr tablets on hand, and the doctor has ordered 15 mg of the drug. You give _____ tablet(s).

108. The doctor ordered $\frac{3}{4}$ gr. The tablets on hand contain 30 mg each. You give _____ tablet(s). (Hint: Find $\frac{3}{4}$ gr = ? mg; then use the WANT/HAVE formula.)

109. An order is for 45 minims of a drug, but you do not have a measuring container marked in minims. You do have a container marked in milliliters. You administer _____ ml.

Translate the medication order and answer the dosage questions.

110. An order reads *"Fer-In-Sol* 18 mg q.d.p.c." One teaspoon supplies 18 mg of iron. The pharmacy sends up an 8-oz bottle of *Fer-In-Sol.*

    a. How many teaspoons are there in an 8-oz bottle (8 oz = ? tsp)? _____

    b. About how many days will the bottle of *Fer-In-Sol* last? _____

Practice calculating dosages for children. The usual adult dose of Dilantin is 100 mg.

111. How much *Dilantin* would you give to a child who is 11 months old? _____

112. How much *Dilantin* would you give to a child who weighs 34 lb? _____

113. How much would you give to a 10-year-old? _____

114. How much would you give to a 16-year-old? _____

Practice calculating IV therapy doses.

115. How many drops per minute will you give if the order is 500 ml of 5 percent D/W in 5 hours? The drop factor is 15 gtt = 1 ml. _____

116. You are ordered to give the patient 500 cc of blood in 5 hours. Calculate the rate of flow. The drop factor is 20 gtt = 1 cc. (Remember, the tubing gives the drop factor, and for blood it can be 20 gtt = 1 cc instead of 15 or 16 gtt = 1 cc.) _____

117. The physician orders 1500 ml of 5 percent D/W in 24 hours. The drop factor is 15 gtt = 1 cc. How many drops per minute will you give? _____

118. Order: give 2000 cc of 5 percent D/W in 20 hours. Calculate the infusion rate if the drop factor is 15 gtt = 1 cc. _____

PharmInfo Net contains news and information from the pharmaceutical and health care industries. Go to http://pharminfo.com. Click on Drug FAQ's. This takes you to a listing of drug names by generic name and trade name. Click on any drug name to learn about common concerns including proper drug dosage.

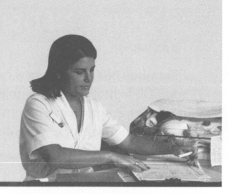

In this chapter you will learn about various forms of medications and the routes by which they are administered. You will learn how to translate medication orders so that you can give medications in the proper form at the correct time and by the right route. You will learn how to do the routine tasks involved in giving medications: how to order, store, and dispose of drugs; how to keep track of medication orders; how to set up medications; and how to chart medications after giving them. You will also learn how to give drugs safely by following the basic rules of medication administration.

OBJECTIVES

After studying this chapter, you should be able to

• list the various forms of medication, ranging from liquids to solids.

• list and describe the routes for administering medications.

• tell who is allowed to give medications by the parenteral route.

• give the meanings of abbreviations for medication forms, routes, administration times, and general medical abbreviations.

• use the military clock.

• name the parts of a medication order.

• identify single-dose and multiple-dose packaging of drugs.

• outline the use of the Kardex, medicine card, and medication record to communicate medication orders.

• set up medications following proper procedure.

• state the rules for giving medications and explain each one.

• describe the problem-oriented medical record and the subjective–objective–assessment–plan method of charting.

• demonstrate accurate, complete, and organized charting.

KEY TERMS

active ingredient: the ingredient in a drug that produces the therapeutic effect

ampule: a small, sealed glass container holding medication for injection; a vial

charting: keeping records of all patient care on appropriate forms

concentration: amount of drug in a certain amount of liquid

controlled substances: drugs regulated by the Controlled Substances Act because of their potential for abuse

enteric-coated: coated with a substance that dissolves in the intestine but not in the stomach (enteric—pertaining to the small intestine)

expiration date: date after which a drug should not be used

incident report: a form used for giving information about a drug error, patient injury, or accident

infusion: placement of a tube into a vein for the purpose of slowly adding fluids to the body (e.g., dextrose, plasma); also called intravenous (IV) drip

inhalation: administration of drugs by way of droplets or mist that the patient breathes in

insertion: placement of an object into a body cavity (e.g., putting a suppository into the rectum)

instillation: placement of drops of liquid into the eyes, ears, nose, or some other body cavity

irrigation: rinsing a body cavity with water or other solutions

Kardex file: portable card file listing daily medication orders and treatments for all patients on a unit

medication administration record (MAR): form documenting drugs that are administered to a particular patient every day; each dose is checked off after it is given

medicine cards: small cards used for setting up medications when a unit-dose system is not used

medicine cart: movable unit for dispensing medications

nurses' notes: form for charting observations, stat and PRN medications, and special treatments given

outpatient: patient who is not hospitalized; a walk-in (ambulatory) patient

patient chart: a permanent record of care received

patient history sheet: a form describing the development of a patient's symptoms and the course of the disease

pharmacy requisition form: form on which to order supplies and medications from the pharmacy

physician's order sheet: form for writing medication orders, located in the patient chart

POMR: problem-oriented medical record

preparation: form in which a drug is available; determines route of administration

PRN order: drug order to administer a drug as needed

routine order: drug order by which the ordered drug is administered until a discontinuation order is written or until a specified termination date is reached

scored: marked with a groove, as a tablet, so as to be easily broken in half

SOAP: structured plan for charting; standards for subjective–objective–assessment–plan

soluble: capable of being dissolved

solution: liquid containing a dissolved drug

standing order: drug order that is to be continued until further notice

stat order: a single drug order that is administered immediately

sterile: free of microorganisms

suspension: liquid containing undissolved particles of a drug

vial: small, glass, single-dose or multiple-dose vacuum-sealed container with a rubber seal that must be punctured with a needle to fill a syringe for injection; an ampule

FORMS OF MEDICATION

Drugs are mixed with various ingredients to make them suitable for patients. There are ingredients to make oral medicines taste good. Elderly as well as young patients take these medications more easily. There are ingredients to thin out a drug mixture so that the dosage can be controlled. Other ingredients allow drugs to be applied on the skin or placed into body parts, such as the eyes, ears, or rectum. These combinations of drugs with various ingredients are called drug **preparations** or products.

Different forms of drugs are appropriate for different routes of administration, so it is important to use the correct form. Failure to administer the drug in the correct form results in medication error. Using an incorrect form can also cause damage to body cells. Therefore, you need to learn about the various drug preparations and their uses. Medication forms are classified as liquids, semiliquids, semisolids, and solids. Table 4.1 lists medication forms and their abbreviations.

TABLE 4.1: Medication Forms and Abbreviations

CLASSIFICATION	FORM	ABBREVIATION	EXAMPLE
Liquid	Solution	soln.	Normal saline
	Syrup	syr.	Robitussin cough syrup
	Fluidextract	fld. ext.	Fluidextract of ipecac
	Spirits	sp.	Spirits of peppermint
	Elixir	elix.	Donnatol elixir
	Fluid	Fl.	IV solutions
Semiliquid	Tincture	tinct., tr.	Tincture of iodine
Solid	Capsule	cap., caps.	Librium
	Tablet	tab.	Lanoxin
Semisolid	Suppository	supp.	Ducolax
	Ointment	oint., ung.	Petroleum jelly

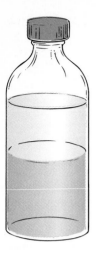

Figure 4.1
A medication that is in the form of a suspension should be shaken before administering.

LIQUIDS AND SEMILIQUIDS

Many drugs are administered in liquid form. They may be given by mouth, rubbed onto the skin, or dropped into eyes, ears, or other parts of the body. Liquid preparations are useful because they allow rapid absorption of the drug. Liquid oral medicines are especially convenient for children and elderly patients who have trouble swallowing solid capsules or tablets.

Some drugs are **soluble,** or able to dissolve in liquids, and others are not. When **active ingredients** are mixed with water, alcohol, or both, the resulting preparations are either solutions or suspensions. In **solutions,** the drug is completely dissolved in alcohol or water. In **suspensions,** the drug is incapable of completely dissolving, and tiny particles or droplets of the drug are held, or suspended, throughout the liquid.

If suspensions are left standing for a while, particles settle to the bottom of the bottle (oils rise to the top). The clear liquid portion is then visible. This situation is normal and can be corrected by shaking the bottle well before giving the medication (Figure 4.1). Solutions, on the other hand, rarely separate when left standing. If they do, it is because they have been stored improperly or are past the **expiration date** for safe usage. Separated solutions must be discarded.

Within the broad categories of solutions and suspensions, there are several specific liquid forms of medication. Tinctures, fluidextracts, elixirs, spirits, and syrups are all types of solutions. Emulsions, magmas, gels, and lotions are types of suspensions.

SOLUTIONS

Tinctures, fluidextracts, elixirs, and spirits are highly **concentrated** forms of drugs. They contain much higher amounts of drug per unit of liquid than do other liquid forms. Therefore, the dose is smaller. These preparations must be measured carefully, using a dropper or a medicine glass. The medicine may be added to water, juice, or another solution suggested by the doctor. The patient then drinks this mixture. These mixtures should never be injected.

Tinctures. Tinctures are solutions made with alcohol or alcohol with water. The active ingredients make up 10 percent to 20 percent of the solution. Tinctures are potent drugs. Examples are tincture of iodine, a strong antiseptic; belladonna tincture, an anticholinergic used to decrease intestinal motility; and camphorated opium tincture, commonly known as paregoric, an antidiarrheal.

Fluidextracts. Fluidextracts are alcohol extracts from plant sources. They are the most concentrated and potent of any liquid preparation. An example is cascara sagrada aromatic fluidextract, used as a laxative.

Elixirs. Elixirs are solutions of alcohol and water containing 10 percent to 20 percent of a drug. Elixirs have special added ingredients to make them sweet-tasting and pleasant-smelling. Because they have a sweet taste, they are better tolerated by children and the elderly. Phenobarbital elixir, an anticonvulsant, and *Benadryl* elixir, an antihistamine, are examples.

> ## CAUTION: Solutions with Alcohol
>
> Tinctures, fluidextracts, elixirs, and spirits contain alcohol. Do not administer them to a diagnosed alcoholic or a patient with diabetes. Storage is important with these alcohol solutions. They must be kept tightly stoppered, so the alcohol cannot evaporate. Store them in a dark place, as stated on the labels. Otherwise, the drug may separate from the alcohol. If this should happen, do not use the preparation. Order another from the pharmacy.

Spirits. Spirits are alcohol solutions of volatile oils, or oils that evaporate. An example is peppermint spirit, used to remove excess gas from the gastrointestinal tract. Spirits contain 5 percent to 20 percent active ingredients.

Syrups. Syrups are heavy solutions of water and sugar, usually with a flavoring added to disguise the unpleasant taste of the drug. They may be as much as 85 percent sugar. They are mixed with a very small amount of a drug. Examples include cough syrups, such as *Robitussin*.

SUSPENSIONS

Emulsions, magmas, and gels are given in small amounts because they contain large portions of active drug ingredients, the ingredients that produce the therapeutic effects. Suspensions must be shaken before use.

Emulsions. Emulsions are suspensions of oils and fats in water with an emulsifying agent. Cod liver oil (a laxative) is an example.

Magmas. A magma contains heavy particles mixed with water that forms a milky liquid. Magmas must be shaken prior to administration. Milk of magnesia (a laxative) is a familiar example of a magma.

Gels. Gels are similar to magmas, but they contain finer particles. An example is *Altern Gel* (an antacid).

Liniments. Liniments are liquid suspensions for external application to the skin to relieve pain and swelling. Liniments are rubbed onto the skin to promote absorption. An example is *Ben-Gay*.

Lotions. Lotions are suspensions of drugs in a water base for external use. Lotions are patted onto the skin rather than rubbed in. They may be protective, emollient (soothing and softening to overcome dryness), astringent (vasoconstricting), or antipruritic (to relieve itching). Lotions tend to settle out and must be shaken before use. Calamine lotion is a common example used for its protective, astringent, and antipruritic effects for poison ivy.

Aerosols. Aerosol medications are commonly delivered by oral inhalers or nebulizers that allow for rapid absorption into the bloodstream (Figure 4.2). An example is *Proventil*, a bronchodilator used in the treatment of obstructive airway disease such as asthma.

SOLIDS AND SEMISOLIDS

Solid forms of drugs are widely used in drug treatment. Except for powders, there is no mixing, shaking, and measuring to be done, as there is with many liquids. The solid forms are also a convenient way to take unpleasant-tasting or irritating drugs.

Ointments. Ointments are drugs mixed in lanolin, a fine oil taken from the skin of sheep, or in petrolatum, a jelly made from petroleum. They are usually applied to skin surfaces, but some ointments can be placed into the eyes. Eye ointments must always bear the label "Sterile—for ophthalmic use."

Pastes. Pastes are semisolid preparations that are thicker and absorbed more slowly than ointments. They are used for skin protection. An example is zinc oxide paste.

Powders. Powders are fine, dry particles of drugs. They may be dissolved in liquids or used as is, depending on the physician's orders. Powders have both internal and external uses. An example is potassium chloride (*Kato Powder*), which is mixed with water or juice and swallowed as a potassium supplement.

Tablets. Tablets are drug powders that have been pressed or molded into small disks. They are designed to be swallowed, either alone or with a liquid. Tablets come in a variety of sizes, shapes, and weights. Some have colored coatings and flavorings and are stamped or printed with the name of the

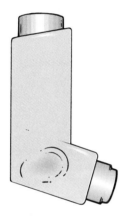

Figure 4.2
Oral nebulizer.

manufacturer. Many tablets are **scored,** which means they have one or more grooves down the middle. The grooves make it possible to break the tablets into halves or quarters if needed.

Capsules. A capsule is a gelatin sheath that contains one dose of medication. The drug inside the capsule can be either a powder, an oil, or a liquid. When the capsule is swallowed, the gelatin quickly dissolves and releases the medicine into the stomach.

Caplets. Caplets are identical to capsules in size and shape, but have the consistency of a tablet.

Sustained-Release Tablets and Capsules. These medication forms contain several doses of a drug. The doses have special coatings that dissolve at different rates, so that medicine is released into the stomach gradually. Some doses are released immediately. Others are released up to 12 hours later. Sustained-release tablets and capsules allow drug effects to continue at the same level over a long period. Delayed release and timed release are other terms used to describe these products. An example is nifedipine *(Procardia XL),* a calcium channel blocker used in the treatment of chest pain and high blood pressure.

CAUTION: Sustained-Release Tablets and Capsules

Never crush, open, or empty a sustained-release tablet or capsule into food or liquid. Using sustained-release medication in this way can cause the patient to receive an overdose.

Enteric-Coated Tablets and Capsules. These are tablets and capsules with a special coating that keeps them from dissolving in the acid secretions of the stomach. They do not dissolve until they reach the alkaline secretions of the intestine. The **enteric coating** prevents an irritating drug from upsetting the stomach. It also prevents the stomach juices from interacting with the drug to change its effect. An example is *Ecotrin*, a nonnarcotic analgesic used for pain, an antipyretic used for fever, and a nonsteroidal anti-inflammatory used in the treatment of arthritis.

PATIENT EDUCATION

Enteric-Coated Tablets

• Explain what signs to watch for to know if the drug is taking effect, because some patients' intestines are not able to dissolve a tablet's enteric coating.

• Do not crush or mix enteric-coated tablets and capsules into food or liquid, because it would destroy the enteric coating and cause the medication to be released in the stomach instead of the intestine.

Troches and Lozenges. Troches and lozenges are tablets designed to dissolve in the mouth rather than be swallowed. They may be flat, round, or rectangular and are used for their local effects. They contain a high concentration of a drug in a sugar base that comes into contact with the mouth and throat as they dissolve. They can help relieve pain or soothe irritation in those areas.

Suppositories. Suppositories are drugs mixed with a firm base, such as cocoa butter, that melts at body temperature. The drug mixture is molded into a shape suitable for insertion into the vagina, rectum, or urethra. After insertion, the suppository dissolves against the warm mucous membranes of these openings and releases the drug. The active ingredients take effect locally or are absorbed into the bloodstream for systemic effects. An example of a vaginal suppository is miconazole nitrate (Monistat), an antifungal used for vaginal fungal infection. An example of a rectal suppository is bisacodyl (Ducolax), a laxative used for relief of constipation.

ROUTES OF ADMINISTRATION

Drugs can be administered to patients through several methods or routes. Each route has its advantages and disadvantages. The route chosen depends on the type of medication, the dosage form, and the desired effects. Table 4.2 lists routes of administration and their abbreviations.

TABLE 4.2: Routes of Administration

ROUTE	MEANING	ABBREVIATION
Buccal	Inside the cheek	buc
Intradermal	Into the skin	ID
Intramuscular	Into the muscle	IM
Intravenous	Into the vein	IV
Oral	By mouth	PO, p.o.
Rectal	By rectum	R
Subcutaneous	Under the skin (into fatty layer)	SC, sub-Q, SQ, subcu
Sublingual	Under the tongue	subling, subl, SL
Topical	On the skin	T
Vaginal	By vagina	p.v., vag

ORAL

Oral administration means that a drug is given by mouth and swallowed, either alone or with a glass of liquid. The drug is then absorbed into the bloodstream through the lining of the stomach and intestine.

Oral administration is the easiest, safest, and most economical way for a patient to take medicine. However, it is also the slowest way for a drug to reach the cells of the body. The drug can be broken down by enzymes in the digestive system. Its absorption can be affected by the presence of food. Irritating medicines may cause nausea and stomach discomfort. Nevertheless, the oral route is well accepted and often used in drug therapy. Oral medications are usually in liquid, tablet, or capsule form.

SUBLINGUAL

Sublingual administration means placing a drug under the tongue, where it dissolves in the patient's saliva. It is quickly absorbed through the mucous membrane that makes up the lining of the mouth. The patient is not permitted to drink or eat until all the medication is dissolved.

Compared to the oral route, the sublingual route has the advantage of faster absorption. It also yields a higher concentration of the drug in the blood, because the drug does not pass through the digestive system first. This is a convenient route as long as drugs are not irritating or bad-tasting.

Medications for sublingual administration are in the form of tablets. They are usually given for their systemic effects. Nitroglycerin, a drug that dilates heart vessels, is often administered sublingually. Ergotamine tartrate (Ergostat) may be given sublingually for migraine headache.

BUCCAL

Buccal administration is similar to sublingual administration, except that the medication is placed in the mouth next to the cheek. The drug is absorbed through the mucous membrane that lines the inside of the cheek. Buccal medications are in the form of tablets. They should not be swallowed, and no food or drink is permitted until after they dissolve. Teach patients to alternate cheeks with each dose to avoid mucosal irritation. *Oxytocin*, a drug that brings on labor in pregnant women, may be administered buccally.

TOPICAL

Topical administration is the method of applying a drug directly to the skin or mucous membrane, usually for a local effect. Medications such as nitroglycerin or estrogen may also be applied by disk or patch. The disk or patch contains the medicine, which is released into the skin. This route of administration has systemic effects. Drugs for topical use are often designed to soothe irritated tissues or to prevent or cure local infections. They are in the form of creams, liniments, lotions, ointments, and liquids. Liquids may be sprayed, swabbed, or painted onto the desired surfaces. Other forms are rubbed or patted on or held against the skin surface with a bandage. Absorption through the skin is slow, whereas absorption through mucous membranes is rapid.

Topical medications can be dropped into the eyes, ears, and nose **(instillation),** and they can be inserted into the vagina, urethra, urinary bladder, and rectum **(insertion).** Any of these areas may also be rinsed with water containing drugs **(irrigation).** These applications are easy to perform, but correct procedure must be followed to avoid damaging the tissue.

RECTAL

Inserting medication into the rectum in the form of a suppository is called rectal administration. Enemas are also administered into the rectum. Absorption through the lining of the rectum is slow and irregular. However, this may be the best route when a patient cannot take medications orally. For example, a vomiting patient or an unconscious patient may require rectal administration.

VAGINAL

The vaginal route of administration requires inserting a cream, foam, tablet, or suppository into the vagina. Medications inserted vaginally are usually given for their local effects, as in the treatment of a vaginal infection with *Mycostatin*.

INHALATION

In **inhalation** administration, medicine is sprayed or inhaled into the nose, throat, and lungs. The drug is absorbed through the mucous membranes in the nose and throat or through the tiny air sacs that fill the lungs. Drugs to be inhaled are in the form of gases or fine droplets (sprays, mists, steam, etc.).

The lungs contain a large surface area, so there is good absorption. However, it is hard to regulate the dose. The inhalation method is also awkward and not suitable for drugs that might irritate the lungs.

Inhalation is widely used for rapid treatment of asthma symptoms. Special devices, such as inhalers, nebulizers, and atomizers, make inhalation therapy relatively convenient. Because microorganisms can easily enter the body through the linings of the lungs, the equipment used for inhalation therapy must be very clean.

PARENTERAL

Parenteral administration involves injecting a drug into the body with a needle and syringe. This method gives much more rapid absorption and distribution than does oral administration. The dosage can also be carefully controlled. The parenteral route is especially useful in emergencies, when a drug effect is needed immediately.

> ### CAUTION: Laws for Administering Medications
>
> Parenteral administration requires special training, special safety precautions, and special equipment. State regulations allow only certain licensed health workers to administer medications parenterally: for example, nurses and nurse practitioners.

There are several disadvantages to the parenteral route. All injection equipment and medicines must be **sterile,** or free of microorganisms. The method is expensive, sometimes painful, and awkward for patients to administer to themselves. Except for the intravenous route, there is the danger of injecting a drug incorrectly into a vein, which could cause serious harm and even death.

Medicine for injection must be in liquid form. Often it must be prepared as a suspension of a powder in distilled water.

The parenteral route is divided into four main categories, according to the location of the injection.

In intradermal (intracutaneous) administration, a small amount of medicine is injected just beneath the outer layer of skin. The dose is usually less than 0.3 ml. The injected drug forms a small bubble (bleb) under the skin. Intradermal injections are used in tuberculin tests, allergy tests, and vaccinations. The drug is absorbed slowly with this type of injection.

In the subcutaneous route, medication is injected into a layer of fatty tissue that lies right below the skin. This is called the subcutaneous (under the skin) tissue. The dose is approximately 1 to 2 ml. Insulin, hormones, and local anesthetics are among the medications administered by subcutaneous injection.

Intramuscular administration is the injection of a drug deep into muscle. Because the muscles are well supplied with blood, absorption from the muscles is faster than absorption from the skin layers. Muscles can also absorb a greater amount of fluid without discomfort to the patient; the usual dose is 1 to 3 ml. The common sites for intramuscular administration include dorsogluteal, vastus lateralis, ventrogluteal, and deltoid muscles (Figure 4.3 on page 60). Intramuscular injection is also preferred for substances that can irritate the skin layers. Penicillin is often injected intramuscularly. The danger of causing tissue damage is less because the injection is entering deep into the muscle. There is, however, a risk of injecting the drug directly into a vein. For example, if penicillin were injected into a vein, it could cause serious side effects or prove fatal. During intramuscular administration, care must be taken to inject only large, healthy muscles and to avoid hitting major nerves, bones, and blood vessels.

Intravenous injection is a method for placing a sterile drug solution directly into a vein. It is the most desirable route when a fast-acting medication is needed quickly, as in emergency situations. However, introducing a drug directly into a vein is the most dangerous method of administering drugs, because there is no time to correct an error.

Intravenous injection differs from intravenous infusion, or IV drip, mainly in speed of action. **Infusion** is the insertion of a tube or a needle into a vein through which fluids are slowly added to the bloodstream over a period of time. Infusion is used often in nursing care to keep the body s fluid level in balance. Drugs can be added to IV fluids for a continuous drug effect. Or they

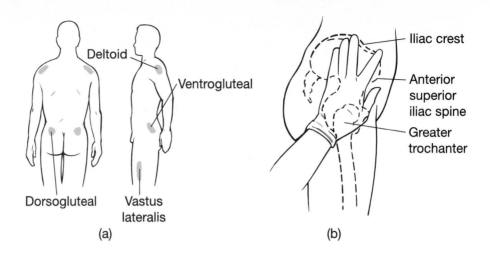

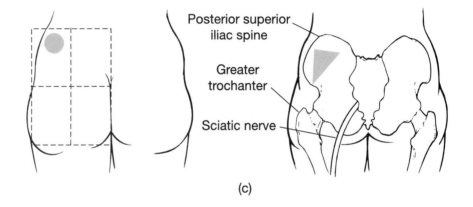

Figure 4.3
(a) IM injection sites; (b) locating the ventrogluteal site; (c) two ways to locate the dorsogluteal site.

can be injected into the IV tube that leads into the vein, which is almost the same as injecting directly into the vein.

Although there are other methods for administering drugs by the intravenous route, all drugs administered intravenously are administered only by a registered nurse, physician, or specially trained individual such as a paramedic.

Intracardiac, intra-arterial, intrathecal or intraspinal, and intraosseous are types of injections that only physicians are permitted to perform. These methods are for injecting a drug into the heart muscle, into an artery, into the spinal spaces, or into a bone, respectively.

THE MEDICATION ORDER

When a physician tells a nurse or another health care worker which drug or drugs to administer to a patient, the physician is giving a medication order. It may be expressed in writing or verbally. It is preferable to give them in writing. Orders should not be given verbally because of the possibility of error. When an order must be given verbally, as in an emergency situation, it should be written down and signed by the physician within 24 hours. Written orders are stated in a special book for doctors' orders or on a **physician's order sheet** in a patient's chart (Figure 4.4).

A prescription blank is used to write medication orders for patients who are being discharged from the hospital or who are seeing the doctor in a medical office or clinic (Figure 4.5). These patients are called **outpatients.**

Physicians are usually the only health care professionals allowed to prescribe medicines, but in some states, nurse practitioners, pharmacists, and

Figure 4.4
Physician's order sheet.

Unless "This Brand Only" appears after a drug order, a brand name other than the one ordered may be used in accordance with formulary policy.

DATE	TIME	ORDERS AND SIGNATURE•USE BALL POINT PEN	REQUEST SENT ✔	TIME	NURSE'S SIGNATURE
6/8	0800	Axid 150mg P.O. BID			
		K-Dur 20meq PO QID			
		Colace 100mg PO @ HS			
		Lanoxin 0.125mg PO daily			
		Chest X ray			
		Barium swallow			
		Stool specimen x 2			
		General diet			
		Activity as tolerated			
		Sam McShane MD			

FORM NO. 2300-00081   (REV. 10/XX)   **PHYSICIAN'S ORDERS**   Addressograph/Label Here
Springfield   CHART COPY
Healthcare System

Figure 4.5
An outpatient prescription blank.

SPRINGFIELD HEALTHCARE SYSTEM 1014862
SPRINGFIELD HOSPITAL   **SPRINGFIELD HOSPITAL WEST**

PATIENT'S NAME _____ DATE _____

ADDRESS _____ AGE _____

℞

LABEL _____ ☐ GENERIC AND/OR EQUIVALENT ALLOWED.

REFILL _____

_____ _____ M.D.
Physician's Signature   (Print Physician's Name)

DEA NO. _____ ADDRESS _____
Form No. 01805308 (Rev. 2/XX)

physician's assistants are permitted to prescribe. They prescribe drugs under the direct supervision of a physician with whom they work.

Who is allowed to take down verbal orders differs according to each agency's policies. Ask about your agency's specific policies regarding the writing and receiving of medication orders. No medication is given without an order.

The medication order includes several important pieces of information. You, the health care worker, must read and understand all this information so that you may correctly prepare and administer the medication. The basic parts of a medication order include patient's name, date, drug name, dosage, route of administration, time and frequency, physician's signature, quantity and number of refills, and, when the prescription is for a controlled substance, the physician's DEA number.

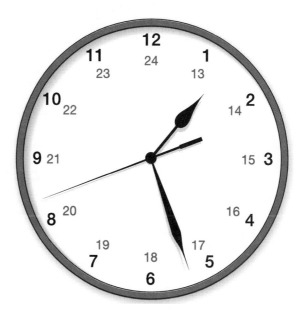

Figure 4.6
Military time—a 24-hour system.

- *Patient's full name.* For proper identification, the patient's first and last names are needed. The patient's admission number is included in some health facilities. The patient's age should be included, especially if the dosage should be checked (e.g., for children and elderly patients).
- *Date of the order.* The day, month, and year are included. Often the time of day is also shown. This practice helps avoid confusion when the staff changes shifts. Many institutions use military time, a 24-hour system, to avoid confusing a.m. and p.m. times that occur in the 12-hour system. For example, 9:15 a.m. would be written as 0915 hours, and 5:45 p.m. would be written as 1745 hours. Figure 4.6 illustrates military time. In the figure, a.m. hours are numbered in the outer circle and p.m. hours in the inner circle. Using military time, the day begins at 0001 (12:01 a.m.) and ends at 2400 hours (12:00 midnight). The number of the hour is used with zeroes as appropriate to indicate both hours and minutes; for example, 0600 (6 a.m.) and 2300 (11:00 p.m.).
- *Name of the drug.* On a prescription blank, the drug name is preceded by "Rx," which means "take thou." The drug's generic name or product name is written out. For reasons of cost, it is becoming more common for doctors to order drugs by their generic names. There may be a special line on the prescription blank for writing in the generic name or one that says "may substitute generic drug." If a drug name is not familiar to you, consult a drug reference such as the USP Drug Information for the Health Care Professional or the PDR.
- *Dosage.* This includes the amount of the drug and the strength of the preparation (e.g., two 100-mg tablets as opposed to 50-mg tablets or 250-mg tablets).

- *Route of administration.* The specified route is important because some medicines can be given by several different routes. If no special route is ordered, notify your supervisor so the physician may be called to identify the correct route of administration. Never assume that a medication is administered by a certain route. Accuracy is essential.
- *Time and frequency.* Both the time to administer the drug and how often must be clearly stated (e.g., BID for 10 days).
- *Physician's signature.* Without the signature of the physician, the medication order is not legal. When a nurse or other staff member must take an order by phone, the nurse signs the order, and the physician co-signs it within 24 hours. When a physician prescribes drugs for clinic outpatients or private patients, the medication order also includes the number of refills and the quantity.
- *Number of refills and quantity.* Some drugs, especially Schedule II drugs, may not be refilled without another prescription. For other drugs, the order may show a certain number of refills, ranging from no refills to PRN (as needed). No prescription or refill is good for more than 1 year. The medication label shows the number of refills following the Latin word *repetatur,* meaning "repeat." Outpatient prescriptions must specify the quantity of the drug to be dispensed to the patient (e.g., 30 tabs).
- *Physician's DEA number.* This registration number from the Drug Enforcement Agency is required on all prescriptions for controlled substances.

State laws and agency policies regulate who may carry out the routine responsibilities in medication administration. Check the policy manual of your health facility to find out who may calculate and measure doses; set up and administer medications; transcribe medication orders; count and handle controlled substances; order, reorder, and receive drugs from the pharmacy; observe patients and chart progress; report to the physician; give patients health instruction; and so on.

TYPES OF DRUG ORDERS

The most common type of drug order is the **routine order,** which means that the ordered drug is administered until a discontinuation order is written or until a specified termination date is reached. Some agencies use automatic stop dates, which are a means to force the physician to reevaluate a patient's medication schedule and either continue current medications or change them, based on the patient's condition.

Another type of order is the **standing order,** which outlines a specific condition in which a drug is to be administered. Standing orders are written and signed by the physician in charge of a patient's care before the drugs are needed. They are frequently used in critical care units, where a patient's condition changes rapidly and immediate action is required, such as administration of a certain drug for an irregular heartbeat. Standing orders are also used in long-term care facilities where a physician is not readily available; for example, "Give *Tylenol* 500 mg q 4 hrs for temperature of 101°F or above."

A **PRN order** is an order written by the physician for a drug to be given when a patient needs it. The majority of drugs written as PRN orders are pain medications; for example, "*Demerol* 75 mg q 3–4 hrs for incisional pain." A single (one-time) order is an order to be given only once at a specified time. These orders are frequently written for preoperative drugs or drugs to be given before diagnostic procedures. An example is "*Valium* 10 mg PO at 0700." A **stat order** is a single order that is administered immediately. Stat orders are usually written for emergencies when a patient's condition suddenly changes; for example, "Give *Procardia* 10 mg SL stat."

You will occasionally have questions about a medication order. Perhaps you cannot read the prescriber's handwriting. The prescribed dosage may seem unusually high. You may find that a patient does not tolerate a certain drug well. Or the patient may have trouble taking the drug by the prescribed route. When these situations arise, it is your duty to check the order with the doctor or supervisor. In no case should you give a medication unless the orders are clearly written.

It is also important to know your agency's policies concerning which staff members are allowed to carry out which procedures. You should not be asked to carry out any procedure that is against agency policy; for example, to administer an adjusted medication dose without a new medication order.

STANDARD MEDICAL ABBREVIATIONS

Abbreviations are a shorthand form used to write medication orders. They are a quick, convenient way to summarize instructions on what drug to give and how to give it. Certain standard abbreviations are familiar to most people in the medical field. Tables 4.3 and 4.4 show some abbreviations commonly used in writing medication orders. You must memorize standard medical

TABLE 4.3: Abbreviations for Times of Administration

ABBREVIATION	MEANING	ABBREVIATION	MEANING
a.c.	Before meals	q.d., QD	Every day
ad lib.	As desired	q.h.	Every hour
AM, a.m.	Morning	q2h, q.2h.	Every two hours
BID, b.i.d.	Twice a day	q3h, q.3h.	Every three hours
h., hr.	Hourly	q4h, q.4h.	Every four hours
h.s.	Hour of sleep, bedtime	QID, q.i.d.	Four times a day
n., noc.	Night	q.o.d.	Every other day
p.c.	After meals	stat	Immediately
PM, p.m.	After noon	TID, t.i.d.	Three times a day
PRN, p.r.n.	As necessary		

TABLE 4.4: Abbreviations of Medical Terms

ABBREVIATION	MEANING	ABBREVIATION	MEANING
a	Before	os	Mouth
AD	Right ear	OS	Left eye
AS	Left ear	OU	Both eyes
AU	Both ears	p	After
c̄.	With	per	By means of
°C	Degrees Celsius (Centigrade)	pH	Hydrogen concentration (acidity and alkalinity)
c/o	Complains of	PO, p.o.	By mouth
dil.	Dilute	q.	Every
°F	Degrees Fahrenheit	q.s.	A sufficient amount
♀	Female	®	Registered product name
M.	Mix	Rx	Take
♂	Male	s.	Without
n.p.o.	Nothing by mouth	sig.	Label
OD	Right eye	ss	One-half
ophth., op.	Ophthalmic		

abbreviations to enable you to read and understand any medication order that you are expected to carry out. At some time, you may also have to translate a prescription into simple language for a patient's family.

There is often variation in the style of drug orders. You may find abbreviations capitalized on some orders and not capitalized on others. You may also find differences in punctuation. The use of capital letters and periods is inconsistent in the profession. Check to see if your agency has its own list of approved abbreviations, and follow that list.

ORDERING DRUGS FROM THE PHARMACY

After a physician writes a medication order for a patient, the proper drugs must be obtained. The way this is done depends on the type of facility in which you work. Most hospitals have a pharmacy within the building. They may also have satellite or minipharmacies on each unit.

Hospital pharmacy requests can be made in several ways. The physician's order sheet has a second page that makes a carbon copy of the medication order. This second page can be torn out and sent to the pharmacy. It tells the pharmacist which drugs, and in which form, to send back to the floor for the patient.

If a copy of the physician's order sheet cannot be used, the nurse must write out the drug orders on a **pharmacy requisition form** (Figure 4.7). This is sent to the pharmacist, and the orders are filled from it. There may be more

---

SPRINGFIELD HOSPITAL DISTRICT

SPRINGFIELD HOSPITAL   SPRINGFIELD HOSPITAL WEST

NURSING/PHARMACY COMMUNICATION SLIP
(Addressograph space)

MEDICATION AS ORDERED/DOSES NEEDED/TIME REQUIRED:
1. _____
2. _____
3. _____

REASON FOR REQUEST:
   ( ) TRANSFERRED TO _____
   ( ) GOING ON PASS – NEED DOSES
   ( ) NEW ALLERGY _____
   ( ) RECEIVED W/O MEDS FROM _____
   ( ) MEDS DAMAGED / DROPPED
   ( ) PRN/REFILL MEDS:
      ( ) NEED 24–HR SUPPLY (AROUND–THE–CLOCK)
      ( ) RETURN TO PAR LEVEL (UP TO 2 DOSES)
   ( ) OFF UNIT – NEED MAKE-UP DOSE(S)
   ( ) MEDS LOST / NOT RECEIVED
   ( ) OTHER _____
NURSE SIGNATURE: _____
   PHARMACY WILL NOT DISPENSE FROM YELLOW COPY
WHITE COPY–PHARMACY   YELLOW COPY–CASSETTE

847–0003–10–91

Figure 4.7
Pharmacy requisition form.

than one drug order on each requisition form. When filling out a pharmacy requisition form, be sure to copy all the information correctly from the doctor s order and to fill in every item on the form.

Using the physician s order sheet for ordering drugs is safer than using a requisition form, because no copying is required. There is less chance of a medication error. When and if there is an error, it is much easier to find the source. State laws have helped to establish this single-entry ordering system wherein the order goes from the doctor directly to the pharmacy.

In a hospital, drugs are requested every day as soon as they are ordered. The pharmacy usually sends up enough of each drug to last 8 hours. At some facilities the pharmacist or pharmacy technician checks the medicine supplies of the unit PRN. In some hospitals, drug orders are entered into a computer, either by the doctor or by a nurse or unit clerk following the doctor s verbal or written orders. In some facilities, drugs are reordered by sending the empty containers to the pharmacy along with appropriate requisition forms.

Some long-term care facilities have their own pharmacies, but most do not. They must order drugs from an outside pharmacy. The ordering system is somewhat different from that used in hospitals. Drugs can be ordered using either a carbon copy of the physician s order sheet or a pharmacy requisition form. These forms are sent to the pharmacy at a certain time each day. The drugs are prepared at the pharmacy and sent back within 24 hours. When they come in, they are checked by comparing the delivery ticket with the doctor s orders.

Reorders are listed on a special reorder sheet. To make up the list, part of the original drug label called the strip label is pulled off each container and pasted onto the reorder form (Figure 4.8). The form then goes to the outside pharmacy where the orders are filled.

Most drugs for long-term care patients are ordered for an indefinite period. In other words, they are standing orders. For that reason, drugs are ordered in large batches and are reordered only every 30 to 90 days.

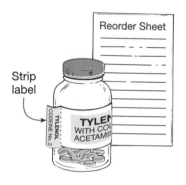

Figure 4.8
To reorder drugs, remove the strip label from the container and affix it to the reorder sheet.

DRUG PACKAGING

The pharmacy supplies drugs in one of two forms: single-dose packages or multiple-dose packages (Figure 4.9).

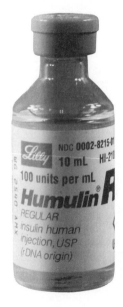

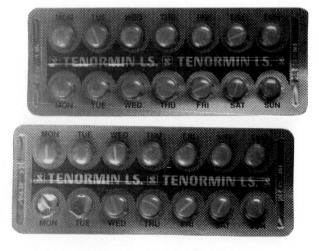

Figure 4.9
Medications come from the pharmacy in unit-dose (left) or multiple-dose (right) packaging.

SINGLE OR UNIT DOSE

In single-dose or unit-dose packaging, each dose of medication is individually wrapped or bottled and supplied for a 24-hour period. Single-dose **ampules,** vials, and prefilled syringes are supplied for some parenteral medications. Each single-dose package contains the proper dose for one administration. It is labeled with the drug name, strength, expiration date, and sometimes the patient's name.

Unit-dose packaging provides the safest and most convenient means of administering medicines. The drugs require little handling and no special preparation before being taken to the patient. Unused doses can be returned to the pharmacy for credit. The individual wrappings ensure that they will not become contaminated in handling.

MULTIPLE DOSE

Many drugs are sent from the pharmacy in multiple-dose bottles or vials. A **vial** is a small vacuum-sealed container with a rubber seal at the top that must be punctured with a needle before administering a dose. The person who is to administer the drug must measure and pour out single doses of liquid medications or count out tablets or capsules from a bottle.

STORAGE AND DISPOSAL OF DRUGS

MEDICINE ROOM

All medications are stored in a medication room, a portable medicine cart, or an individual storage unit adjacent to the patient's room.

The medication room contains a sink, a refrigerator, and storage cabinets. The refrigerator is necessary because some drugs must be stored in a cool place so as not to lose their effectiveness. Drugs that need refrigeration are so labeled. Among them are antibiotics and tetanus vaccine.

There is a special cabinet in the medicine room for controlled substances. It is kept locked so that the use of these restricted drugs can be monitored. A designated nurse or the charge nurse keeps the narcotics keys throughout the shift.

Another cabinet may hold stock supply drugs, or drugs commonly used by many patients. Some stock supply drugs are also kept in the refrigerator. Drugs like aspirin, *Tylenol*, milk of magnesia, and *Maalox* are often part of the stock supply. If a facility has stock emergency drugs, they are generally kept in a cabinet separately from other stock drugs. Stock supply drugs are declining in use because of the potential for medication errors caused by the large assortment of stock medications to choose from. Other problems include financial loss resulting from misplaced or forgotten charges, expired drugs, the need for frequent inventorying of the drugs, and lack of available storage space. The stock supply system thus costs more and is less safe for the patient. The national trend is toward the unit dose system.

Cabinets in the medicine room should be kept closed. Drugs that are for external use only are always kept in separate cabinets or compartments. Keep the medicine room and refrigerator clean and tidy at all times. This is vital in helping to prevent medication errors.

MEDICINE CART

For convenience, doses of routine drugs are often stored in a **medicine cart.** There may be more than one medication cart, depending on the size of the unit or facility. Each medication cart covers a set number of rooms. In some facilities, medication carts may be kept in the halls near the rooms they serve. They may be kept locked when not in use. The carts have drawers marked off for different patients. A 24-hour supply of unit-dose packages is kept in each patient's drawer. When it is time to administer a dose, the cart can be wheeled from room to room. The medications are then dispensed right out of the drawers. The pharmacist or pharmacy technician refills each patient's drawer at a designated time of day. A limited number of PRN medications are also placed in each patient's drawer (Figure 4.10).

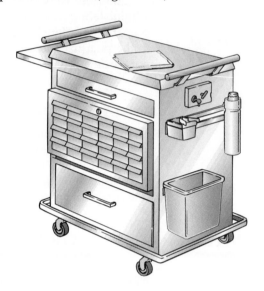

Figure 4.10
Medicine cart.

A special locked drawer in the cart contains the Schedule II, III, and IV drugs. The health care worker unlocks this drawer only when a dose of a controlled substance is needed. The drawer is relocked immediately, before giving the medication to the patient.

A folder or chart on top of the medicine cart contains each patient's medication record, which tells which drugs are to be administered at which times.

COMPUTER-CONTROLLED DISPENSING SYSTEM

Computer-controlled dispensing systems are used successfully throughout the country. They are especially beneficial to the control of narcotics. Each designated member of the health care team has a security code that permits access to the unit. After entering the patient's identification number, the team member selects the specific drug, dose, and route. In addition to delivering the medication, this system records it and charges it to the patient's account.

MEDICINE TRAY

Another way to carry drugs from room to room at administration time is by means of a medicine tray. There are two types of trays. One is a flat tray on which the medicine cups are placed, with a medicine card next to each cup. The other is a plastic tray with molded recesses for holding cups and medicine cards. A molded tray is better than a flat tray because the cards and cups cannot move about and get mixed up (Figure 4.11).

DISPOSING OF UNUSED DRUGS

Never return unused doses of medications to stock supply bottles. Discard the unused doses in the proper manner. Each health facility has its own policy regarding drug disposal. Usually the drugs must be returned to the pharmacy. In some cases, they must go to a certain person or to a storage area. They are then held until there is a batch of drugs to return to the pharmacy.

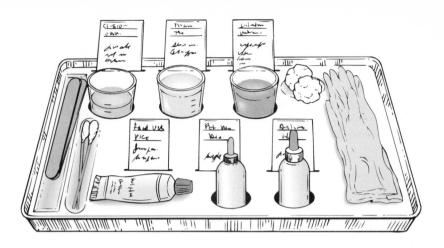

Figure 4.11
Medicine tray.

Disposal of controlled substances must be witnessed by another staff member. The amount wasted must then be documented on the narcotic sign-out sheet.

KEEPING TRACK OF MEDICATION ORDERS

Whenever more than one patient is being cared for, it is necessary to keep track of which patient is to get which medicine at what time. In a unit of 20 patients, some of whom are to receive several drugs, careful preparation is needed to keep their medications straight. Medical facilities and long-term care facilities have various ways of handling this problem. Three common methods are the Kardex file, medicine cards, and the medication record.

KARDEX

The **Kardex file** is a card-filing system that serves as a quick reference to the needs of a patient. Each card is folded once. The card for each patient gives up-to-date information about medications, treatments, and care. All information that can be changed or updated must be written in pencil, so that each time new orders are given, the old ones can be erased and the new ones penciled in. Health care workers can use the Kardex to organize their work day.

MEDICINE CARDS

Medicine cards are used less frequently because the unit-dose system has cut down on the need for them. Where they are still used, information is transcribed or copied onto a set of medicine cards from the Kardex. One medicine card is written for each type of drug a patient is to receive. Each card states the patient's name; room and bed number; and name of the drug, dose, route, and time at which the drug is to be given. Sometimes the card also includes the signature of the nurse or clerk who copied the information from the Kardex.

If the information on a medicine card seems unclear to you, be sure to recheck the Kardex and the physician's order sheet. A mistake may have been made in copying this information. Never try to read through a card that has had medicine spilled on it. You may make a medication error. Go back to the patient's chart and the Kardex and make a new medicine card. Be sure, however, to copy the information correctly onto the new card. If you need more help, consult the nurse in charge or the drug reference books on your unit.

MEDICATION RECORD																																					

Family Name		First Name		Middle Name		Month		Year	Room No.	Bed No.	Admission No.
Shrock		Tammy		Anne		Sept		XXXX	517	1	874321

Attending Physician	Supervising Nurse
N. Morris	P.T. Brown

MEDICATIONS	Hour	1	2	3	4	5	6	7	8	9	10	11	12	13	14	15	16	17	18	19	20	21	22	23	24	25	26	27	28	29	30	31
Dilantin 100mg. p.o.	0900	LE	LE	LE	AW	AW	LE																										
t.i.d.	1300	LE	LE	LE	AW	AW	LE																										
	1700	CS	CS	CS	CS	HF	HF																										
Chloromycetin ophth.	0900	LE	LE	LE	AW	AW	LE				X																						
oint. q.i.d.	1200	LE	LE	LE	AW	AW	LE				X																						
	1500	CS	CS	CS	CS	HF	HF			X																							
	1800	CS	CS	CS	CS	HF	HF			X																							
								last dose 1200 (D)																										

INSULIN TYPE	Hour Given	Amount Given	U 16	U 16	U 16	U 16	U 17	U 17																					
NPH	0600	Amount Given	16	16	16	16	17	17																					
CODE	R-Refused D-Discontinued O-Ordered	Sugar	N	N	N	+	+	N																					
		Acetone	N	N	N	+	+	+																					

Initial medications and identify initials below with signature

NURSES	INITIALS	SIGNATURES	NURSES	INITIALS	SIGNATURES	NURSES	INITIALS	SIGNATURES
A.M. Nurse	LE	*Lorna Emmett*	P.M. Nurse	CS	*Carl Simms*	Night Nurse	KB	*Karen Black*
A.M. Relief	AW	*Alice Wright*	P.M. Relief	HF	*Hilma Francis*	Night Relief	TT	*Tillie Tate*

Figure 4.12
Medication record showing routine medications at the top of the form and PRN medications at the bottom part of the form.

MEDICATION ADMINISTRATION RECORD

The **medication administration record (MAR)** is a convenient way to document all the drugs administered to a patient every day. It is especially helpful when several drugs must be given at different times. The name of each drug is written once on a patient's medication record (Figure 4.12). Routine medications are usually written at the top of the medication record and PRN medications at the bottom or on a separate form. The amount, strength, and route are recorded.

If a drug is to be given regularly, a complete schedule is written for all administration times. Then, each time a dose is administered, the health care worker checks off the time it was given and initials it. Never sign off on a drug before actually giving it. The full name of each person who dispenses medications is listed somewhere on the sheet so the initials can be identified, if necessary.

The medication record is prepared by the clerk, pharmacist, or other health care worker as drugs are ordered. The nurse then checks the form against the doctor's order and signs it. The current day's medication records for all patients are kept in a special folder or chart on the medicine cart or in the medication room. The MARs from previous days are placed in the individual patients' charts.

SELF-TERMINATING ORDERS

Self-terminating or automatic stop orders mean that a drug is to be given only until a certain date or time. When this type of order is copied from the physi-

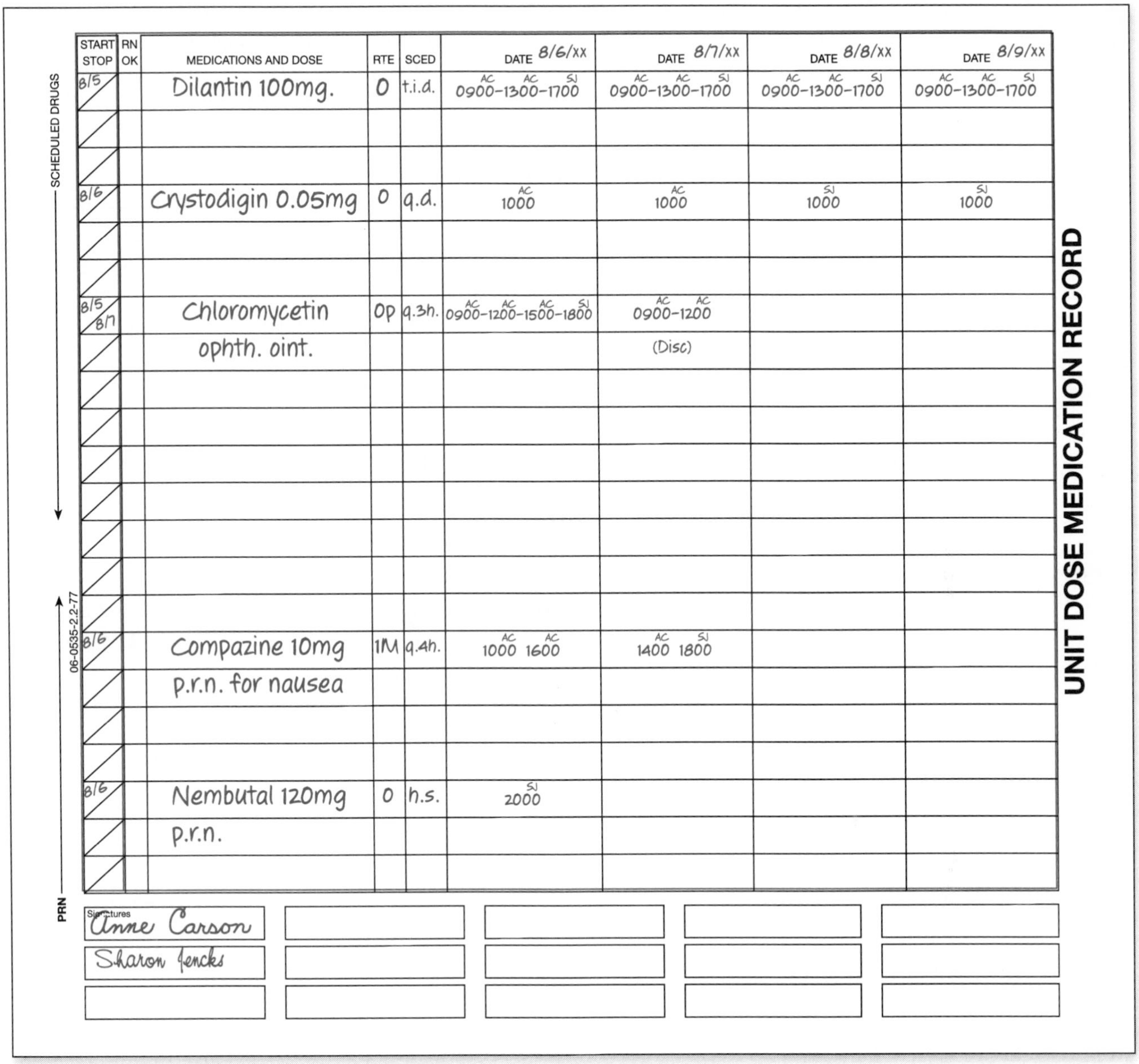

UNIT DOSE MEDICATION RECORD

START STOP	RN OK	MEDICATIONS AND DOSE	RTE	SCED	DATE 8/6/xx	DATE 8/7/xx	DATE 8/8/xx	DATE 8/9/xx
8/5		Dilantin 100mg.	O	t.i.d.	AC AC SJ 0900-1300-1700	AC AC SJ 0900-1300-1700	AC AC SJ 0900-1300-1700	AC AC SJ 0900-1300-1700
8/6		Crystodigin 0.05mg	O	q.d.	AC 1000	AC 1000	SJ 1000	SJ 1000
8/5 8/7		Chloromycetin ophth. oint.	OP	q.3h.	AC AC AC SJ 0900-1200-1500-1800	AC AC 0900-1200 (Disc)		
8/6		Compazine 10mg p.r.n. for nausea	1M	q.4h.	AC AC 1000 1600	AC SJ 1400 1800		
8/6		Nembutal 120mg p.r.n.	O	h.s.	SJ 2000			

Signatures: *Anne Carson* / *Sharon Jencks*

(06-0535-2.2-77 — SCHEDULED DRUGS / PRN)

Figure 4.13
Medication record showing a self-terminating drug order.

cian s order sheet, the nurse or clerk makes a special note or mark on the Kardex, medicine card, or medication record. This notation shows the date and time after which the drug should no longer be given. In Figure 4.13, the order for chloromycetin shows such a note. When that time comes, the nurse or clerk notifies the patient s doctor that the order has terminated. If the doctor decides the patient should continue receiving the drug, a new order is written. Automatic stop orders usually cover antibiotics, narcotics, corticosteroids, anticoagulants, and barbiturates.

CONTROLLED SUBSTANCES

Controlled substances are drugs whose use is restricted. This group of drugs includes narcotics, stimulants, and depressants. Because of legal restrictions, these medications must be counted or measured at the beginning of each shift. As the shift changes, the person coming off duty and the person coming on duty count the narcotics together. They record the quantity of each controlled substance on the narcotics form. They then sign a special form so that there is a record of who counted the drugs on each shift. If the count is found to be incorrect at a later shift, the error can be traced to the proper personnel.

Controlled substances are packaged in either single doses or multiple doses. For example, *Demerol* 50 mg for injection is packaged in a box of 10 prefilled syringes. Oral narcotics such as *Percodan* may come in single-dose packages in a box of 25. The packages are given a special seal at the pharmacy.

Each time a controlled substance is administered from the stock supply, the health care worker must sign a proof-of-use record, such as the one shown in Figure 4.14. Each health facility has its own form for this purpose. The form usually shows the number of doses sent to the unit's stock supply from the pharmacy. As each dose is used, the date, time, patient, room number, amount given, physician, and person administering the dose must be recorded. If a dose less than the prepared individual dose is given, the amount actually given is noted. The unused portion must be destroyed in front of a witness, who must also sign the form.

Many health care facilities use the computer-controlled dispensing system for dispensing narcotics. After the designated health care member enters the security code and the patient's identification number, the specified drug is delivered—for example, *Demerol* 100 mg IM q 4 hr for Mrs. Decoda, Room 412B.

NARCOTIC/BARBITURATE PROOF OF USE RECORD
SPRINGFIELD HOSPITAL WEST

CHECK ONE
☐ DO NOT REISSUE
☑ REISSUE
☐ MED DISCONTINUED
☐ PAT. DISCHARGED
☐ OTHER

RETURNED BY: *Greg Storms, Pharm. Aide* DATE: 8/11
RECEIVED BY: *P. Long, R.N.* DATE: 8/11

ALL PREPS LOST, DESTROYED OR UNACCOUNTED FOR MUST BE EXPLAINED.

NO	DATE	TIME	PATIENT	BED	AM'T mgs	PHYSICIAN	ADMIN. BY	AMOUNT & WITNESS
25	8/11	1600	Carol McCullum	921	100 mg	T. Mann	P. Long	
24	8/12	0800	Shirley Dugan	912	75 mg	P. Zipp	J. Cox	25 mg/J. Jones
23	8/14	1400	Rickey Hornett	924	100 mg	D. Perkins	C. Kelly	
22	8/19	1300	Robert Lance	916	100 mg	P. Zipp	C. Kelly	
21	8/21	0630	Kelly Radner	910	50 mg	C. Ruff	P. Long	50 mg/H. Holly
20								
19								
18								
17								
16								
15								
14								
13								
12								
11								
10								
9								
8								
7								
6								
5								
4								
3								
2								
1								

USE LINES BELOW FOR CORRECTION OF ERRORS WHEN APPLICABLE

ISSUED TO:

Unit C
UNIT OR PATIENT NAME & BED NO.
ISSUED BY: *M. Chrenay, R.PH*
RECEIVED BY: *Greg Storms, Pharm. Aide*

SERIAL NO. 461   NO. ISSUED 25   DATE 8/11

DRUG NAME	STRENGTH	FORM	SIZE
Demerol	100 mg	ampuls	2ml

Figure 4.14 Administering controlled substances requires documentation on a proof-of-use record.

Medications are ordered by the physician, requested from the pharmacy, and stored in the proper area. Now comes the time when you, the giver of medications, must be most alert—setting up medications. Setting up medications means taking information from the Kardex, medication record, or medicine card and preparing an actual dose of medication for a patient. You will be setting up several drugs at a time, and you must be aware of all of the possibilities for error. Here are some guidelines to help you prepare a medicine tray or drug cart for your rounds.

1. Clear your mind of everything except getting the medications set up properly. Do not try to carry on a conversation with someone while you work; the task at hand needs your full attention.

2. Before handling any medications, think about cleanliness. Microorganisms can be transmitted to patients on tablets and other medications, so follow aseptic procedure (discussed in Chapter 6). Wash your hands before touching any drug product. Try not to touch the drugs at all; pour them directly into paper or plastic medicine cups. Never give a pill that has fallen on the floor; throw it away. Do not cough or sneeze on the medications. Keep unit doses sealed until you are ready to give them.

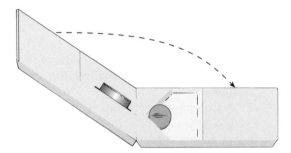

Figure 4.15
Pill cutter.

3. Setting up is the time when you need to decide whether you must calculate a dose. You will notice whether the pharmacist's order is in a unit of measurement different from that of the physician's order. At this point you will utilize the skills you learned in Chapter 3. Use the appropriate conversion tables and have your work checked if you have any doubts at all. If you need to divide a tablet, use a pill cutter, if available (Figure 4.15). Place the pill in the pill cutter form and close the lid. The pill form holds the pill firmly in place. As you close the lid, a knife in the top lid divides the pill in half. If a pill cutter is not available, use a knife edge to press down hard on the scored part of the tablet to make a quick, clean break, or cover the pill in a tissue and hold it with the fingers to break it.

4. When you pour liquid medication from a bottle, pour it from the side away from the label. Remove the cap from the bottle and place it upside down to prevent contamination. Hold the bottle with the label against the palm of the hand while pouring, to prevent liquid from running down the bottle and destroying the label. Place the medication cup on a surface at eye level to ensure accuracy of the dose (Figure 4.16). Do not hold the cup at eye level, because it is difficult to make sure the cup is level and not tipped.

5. If preparing a unit-dose tablet, place the packaged tablet directly into the medicine cup. Never open the package until administering the medication to the patient.

6. If preparing a dose from a bottle, pour the required number of tablets into the bottle cap and transfer them to a medicine cup. Never touch the tablets with your fingers.

7. Decide whether the medication is to be mixed with a liquid or food. Drugs are sometimes mixed with a soft, palatable food such as applesauce or fluid such as juice to hide their taste. Tablets may be crushed and capsules

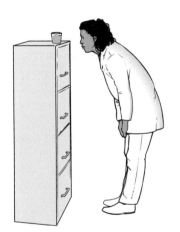

Figure 4.16
Medication should be measured at eye level on a stable surface.

opened and mixed to make them easier for a patient to swallow. Check a drug reference book to make sure the medication can be crushed. Never crush enteric-coated or sustained-action medications.

THE FIVE RIGHTS: RULES FOR GIVING MEDICATIONS

The rules, or "five rights," for giving medications are the same no matter who is giving them. The five rights of medication administration are the

- right drug
- right dose
- right patient
- right route
- right time

RIGHT DRUG

Give only medicine that you have prepared yourself. Never give any medication that someone else has prepared. Give drugs only from labeled containers. Keep unit-dose packages wrapped until you are ready to administer the drug to the patient so the label stays with the medication. When administering drugs, compare the label three times with the medication card or unit-dose recording form:

1. Compare before taking it from the shelf or drawer where it is stored.

2. Compare as you remove the ordered amount of the drug from the container.

3. Compare before you return the container to the shelf or drawer.

If a patient refuses medication that has been removed from its package, never return it to the original container. If a single-unit dose package is unopened, you may return it to the patient's drawer.

Be aware of the different names for the same drug—the generic name and the trade name. For example, furosemide is the generic name for a common diuretic. *Lasix* is the trade name. Also be aware that very different drugs can have similar names. *Orinase* and *Ornade*, for example, might be mistaken for each other, but one is for diabetes and the other is for a stuffy nose. You should carefully note the spelling of a drug's name and be sure to verify an order if the handwriting is unclear.

Know the abbreviations for the different dosage forms.

Recheck any medicine that the patient feels is wrong. Be sure the label corresponds to the name of the drug written on the medicine card or medication record.

RIGHT DOSE

Medication errors are significantly reduced by the unit-dose system, because the medications are already in the correct dose. When calculations are required to achieve a correct dose, have another member of the health care team check them. Many facilities require the health care worker who sets up insulin or anticoagulants to check them with another worker.

Know the correct dosage symbols and abbreviations. Use properly marked measuring containers: a minim glass for minims, medicine glasses marked with metric or apothecary units, and a medicine dropper, if drops are ordered.

Be sure that the amount the patient receives matches the amount stated on the medicine card or chart. Stay with each patient until he or she takes the medicine.

Help weak patients take medication to be sure they get the full amount.

Correctly divide or crush a tablet, as previously discussed.

RIGHT PATIENT

An essential step to safe medication administration is to give the right medication to the right patient. Always identify the patient in some way. Make absolutely certain that you know who the patient is. Read the identification wristband that all hospital patients wear. Avoid calling a patient by name, because a confused patient may respond to someone else s name. Ask patients their names, reassuring them that it is routine procedure to have them state their name.

Check the patient s name against the name on the medicine card or medication record each time you administer medication.

RIGHT ROUTE

Always write the route on the medicine card or medication record. Package inserts, drug references, and the patient chart reveal information about the right route. Call the nurse in charge if you still have questions after checking these references. The physician should be contacted if the route is not specified on the medication order. Know the correct abbreviations for the routes. (Refer to Table 4.2.)

Be aware of factors or changes in the patient s condition that can affect the route of administration. For example, the rectal or parenteral routes probably make more sense than the oral route for a patient who is vomiting. Ask the doctor to write a different order when these changes arise.

RIGHT TIME

Know the correct abbreviations for times of administration (Table 4.3). Check the medication record or medicine card for the correct time to give a medication. All routine medications should be given within thirty minutes of the scheduled time.

Never leave a drug at the patient s bedside. To make sure all medications are taken, observe while the patient takes the medication.

Organize your work time at the beginning of each shift so that you can get medications to each patient on schedule. Review all of the day s nursing activities and your own duties. Plan accordingly, taking into account the times when patients are to receive medications.

Check whether an oral drug should be taken on an empty stomach or with food. Drugs to be taken on an empty stomach should be given 1 hour before meals or 2 hours afterward. Drugs given after meals should be given within 30 minutes of the ordered time. Drugs such as insulin must be given exactly as ordered before a meal. Administer medications that cause sleepiness at bedtime. Administer diuretics, or water pills, in the early part of the day.

CHARTING MEDICATIONS

Whenever a patient receives some form of treatment, such as medication, a record is kept of that treatment. Special problems or circumstances are also recorded, such as new symptoms, the patient s own statements, laboratory tests performed, and so on. All the events in the course of a patient s treatment are written in the **patient chart** or medical record, which is a permanent record of care received.

The chart is important because it is a form of communication among the patient, doctor, and other members of the health care team. The patient chart is also a legal document. It is the official record of the care a patient receives. The patient or the patient s family may question the quality of treatment. The health facility can evaluate quality by referring to the chart. In the event of a lawsuit, the chart can be used in court to decide whether the patient received competent or incompetent care. The chart is taken as proof of the care the patient received.

Researchers may also use the chart to study certain diseases or drugs. The chart may serve as a teaching tool for medical students. Or it may be used to gather facts and figures about the overall performance of a health facility.

For all these reasons, it is important to learn how to write the necessary information on a patient chart. This is called **charting** or documenting. All documentation and reports become part of the patient's medical record and must be factual, accurate, complete, current, organized, and confidential.

First, you should know that not all charts look alike. Different health facilities have their own forms for keeping records. The traditional patient chart consists of a collection of different forms. Individual staff members chart the problems for which they are responsible and the treatment or care they give. Other team members refer to these specific reports as needed.

The traditional patient chart contains the physician's order sheet. The patient's doctor fills it out, or in the case of verbal or telephone orders, a registered nurse. It contains orders for tests, procedures, and drugs to treat the patient's condition. The doctor also fills out a **patient history sheet** describing the patient's medical problems in more detail. Various other forms are used to record such things as laboratory tests, X rays, reports of specialists, and the patient's progress. Two forms you will deal with in administering medications are the medication record and the nurses' notes.

MEDICATION RECORD

You have learned what the medication record is. Now you will learn how to chart after administering a medication. You must include these facts on the medication record:

- Name of the drug
- Strength and/or amount of the drug
- Times at which the drug is given
- Route by which the drug is given
- Initials and signature of the health worker who administers the drug

For routine medications, most of this information is written or printed from the computer ahead of time. You need chart only your initials each time you administer a drug.

In case a dose of medicine is not given at a scheduled time, you should record both the time for the missed dose and the time the medication was administered. Usually this is done by circling the skipped time on the medication record. You should also explain why the drug was not given, either on the nurses' notes or medication administration record or on both, depending on facility policy. Some reasons that you may not be able to give a drug on time are that the patient may be having an X ray taken, or abnormal laboratory results have been reported, or there may have been a rise or fall in the patient's pulse, respiration, or blood pressure.

If the medication record has a section for PRN medications, chart the time and reason for administration and your initials. Many facilities also require documentation of PRN medications in the nurses' notes.

NURSES' NOTES

The traditional form known as **nurses' notes** is called by several names, including progress notes and nurses' progress notes. The nurse uses these notes to chart observations of the patient and the nursing care provided (Figure 4.17). Stat medications, and sometimes PRN medications, are also charted on the nurses' notes.

NURSES' NOTES

Family Name	First Name	Attending Physician	Room No.	Hosp. No.
Powers	G. Frederick	Dr. Stephens	321	43-586

Date	Time	REMARKS - TREATMENT	Nurses' Signature
8/1	0100	Demerol 100 mg given IM for c/o severe right knee pain ———	B. Cassel, LPN
8/1	1800	Refused Motrin 400 mg P.O. Pt states "it upsets my stomach." Supervisor notified. ———	J. Hart, Med Aide
8/2	1015	Procardia 10 mg. given SL stat for B/P $^{196}/_{104}$ ———	F. Strum, LPN Student

Figure 4.17
Nurses' notes.

The following information must be charted in the nurses' notes each time a stat or a PRN medication is given:

- Name of the drug
- Strength and/or amount of the drug administered
- Route
- Time of administration
- Results of checking vital signs (blood pressure, temperature, respiration, pulse) if required for specific drugs
- Any special information regarding the drug or the patient (e.g., problems in getting the patient to take the drug, unusual reactions)
- Signature (first initial and last name) and title of the person who administers the drug

In addition to recording stat and PRN medications, the form includes other information. Whenever you do not give a medication or notice something unusual with any medication, chart it on the nurses' notes. You should also make a note on the nurses' notes any time a scheduled medication is not given. The second entry in Figure 4.17 shows a case like this.

THE POMR

One method of documenting is called the **POMR** (problem-oriented medical record). In this system the chart is organized according to a numbered list of problems or diagnoses (Figure 4.18 on page 78). All health team members chart on the same form. They chart their observations, plans of action, treatments, and results, with a number telling which particular problem they are working on.

SPRINGFIELD HOSPITAL AND HEALTH CARE CENTER
Patient Record

7209
347841-6 m 28-447
TIMMONS, RALPH
DR. THOMAS MOORE
1 - PROT 5/6/20

ALLERGIES	BLOOD TYPE
Penicillin	AB+

PROBLEM NUMBER	DATE	PROBLEM DESCRIPTION	DATE RESOLVED
#1	3/25	Diabetes mellitus, insulin-controlled	
#2	3/25	Midline abdominal incision	
#3	3/25	Wife seriously ill	

Progress Notes

PROBLEM NO. & DESCRIPTION	SUBJECTIVE(S)-OBJECTIVE(O)-ASSESSMENT(A)-PLAN(P)
#2 - Incision	S: Complains of incisional pain
	O: Generalized redness around incision line;
	sm. amt. greenish drainage; T 101.4° F
	A: Possible wound infection
	P: Obtain culture; notify Dr. Moore
	L Parker, LPN

Figure 4.18
The POMR (problem-oriented medical record) shown at the top and the SOAP (subjective–objective–assessment–plan) notes shown at the bottom allow members of the health care team to chart what they do for the patient's individual problems.

The list of problems includes any social and psychological factors in the patient's life that may have an effect on treatment. The POMR is designed to make sure that all members of the health care team are aware of what the others are doing and planning for the patient. In this way, the patient receives coordinated care.

Where the POMR is in use, patient progress is often charted by **SOAP** (subjective–objective–assessment–plan) or PIE (problem–interventions–evaluations) notes. These are ways to organize information for charting. When you want to make an entry using SOAP, include the following:

- **S**ubjective data—the patient's complaints and feelings in his or her own words
- **O**bjective data—your own observations or measurements (e.g., blood pressure, appetite)
- **A**ssessment—an interpretation of the patient's condition
- **P**lan—specific orders, such as treatments, diagnostic tests, medications, or patient education, that will help the patient's current problem

To make an entry using PIE, include the following:

- **Problem**—a problem pertinent to the patient
- **Interventions**—your actions to address the problem
- **Evaluation**—your assessment of interventions and the patient's response to therapy

Another method of charting is charting by exception. It is designed to decrease the amount of time spent charting. With this method, the health care team establishes normal assessment findings and standardized interventions for each patient. Then, a team member has only to write a note when a patient's condition does not meet the standardization.

CHARTING IN LONG-TERM CARE FACILITIES

The forms used for charting in a long-term care facility are different from those used on a hospital unit. Usually there is no medication record. Rather, any drugs administered are charted on a patient history sheet or on the nurses' notes. Again, all important information must be charted: drug name, strength and/or amount, route, time of administration, your signature and title, and any other notes about the patient or the drug.

PRINCIPLES OF CHARTING

Because the chart is a record of a patient's treatment, it must record only facts. You must write only things you did or saw or heard the patient say. Your own conclusions and opinions about a patient's behavior are not to be charted. The only exception to this rule is in the SOAP method of charting, which calls for your assessment of the patient's problem. In this case, it is clear that you are stating your own conclusions.

All charted information must be factual. Why are facts better than opinion in charting? Let us take an example. If you found Mrs. Smith in her room crying, you would not write on the chart "seems depressed about upcoming operation." Instead, you would write "was crying," since there could be many reasons that Mrs. Smith is crying. Suppose that Mr. Jones gagged on a tablet this morning. If you wrote "doesn't like medicine" on the chart (your opinion of the situation), your information would be misleading. Perhaps a physical problem caused Mr. Jones to have trouble swallowing. The chart shows the problem more clearly if you write simply "difficulty noted in swallowing tablet." Avoid terms like "appear" or "seems,"which can lead you to draw assumptions without objective data to support them.

Another important feature of charting is that it is a summary of events. It must be accurate, complete, current, and organized. For example, "incision to chest not healing" is not accurate, complete, or based on facts. It allows for assumptions that are not legally sound in health care. Instead, chart "generalized redness noted length of chest incision and warm to touch." Use abbreviations when appropriate. They allow you to say a great deal in a small space. Learn them well and use them carefully so that others can understand your notes. It is also useful to learn the proper medical terms for symptoms and body functions. Most people in the health care field understand these, and they are a kind of shorthand for complicated explanations. Be careful of similar spellings of words with very different meanings that would be confusing; for example, *dram* and *gram*.

Charting is not difficult, but it requires some practice. Your own charting will be appropriate if you follow a few simple rules:

- Before you begin, make sure you have the right chart.
- Chart medications directly from a medicine card or medication record. If neither one is being used, chart directly from the patient chart.

- Chart only after you give a drug, never before.
- Be specific. Do not write "Gave *Demerol* for pain in the evening." Instead, write "[date], *Demerol* 100 mg given I.M. in right upper outer quadrant of gluteus maximus for c/o sharp pain in left arm."
- Document the effect of PRN medication 30 minutes after you give the drug.
- Record events in the order they occur.
- Mark D/C, for discontinued, after the last dose of a drug is given, or cross out the remaining scheduled times, as required by your agency. The doctor will have specified the day and time of the last dose.
- Do not leave gaps or skip lines. If a note does not fill up a complete line, draw a straight line to fill the gap. Put your signature at the right-hand side directly after the note. (Refer to the nurses' notes in Figure 4.17.)
- If you make an error, do not erase it. Draw one line through the mistake. It should still be visible; do not black it out. Initial it, and write the word *error* on the line. Then rechart the information correctly.
- Never use ditto marks.
- Write only in ink, never in pencil. Only ink ensures a permanent record. Most agencies require you to use a certain color ink. Black ink is the most widely used, but check the policy at your agency. Always print or write legibly when charting. You may print or you may write neatly in longhand.
- Always use proper abbreviations and symbols. Many agencies have lists of the abbreviations they prefer. Check with your agency.
- Consult the nurse in charge when in doubt about a charting rule.

The patient chart is kept strictly confidential. Do your part to make sure that only authorized people see the chart or discuss its contents. Never discuss a patient with another health care worker in a public setting, such as the elevator or cafeteria. This is a breach of confidentiality for which you could be held legally responsible.

REPORTING MEDICATION ERRORS

Medication errors are serious and can be fatal to a patient. A medication error occurs when you violate one or more of the "five rights."

- Give the wrong drug
- Give the wrong dose
- Give a drug to the wrong patient
- Give the drug by the wrong route
- Give the drug at the wrong time

Any of these five situations must be reported immediately to the nurse in charge. You must also complete an **incident report** or a medication error form (Figure 4.19). The incident report is an objective, factual account of what took place. The incident report does not become part of the chart. Agencies use incident reports to monitor the frequency of medication errors so as to take corrective measures to prevent them in the future. The incident report is signed by the health worker who made the error and by the nurse in charge. Many health facilities require that the physician be notified and the patient seen after the medication error. The doctor's orders for further patient care must be followed carefully. It is your legal duty to report an error. Not reporting an error can seriously harm your patient and your future in the health care field.

As a final step, review the events that led to the error. Medication errors can be prevented by carefully reading medication labels. Pay attention to the name and dose of the medication and to the name of the patient. Some drugs have similar names (e.g., *Keflex* and *Keflin*). Have all your calculations checked by another health team member. Many errors occur as the result of incorrect placement of the decimal point. If a medication order is illegible, notify your supervisor so the physician can be called for clarification.

INCIDENT REPORT

SPRINGFIELD HOSPITAL	SPRINGFIELD HOSPITAL WEST	SPRINGFIELD SENIOR CARE	OTHER

NAME: AGE _____ SEX _____   DIAGNOSIS:

MR#:   ADM. DATE: PT. LOCATION:

USE THIS FORM TO REPORT:
1) ANY IDENTIFIED HAZARD: A CONDITION THAT MIGHT CAUSE AN INJURY.
2) AN INJURY OR DEATH THAT IS UNEXPECTED, AND IS MORE RELATED TO CARE, OR LACK OF CARE, THAN TO THE PATIENT'S UNDERLYING CONDITION.
DO NOT MAKE COPIES OF THIS REPORT.

DETAILS OF THE EVENT

Date: Time: _____ am/pm   Location of Incident:

DESCRIPTION OF HAZARD OR DESCRIPTION OF INJURY AND SURROUNDING CIRCUMSTANCES:

Persons involved (Name, Title):

Address/Phone#/Ext.:

CORRECTIVE ACTION TAKEN IN RESPONSE TO THIS INCIDENT:

Name of doctor who examined the patient:

Treatment for injury:

Names of witnesses (Use back of form if space needed):

Address/Phone #/Ext. of witnesses:

Name/Title and Signature of person submitting this report:

Date/Time report written:

Signature of supervisor:

Figure 4.19
Any medication error requires completion of an incident report.

PRACTICE PROCEDURE 4.1

Transcribe Medication Orders

■ **EQUIPMENT**

Physician's order sheet with drugs ordered

Kardex and medicine cards or medication record (the forms used by your agency)

■ **PROCEDURE**

1. Read the medication orders on the physician's order sheet.

2. Transcribe each medication order exactly as it appears on the physician's order sheet onto the Kardex, if used by your agency. Use proper medical terms and abbreviations. Be sure to record all necessary information, including:

Continued

- Name of patient, room number, and bed number
- Name of drug
- Route
- Dosage (strength and frequency of administration)
- Time(s) of administration
- Special administration or nursing instructions, if any

3. Following the Kardex, transcribe each order onto a medicine card or medication record. Include the same information as in Step 2.

4. Check off each order as you finish transcribing it onto the medication record or medicine card.

5. Sign or initial the doctor's order after each set of orders is transcribed.

Show your work to your instructor.

PRACTICE PROCEDURE 4.2

Count Controlled Substances

In a laboratory setting, practice this procedure with a partner. Pretend that one of you is going off duty and the other is coming on duty.

■ **EQUIPMENT**

Controlled substance folder with the forms used by your agency (sign-in/out form, proof-of-use records for several drugs)

Locked box, cabinet, or drawer, and keys

Sample containers of controlled substances (divided containers, multiple-dose bottles [tablet or capsules and liquids], unit-dose packages, etc.)

■ **PROCEDURE**

1. The person coming on duty obtains the key to the controlled-substance storage area from the person going off duty. (Some areas have double doors and require two keys.)

2. Unlock the controlled-substance cabinet, box, or drawer in the medicine room. Remove the containers.

3. Count the amount of medicine in each container.

   - *Divided containers (tablets or capsules).* Look for the slot that has the last tablet or capsule in it. The number of this slot is the number of tablets left.
   - *Unit-dose packages.* Unit doses are numbered. The package with the highest number tells how many doses are left.
   - *Multiple-dose bottles (tablets or capsules).* Tip the bottle on its side and count the contents.
   - *Multiple-dose bottles (liquids).* The bottle should be marked off in cubic centimeters or milliliters. Hold the bottle at eye level and note how many cubic centimeters or milliliters remain.

4. As you count each drug, write the quantity on the appropriate form. Each drug has a form to accompany it. If the form is a proof-of-use record, check that your count matches the amount of drug shown as still available. Different facilities have different ways of verification. Sign your name where requested.

82 Chapter 4

Continued

5. If your count differs from the number shown in the records, do a recount. If there is still a difference, look at the Kardex and other forms to locate the source of error. Notify the nurse in charge if you cannot find the source of error.

6. Correct errors on your forms according to the policy of your health facility.

7. Sign any of the forms required by your agency (sign-in/out, key count, etc.).

8. Return medications to the lock-box and close and lock the doors. Return the controlled-substance folder to the place where it is kept.

9. The person who has just come on duty keeps the key(s) for use in administering controlled substances during the next shift.

Show your work to your instructor.

PRACTICE PROCEDURE 4.3

Record the Use of Controlled Substances

■ **EQUIPMENT**

Locked storage area (box, cabinet, or drawer) and keys

Medication record, medicine cards, or Kardex with several orders for controlled substances

Proof-of-use records for several controlled substances

Sample containers of controlled substances (unit dose, multiple dose)

■ **PROCEDURE**

1. Unlock storage area and read medication orders. Follow Steps 2 through 7 for one medication at a time.

2. Read the label as you remove a container from the storage area.

3. Choose the proof-of-use form that goes with that drug. Fill out the form, giving the date of administration, time of administration, patient's full name, room and bed number, amount of medication taken from the container, patient's physician, name of the person giving the medication, and the amount of medication given to the patient.

4. Have someone act as a witness if you must discard some of the medication. You may have to discard medication if:

   • You must give a smaller amount than the smallest unit-dose size.
   • You suspect that a drug is contaminated or you contaminate the drug when setting it up.

   The witness should sign the proof-of-use record and state how much of the drug was destroyed.

5. Set up the medication as you would any other. Be sure to read the label again as you open the container.

6. Replace the container in the storage area. Read the label one last time as you do so.

7. Repeat these steps for the remaining controlled substances.

8. Lock the storage area and replace the controlled-substance folder. Keep the keys in your pocket for use on duty.

Show your work to your instructor or the nurse in charge.

This procedure may be used to set up a medicine cart when you have multiple-dose packages. If the drawers of the cart are marked with patients' names, you may set up from a medication record rather than from medicine cards.

■ EQUIPMENT

Medicine cards

Medicine tray (flat or molded)

Containers of medicine (unit dose and multiple dose)

Paper cups for tablets or capsules, plastic cups for liquids

Supplies (water and water cups, tongue blades, spoons, blood pressure cuff, applesauce or juice for mixing medications, if necessary)

■ PROCEDURE

1. Set up one medication at a time. Place one card on the tray. You need the medicine card to be able to tell which medicine to give to which patient.

2. Read the label as you take the appropriate medicine container from the cabinet, refrigerator, or medicine cart. Hold the label at eye level.

3. Before opening the container, check the label against the medicine card.

4. Pour or count out the drug into plastic or paper cups. Double-check the dose against the medicine card after you have poured or counted out the medication.

5. Set the medicine cup on the tray next to its medicine card. By setting up only one drug at a time, you make sure that you will put the right card with the right medication. (Refer to Figure 4.11 to see how a typical tray is set up.)

6. Measure liquids at eye level. Pour with the label away from the side on which you are pouring.

7. After measuring out dose, place on eye-level shelf to assure accuracy of dose.

8. Read the label again as you put away the container. Be sure to wipe off any spilled medication.

9. Place any needed supplies on the tray for administering the medications.

10. Follow Steps 1 through 9 as you set up the remaining medications, one at a time.

Show your work to your instructor.

PRACTICE PROCEDURE 4.5

Dispense Unit-Dose Medications From a Cart

■ EQUIPMENT

Folder with medication records

Medicine cart, drawers labeled with names of patients

Continued

Unit doses of medicine placed in appropriate drawers of medicine cart

Medicine cart supplies (water, cups, spoons, etc.)

■ PROCEDURE

1. Open folder to first patient's medication record.

2. Go to that patient's room and identify the patient by:

   • Checking the name on the wristband or on the bed.
   • Asking the patient his or her name. (Never use this method as the only way to identify a patient.)
   • Asking personnel to help you identify any patient who seems confused or who does not have a wristband or a bed tag.

3. Open the appropriate patient's drawer, identify the right medication, and give it to the patient, following these steps:

   • Read the medication record and identify the medication.
   • Read the label of the unit-dose package and compare it with the medication record.
   • Read the label of the unit-dose package as you give it to the patient.
   • Read the label of the unit-dose package as you discard it.

4. Chart administration of each drug on the medication record.

5. Make the patient comfortable.

6. Go to the next patient's room. This should be the patient whose medication record is next in the medication folder.

Show your work to your instructor.

PRACTICE PROCEDURE 4.6

Fill Out an Incident Report Form

■ EQUIPMENT

Incident report form

Written or oral summary of an actual or made-up medication error (a tape recording or a written story)

■ PROCEDURE

1. Read or listen to the report of a medication error.

2. Record all information requested on the appropriate incident/accident form. Usually this includes:

   • Patient's name, room number, and bed
   • Date, time, and location of the incident
   • Name of the doctor or supervisor who was notified of the incident
   • Nature of the incident or accident and injuries received
   • Diagram of the location of the injury on the body
   • Date and time of this report
   • Your signature

3. Obtain signatures of all persons involved as required on the form.

Show your work to your instructor or the nurse in charge.

Define each term.

1. Active ingredient _____

_____

2. Irrigation _____

_____

3. Inhalation _____

_____

4. Instillation _____

_____

5. Outpatient _____

_____

6. Physician s order sheet _____

_____

7. Routine order _____

_____

8. Standing order _____

_____

9. PRN order _____

_____

10. Stat order _____

_____

Match the forms of medication to their descriptions.

_____ 11. Heavy sugar and water solution with flavoring		**a. ointment**
_____ 12. Alcohol mixed with a volatile oil		**b. gel**
_____ 13. 10—20% drug solution in alcohol and/or water		**c. emulsion**
_____ 14. Highly concentrated alcohol solution		**d. fluidextract**
_____ 15. Sweetened, alcoholic, and aromatic preparation		**e. spirit**
_____ 16. Oils and fats suspended in water		**f. syrup**
_____ 17. Mixture of heavy particles with water; looks like milk		**g. tincture**
_____ 18. Thick mixture of fine particles with water		**h. elixir**
_____ 19. A soothing or counterirritant preparation for external use, designed to be patted on		**i. magma**
_____ 20. Gelatin sheath that contains 1 dose of medication		**j. capsule**
_____ 21. A topical or ophthalmic preparation in a base of lanolin or **petrolatum**		**k. lotion**

Continued

Match the route to the proper abbreviation.

_____ 22. Under the tongue   a. buc

_____ 23. Under the skin   b. PO

_____ 24. Into the skin   c. ID

_____ 25. Into the muscle   d. IV

_____ 26. Into the vein   e. subl

_____ 27. By mouth   f. subcu

_____ 28. Inside the cheek   g. IM

Match the appropriate abbreviation to each phrase.

_____ 29. Eye medication orders   a. stat

_____ 30. Medications given as necessary b. BID, QID, q4h, h.s., a.m.

_____ 31. Administration times   c. a.c., p.c.

_____ 32. Before or after meals   d. HCl, NaCl, H_2O

_____ 33. Medications given once a day   e. ad lib., PRN

_____ 34. Immediate, one-time order   f. q. d.

_____ 35. Nothing by mouth   g. NPO

_____ 36. Chemical symbols   h. OD, OS, OU, ophth.

Write the term that the abbreviation stands for.

37. Ext. _____

38. Syr. _____

39. Tinc. _____

40. Supp. _____

41. Sp. _____

42. Fld. ext. _____

43. Cap. _____

44. Elix. _____

45. Tab. _____

46. Soln. _____

47. Susp. _____

Describe the following solid forms.

48. Troche _____

_____

_____

49. Suppository _____

_____

50. Sustained-release capsule _____

_____

51. Scored tablet _____

_____

Fill in the blanks with the word or phrase that best completes each statement.

52. Because of their high drug concentrations, spirits, tinctures, and fluidextracts must be measured with a(n) _____.

53. To prevent alcohol solutions from separating, store them in _____.

54. Bottles containing tinctures, fluidextracts, elixirs, and spirits are kept tightly closed so that the _____ cannot evaporate.

55. All suspensions must be _____ before use.

56. When a drug dissolves in water or alcohol, the result is called a(n) _____.

57. When a drug does not dissolve in liquid, the preparation is called a(n) _____.

58. _____ coated capsules and tablets prevent stomach irritation by dissolving only when they reach the intestine.

59. Liquid suspensions for external application to the skin to relieve pain and swelling are known as _____.

60. Suppositories may be inserted into the _____, the _____, or the _____.

61. A diagnosed alcoholic should not be given any _____ solutions.

62. Sustained-release capsules are also called _____.

63. Oral medicines are made to taste good to help the _____ as well as the _____ take them.

64. Elixirs of phenobarbital or *Benadryl* are _____ to help children and the elderly take them better.

65. In sublingual and buccal administrations, no _____ is permitted until the medication is dissolved.

66. Applying local medications to the skin or the mucous membranes is known as the _____ route.

67. Injecting medications into the body with a needle and syringe is known as the _____ route.

68. Parenteral medications and equipment must be _____; otherwise, there is danger of infection.

Convert from the military-time clock to the regular clock and vice versa.

	Regular Clock	Military Clock
69.	7:00 a.m.	_____
70.	_____	1100 hours
71.	_____	1330 hours
72.	2:00 p.m.	_____
73.	_____	2000 hours

Answer the questions below in the spaces provided.

74. What should you do if you have a question about a medication order? _____

_____

75. What two new members of the health team, as well as doctors, are allowed to prescribe medications in some states? _____

_____

76. What is the important rule to remember when administering delayed-release tablets and capsules? Why is this rule important? _____

_____

_____

77. List seven items of information that must be included on any written medication order. _____

_____

_____

_____

_____

_____

_____

Translate these doctors' orders. Use your knowledge of medical abbreviations to give the meanings of the following orders.

78. *Darvon* caps 65 mg q4h PRN for pain _____

_____

_____

79. *Phenobarbital* elix. 1 tsp (20 mg) h. s. _____

_____

_____

80. *Keflex* 250 mg caps q6h PO _____

_____

_____

81. *Lotrimin* 1% cream bid × 2 weeks _____

_____

_____

82. *Bacitracin* ophth. oint. OD TID for conjunctivitis _____

_____

83. *Pro-Banthine* tabs. 15 mg a. c. _____

_____

84. *Heparin* 5000 units IV stat _____

_____

85. *Acetaminophen* 120 mg R supp. QID _____

_____

Match the medical forms to their descriptions.

_____ 86. Form for charting medications administered on a regular schedule

a. POMR

_____ 87. One form used to chart care given by all health team members

b. prescription blank

_____ 88. Doctor's orders for an outpatient

c. incident report form

_____ 89. Summary of daily medications and treatments for all patients on the unit

d. Kardex file

_____ 90. Used to record medication errors

e. medication record

Answer the following questions in the spaces provided.

91. How many doses of medication are contained in a unit-dose package? _____

_____

92. How many doses of medication are contained in a multiple-dose package? _____

_____

93. What must be counted or measured at the beginning of each shift? _____

_____

94. List two examples of controlled substances. _____

_____

95. Where should controlled substances be stored? _____

_____

96. List two advantages of single-dose packaging. _____

_____

_____

97. Where should drugs labeled "for external use only" be kept? _____

_____

Continued

98. How can you best make a clean break when dividing a scored tablet? _____
_____

99. List the five rights of medication administration. _____
_____
_____
_____
_____
_____

100. List two rules for giving the correct medication. _____
_____
_____

101. List three reasons why the patient chart is an important document. _____
_____
_____
_____

102. What is the SOAP system of charting? _____
_____
_____

103. On a medication record, how would you show that a dose of medicine was not given when scheduled? (Check the procedure in your own agency.)
_____
_____
_____

104. How would you show that you gave a dose of medicine? (Check the procedure in your own agency.)
_____
_____

■ CASE STUDIES FOR CRITICAL THINKING

Show how you would chart the following events in the nurses' notes. Be sure to include all of the required information. Remember that only facts are to be charted, not assumptions or opinions.

Mr. Schwartz is under treatment for a blood clot in the leg. He has been taking *Coumadin,* an anticoagulant, for several days. He is also taking *Diuril,* a diuretic, to reduce the swelling in his leg. The doctor has confined Mr. Schwartz to bed. This is because any movement of the leg might cause the clot to break off and travel in the bloodstream, which could be dangerous.

105. At 0800 on October 5 you give Mr. Schwartz two 5-mg tablets of *Coumadin* to swallow with a glass of water. You chart it on the medication record. As you refill the water pitcher, Mr. Schwartz asks if you happen to have something for an upset stomach. He says his stomach hurts the way it did when he had an ulcer 20 years ago. Because the anticoagulant can cause internal bleeding (e.g., from an old ulcer), you have been alert for signs of this side effect. You

notify your supervisor, who asks the doctor to order a test for internal bleeding. The test results are negative. The supervisor then directs you to give Mr. Schwartz 2 tsp of *Maalox* to calm his stomach.

_____

_____

_____

106. It is 1200 hours and time for Mr. Schwartz's next dose of *Diuril*. Mr. Schwartz complains again about his upset stomach, but this time he tells you it is worse right after he takes the *Diuril*. You skip this dose of *Diuril* and notify the supervisor. The supervisor tells you to continue giving the *Diuril* but to keep an eye out for signs of internal bleeding.

_____

_____

_____

107. It is 2000 hours the next evening and time to give Mr. Schwartz a laxative. The laxative *(Dulcolax)* has been ordered by the doctor because bedridden patients often develop constipation, which can lead to impaction (blocking of the intestine). Straining during a bowel movement might cause the blood clot to break off and become an embolism (a traveling clot). Mr. Schwartz tells you that he has been having regular bowel movements and doesn't want the laxative. He asks why he needs it when he has been in bed for only 2 days. You explain that it is preventive medicine to avoid the problems of impaction and embolism. Mr. Schwartz becomes tearful and tells you that he is afraid he will die. He refuses the laxative. You then notify the supervisor. After consulting with the doctor, the supervisor instructs you to give Mr. Schwartz 10 mg of *Valium* intramuscularly right away. *Valium* is a tranquilizer that will ease Mr. Schwartz's anxiety so that he can relax.

_____

_____

_____

_____

_____

_____

■ APPLICATIONS

Obtain a current copy of the PDR® from your school, nursing unit, or clinic. Use it to answer the questions that follow.

108. What is the name of the section where the listing of unit-dose systems is given? _____

_____

109. In this section, locate the drug spironolactone *(Aldactone).* How is this drug supplied as a unit dose?

_____

_____

110. In the same section, locate diazepam *(Valium).* What information does the manufacturer give about unit-dose systems?

_____

Vitamins, Minerals, and Herbs

In this chapter you will learn about vitamins and minerals and their importance in the diet for normal growth and development. You will also learn the functions, food sources, recommended daily requirement, and symptoms of deficiency or excess for each. You will be able to identify the conditions in which appropriate supplementation is necessary. You will also learn about the growing interest in herbs and the potential dangers of some herbal remedies.

OBJECTIVES

After studying this chapter, you should be able to

- differentiate among the fat-soluble and water-soluble vitamins, macrominerals, and microminerals.
- name the various vitamins and minerals.
- list the function of each vitamin and mineral.
- state the recommended daily allowance of the major vitamins and minerals.
- identify at least two food sources of each vitamin and mineral.
- recognize deficiency symptoms of each vitamin and mineral.
- describe the symptoms resulting from taking large amounts of vitamins over a period of time.
- recognize symptoms associated with elevated levels of certain minerals in the body.
- outline the treatment for conditions resulting from too much or not enough vitamins and minerals in the body.
- discuss the importance of patient education in the appropriate use of vitamin and mineral supplementation.
- describe at least four herbal supplements and their uses.
- describe the potential danger of at least four herbal remedies.

KEY TERMS

anion: negatively charged ion

avitaminosis: a condition that results from a deficiency or lack of absorption of vitamins in the diet; also called hypovitaminosis

cation: positively charged ion

electrolyte: a solution that carries an electrical charge

fat-soluble vitamins: vitamins that are soluble in fat; vitamins A, D, E, and K

homeostasis: state of fluid balance within the body

hypervitaminosis: a condition that results from taking large doses of vitamins over a period of time

hypovitaminosis: a condition that results from a diet lacking in vitamins; also called avitaminosis

inorganic: compounds that do not contain carbon, such as minerals and water

ion: a particle that carries an electrical charge

macrominerals: minerals needed with a daily requirement of 100 mg or more

microminerals: minerals needed with a daily requirement of less than 100 mg; also called trace elements

minerals: inorganic elements essential to the body; classified as macrominerals or microminerals

organic: compounds that contain carbon, such as vitamins, carbohydrates, proteins, and fats

recommended daily allowance (RDA): daily level of intake for essential nutrients considered to be adequate to meet the nutritional needs of healthy individuals

vitamins: organic substances essential for normal metabolism; classified as fat-soluble or water-soluble

water-soluble vitamins: vitamins that are soluble in water; vitamin B complex and C

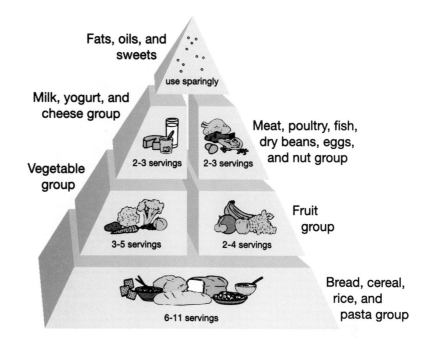

Figure 5.1
Food guide pyramid. (U.S. Dept. of Agriculture)

Food is essential to life, and the food selections we make are important in maintaining health and preventing disease. Today, with a growing interest in health promotion and disease prevention, this interest has led to an awareness of the connection between nutrition and the onset of disease. Vitamins and minerals have a significant role in controlling many of the body's functions. An individual who consumes a well-balanced diet should have no need for supplementation. The United States Department of Agriculture (USDA) developed a food guide pyramid to assist in food buying and preparation (Figure 5.1). It is based on an average diet ranging from 1600 to 1800 calories per day. If an individual follows the guidelines set by the USDA in the food pyramid, the recommended daily allowance (RDA) requirements for vitamins and minerals will be met. However, there are certain conditions in which supplementation may be necessary. A daily diet consisting of less than 1200 calories, increased physical activity, pregnancy, illness, and medication interaction may require vitamin supplementation. Based on the RDA for vitamins and minerals, children will require less.

RECOMMENDED DAILY ALLOWANCE (RDA)

An individual's vitamin need depends on age, sex, weight, level of activity, and overall state of health. The **recommended daily allowance (RDA)** is the level of intake for essential nutrients considered to be adequate to meet the nutritional needs of healthy individuals. The RDA is published by the National Academy of Science and revised approximately every five years. It provides the only available and reliable recommendation for nutrients. The RDA for each nutrient is expressed in international units, or IUs. It is important to understand that the RDA includes not only the amount of food one eats, but also the amount present in supplementation. It is essential to teach patients this fact to prevent toxicity from taking unnecessary megadoses. Always remind patients that the RDA for vitamins and minerals is based on the average, normal, healthy adult (Figure 5.2 on page 96).

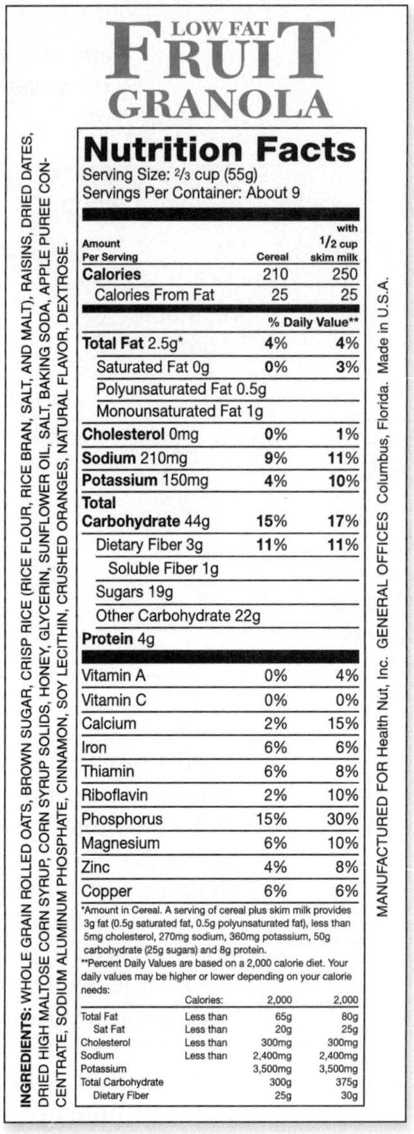

LOW FAT
FRUIT GRANOLA

Nutrition Facts

Serving Size: ²/₃ cup (55g)
Servings Per Container: About 9

Amount Per Serving	Cereal	with ¹/₂ cup skim milk
Calories	210	250
Calories From Fat	25	25
	% Daily Value**	
Total Fat 2.5g*	4%	4%
Saturated Fat 0g	0%	3%
Polyunsaturated Fat 0.5g		
Monounsaturated Fat 1g		
Cholesterol 0mg	0%	1%
Sodium 210mg	9%	11%
Potassium 150mg	4%	10%
Total Carbohydrate 44g	15%	17%
Dietary Fiber 3g	11%	11%
Soluble Fiber 1g		
Sugars 19g		
Other Carbohydrate 22g		
Protein 4g		
Vitamin A	0%	4%
Vitamin C	0%	0%
Calcium	2%	15%
Iron	6%	6%
Thiamin	6%	8%
Riboflavin	2%	10%
Phosphorus	15%	30%
Magnesium	6%	10%
Zinc	4%	8%
Copper	6%	6%

*Amount in Cereal. A serving of cereal plus skim milk provides 3g fat (0.5g saturated fat, 0.5g polyunsaturated fat), less than 5mg cholesterol, 270mg sodium, 360mg potassium, 50g carbohydrate (25g sugars) and 8g protein.

**Percent Daily Values are based on a 2,000 calorie diet. Your daily values may be higher or lower depending on your calorie needs:

	Calories:	2,000	2,000
Total Fat	Less than	65g	80g
Sat Fat	Less than	20g	25g
Cholesterol	Less than	300mg	300mg
Sodium	Less than	2,400mg	2,400mg
Potassium		3,500mg	3,500mg
Total Carbohydrate		300g	375g
Dietary Fiber		25g	30g

INGREDIENTS: WHOLE GRAIN ROLLED OATS, BROWN SUGAR, CRISP RICE (RICE FLOUR, RICE BRAN, SALT, AND MALT), RAISINS, DRIED DATES, DRIED HIGH MALTOSE CORN SYRUP, CORN SYRUP SOLIDS, HONEY, GLYCERIN, SUNFLOWER OIL, SALT, BAKING SODA, APPLE PUREE CONCENTRATE, SODIUM ALUMINUM PHOSPHATE, CINNAMON, SOY LECITHIN, CRUSHED ORANGES, NATURAL FLAVOR, DEXTROSE.

MANUFACTURED FOR Health Nut, Inc. GENERAL OFFICES Columbus, Florida. Made in U.S.A.

Figure 5.2
Nutrition labels show the percent daily values of recommended daily allowance (RDA).

VITAMINS

Vitamins are **organic,** or carbon-containing, substances that are necessary for metabolism and normal growth and development. They must be supplied through the diet because they are either not made in the body or made in insufficient quantity. **Avitaminosis** is a condition that results from a deficiency or lack of vitamin absorption in the diet. It is also called **hypovitaminosis.** A decreased intake of vitamins may occur from an inadequate diet resulting from cultural, religious, or personal practices, fad diets, alcoholism, poverty, or lack of available food. In the United States, avitaminosis most likely results from alcoholism or fad diets. Vitamins may also be adversely affected in the processing, storage, and preparation of food. Foods that are used quickly and have not been exposed to air or the heat and water used in cooking have the highest vitamin content. Vitamins are classified as being either **fat soluble** (A, D, E, and K) or **water soluble** (B complex and C). Understanding their individual functions, food sources, RDA, and symptoms of deficiency and excess are important to determining if a need for supplementation exists.

FAT-SOLUBLE VITAMINS

Fat-soluble vitamins consist of the A, D, E, and K vitamins and are less widely distributed in nature. They are found mostly in fortified milk, whole milk products, green leafy vegetables, yellow fruits and vegetables, fish, liver oil, and sunlight (Table 5.1). Because they are not soluble in water, they are not easily eliminated from the body. A deficiency would take many months to develop. Vitamin deficiencies are rare in most developed countries. When present, a deficiency involves several vitamins. In the United States, RDA can be met by eating a diet from the food guide pyramid. When vitamin deficiencies occur, they are usually found in alcoholics, drug addicts, poor or homeless people, and those who follow poor dietary patterns. Toxicity can also occur over time when there is a consistent intake of megadoses of synthetic vitamins. A condition called **hypervitaminosis** results from taking large doses of vitamins over a period of time.

TABLE 5.1: Fat-Soluble Vitamins

VITAMIN	FUNCTIONS	SOURCES	RDA	SYMPTOMS OF DEFICIENCY	SYMPTOMS OF EXCESS
Vitamin A (retinol)	Formation and maintenance of skin and mucous membranes; bone growth; development of teeth; vision; immune functions	Whole milk; whole milk products; eggs; yellow and green leafy vegetables; yellow fruits; liver; liver oil; fish	5000 IU	Night blindness; rough skin; dry mucous membranes; lack of bone growth; susceptibility to infection	*Mild:* nausea; vomiting; abdominal pain *Severe:* growth retardation; damage to liver and spleen; hair loss
Vitamin D (cholecalciferol, ergosterol)	Maintenance of healthy bones and teeth	Sunlight; fortified milk and dairy products; fish; liver oil	400 IU	Rickets (in children); retarded growth; bowed legs; protruding abdomen; osteomalacia (in adults); bone softening; bone fragility; muscle twitching and spasms	*Mild:* anorexia; nausea; weight loss *Severe:* calcium drawn from bony tissues and deposited in soft tissues, blood vessels, and kidneys
Vitamin E (tocopherol)	Prevents oxidation of fatty acids	Vegetable oils; green leafy vegetables; milk; eggs; cereal	30 IU	Breakdown of red blood vessels	Increased bleeding; intestinal upset; headache; tiredness
Vitamin K	Formation of prothombin (for blood clotting)	Green leafy vegetables; manufactured in intestinal tract	Amount difficult to determine because manufactured in intestinal tract	Hemorrhage in newborns; increased clotting time in adults	Anemia and jaundice in newborns; blood clot and vomiting in adults

WATER-SOLUBLE VITAMINS

Water-soluble vitamins are widely found in plant and animal food sources (Table 5.2 on page 98). They consist of the B complex and C vitamins. Because they cannot be stored in the body, they must be supplied through daily food intake. Some of them can be destroyed by cooking. Because these vitamins are water soluble, they are eliminated from the body in sweat and urine. Although water-soluble vitamins cannot be stored in the body, recent evidence proves that individuals who take megadoses or excessively large quantities of riboflavin (B_2), niacin, and vitamin C can develop a toxicity. Water-soluble vitamins act as catalysts in protein, fat, and carbohydrate metabolism. When the body contains a sufficient supply of the vitamins to assist in protein, fat, and carbohydrate metabolism, additional amounts can be toxic.

TABLE 5.2: Water-Soluble Vitamins

VITAMIN	FUNCTIONS	SOURCES	RDA	SYMPTOMS OF DEFICIENCY	SYMPTOMS OF EXCESS
Vitamin B$_1$ (thiamine)	Necessary for normal nerve conduction and heart function	Pork; fish; poultry; eggs; whole grains; pasta; yeast; wheat germ	1.5 mg	Tingling in extremities; muscle weakness; numbness; mental confusion; disturbances in heart rate; beriberi (rare)	Rapid heart rate; difficulty sleeping; headaches
Vitamin B$_2$ (riboflavin)	Metabolism of proteins, carbohydrates, and fats; growth	Liver; whole grains; dark vegetables; milk	1.7 mg	Cracks at corners of mouth; sore tongue; sensitivity to light	Rare
Niacin	Utilization of protein; breakdown of fat	Meat; poultry; tuna; whole grains; cereals	20 mg	Pellegra; skin disorders, esp. when exposed to sun; diarrhea; confusion	Flushing; headache; nausea; itching; diarrhea
Vitamin B$_6$ (pyridoxine)	Metabolism of proteins, carbohydrates, and fats; formation of red blood cells	Liver; whole grains; green beans; potatoes; nuts	2 mg	Cracks at corners of mouth; anemia; skin lesions	Bloating; headache; fatigue
Folic acid (folacin, folate)	Assists in forming body proteins and genetic material; formation of red blood cells	Liver; kidneys; green leafy vegetables; whole grains	0.4 mg	Anemia; fatigue; sore tongue	May obscure existence of pernicious anemia (vitamin B$_{12}$ deficiency); diarrhea; irritability
Vitamin B$_{12}$ (cobalamin)	Building of genetic material; formation of red blood cells; necessary for normal functioning of nervous system	Liver; kidneys; meat; fish; eggs; milk	6 μg	Pernicious anemia; degeneration of peripheral nerves	None reported
Pantothenic acid	Metabolism of proteins, carbohydrates, and fats; formation of hormones	Meats; whole grains; nuts	10 mg	None reported	None reported
Biotin	Formation of fatty acids; metabolism of protein	Liver; egg yolks; dark green vegetables; green beans	0.3 mg	None reported	None reported
Vitamin C (ascorbic acid)	Maintain healthy bones, teeth, and blood vessels; formation of collagen	Citrus fruits; strawberries; melon; dark green vegetables	60 mg	Scurvy; wounds that will not heal; bleeding gums; bruising; loose teeth	Kidney stones; urinary tract infection; when megadose discontinued, deficiency symptoms may appear briefly until body adapts

A megadose refers to the administration of high doses of a vitamin, usually 10 to 20 times the RDA. If a serious vitamin deficiency exists, it can involve one or even several vitamins. Caution must be used to avoid toxicity. For example, vitamin C increases the renal excretion of uric acid and may cause formation of kidney stones in susceptible people taking megadoses. Taken in large doses, vitamins are classified as drugs rather than nutrients and may cause toxic

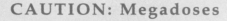

CAUTION: Megadoses

Never take megadoses of any vitamin unless under the supervision of a physician.

effects. The fat-soluble vitamins are stored and may accumulate to toxic levels. Because vitamins are bought without a prescription, fat-soluble vitamins may cause serious health problems because these vitamins cannot be eliminated.

MINERALS

Minerals are **inorganic** elements (they do not contain carbon) essential to the body for health and growth. They serve many important functions in the body. Among these are the formation of bones and teeth, regulation of body fluids and hormone production, muscle contraction, and metabolism of nutrients in foods. Minerals are classified as **macrominerals,** minerals with a daily requirement of 100 mg or more, and **microminerals,** minerals with a daily requirement of less than 100 mg. Calcium, phosphorus, magnesium, sodium, potassium, chloride, and sulfur are examples of macrominerals (Table 5.3). Microminerals, also called

TABLE 5.3: Macrominerals

MACROMINERAL	FUNCTIONS	SOURCES	RDA	SYMPTOMS OF DEFICIENCY	SYMPTOMS OF EXCESS
Calcium	Formation of bones and teeth; blood clotting; transmission of nerve impulses	Milk; milk products; leafy green vegetables; sardines; clams; oysters	1 g	Hypocalcemia; stunted growth in children; osteoporosis in adults; pathological fractures; tingling in fingers; tetany; convulsions	Hypercalcemia; relaxed skeletal muscles; kidney stones; cardiac irregularities
Sodium	Maintenance of acid base balance; control of body's fluid balance; regulation of heart, muscle, and nerve activity	Most foods	—	Hyponatremia; muscle cramps; depression; decreased appetite; weakness	Hypernatremia; confusion; fluid retention
Potassium	Maintenance of acid base balance; maintenance of body's fluid balance; nerve impulse conduction; muscle irritability; regulation of heart rate	Cereals; meats; legumes; fresh vegetables (potatoes); fresh fruits (bananas, oranges, prunes, raisins)	2000 mg	Hypokalemia; muscle weakness; thirst; cardiac abnormalities; confusion; dizziness	Hyperkalemia; confusion; cardiac abnormalities; weakness; decreased blood pressure
Magnesium	Maintenance of electrical activity in nerves and muscles; regulation of body temperature; fat metabolism; protein synthesis	Whole grains; nuts; legumes; green vegetables	400 mg	Hypomagnesemia; neuromuscular irritability; failure to grow; behavioral disturbances; weakness; confusion	Hypermagnesemia; diarrhea; lethargy; cardiac and respiratory disturbances
Phosphorus	Formation of bones and teeth; regulation of acid base balance; metabolism of proteins, carbohydrates, and fats	Milk and milk products; meat; fish; poultry; grains; legumes; nuts	1 g	Hypophosphatemia; bone demineralization; bone pain; pathological fractures	Hyperphosphatemia; calcium loss

trace minerals, include iron, manganese, copper, iodine, zinc, cobalt, fluoride, and selenium (Table 5.4). Although minerals are essential to good health, they can be harmful in excess. Excessive amounts of minerals can pose a risk for children, the elderly, pregnant women, and individuals with a poor diet or with certain diseases. Their functions, food sources, RDA, symptoms of deficiency and excess are essential in determining the need for supplementation.

TABLE 5.4: Microminerals

MICROMINERAL	FUNCTIONS	SOURCES	RDA	SYMPTOMS OF DEFICIENCY	SYMPTOMS OF EXCESS
Iron	Formation of hemoglobin; synthesis of vitamins	Liver; lean meats; legumes; whole grains; dark green vegetables; eggs	18 mg	Anemia; weakness; dizziness; pallor; lowered resistance to infection; fatigue	Nausea; vomiting; black stools; abdominal pain
Iodine	Component of thyroid hormone; important in development and functioning of thyroid gland	Iodized salt; seafood; food additives	150 µg	Cretinism (decrease in stature, mental capacity, and muscle coordination) in infants; decreased thyroid function in adults	Toxic goiter
Zinc	Aids in enzyme activity involved in digestion; helps in wound healing and immune response	Meats; liver; oysters; poultry; legumes	15 mg	Decreased wound healing; failure to grow; decrease in taste and smell; skin lesions	Fever; nausea; vomiting; diarrhea; interference with calcium absorption; muscle pain and weakness
Copper	Helps in formation of red blood cells; aids in enzyme activity involved in digestion	Liver; kidneys; shellfish; nuts; raisins	2 mg	Anemia; bone demineralization	Headache; dizziness; gastrointestinal upset

Minerals are found in both plant and animal foods. Unlike vitamins, minerals are not damaged by heat or light, but some are lost in cooking excessively in water. It is important to educate patients about the appropriate use of vitamins and minerals.

PATIENT EDUCATION

Vitamins and Minerals

- Avoid taking vitamin or mineral supplementation without the direction of a physician.

- The best way to avoid vitamin or mineral deficiency is through a well-balanced diet.
- The food guide pyramid outlines the basic food requirements.
- Megadoses of vitamins can be dangerous.

ELECTROLYTES

Water makes up 45 percent to 75 percent of total body weight, depending on an individual's percentage of body fat. Infants and children have a greater percentage of water content than does the average adult. Within the body's water content are **electrolytes,** or solutions that carry an electrical charge. Macrominerals such as calcium, potassium, sodium, and magnesium are electrolytes. **Ions** are particles that release an electrical charge. Some ions, **cations,** have a positive electrical charge, while others, **anions,** have a negative charge. There must be an equal number of cations and anions in all of the body's fluids to maintain **homeostasis,** or a state of fluid balance.

HERBS

Long before the advent of modern medicine, even before the discovery of vitamins and minerals, people relied on herbs to cure their ills. Many cultures still believe that a simple herb can cure or prevent health problems. Today, there is an explosion of interest in "natural" products, which has dramatically increased the use of herbal remedies. This "back-to-nature" phenomenon developed because of warnings about food preservatives and additives or products that are said to be carcinogenic or cancer-causing. The emphasis on *natural* and *nature* has generated a multimillion-dollar enterprise. There has been a great increase in the number of health food stores selling natural organic vegetables, vitamins, and cosmetics. These products no longer appeal only to certain cultural or ethnic groups, but to the general population. A summary of popular herbs is found in Table 5.5. As a health care team member in a doctor's office, clinic, or hospital, you are in a position to warn patients about certain herbal remedies that can be harmful (Table 5.6).

Several familiar and much-needed medications come from plant sources. Digitalis (*Lanoxin*), used in the treatment of heart disease, comes from the foxglove plant. Vincristine (*Oncovin*) and vinblastine (*Velban*), made from the

TABLE 5.5: Popular Herbs

HERB	PROPOSED USE
Cat's claw	Improve function of digestive and immune systems
Cranberry	Maintain healthy urinary tract
Elderberry	Antioxidant protection against cellular aging
Ginger	Aid in function of gastrointestinal tract
Ginkgo	Maintain brain function; antioxidant properties promote cellular repair
Ginseng	Support body functions under stress
Green tea	Antioxidant properties
Hawthorn	Antioxidant properties; stabilize collagen in joints; maintain heart and circulatory functions
St. John's wort	Promote positive feeling of well-being
Valerian root	Aid for restlessness and inability to sleep

TABLE 5.6: Unsafe Herbs

NAME OF PLANT	COMMON NAME	TOXIC EFFECTS
Aesculus hippocasteranum	Buckeye, horse chestnut	Interferes with blood clotting
Arnica montana	Wolfsbane, mountain tobacco	Extremely irritating to gastrointestinal tract, nervous and muscular systems; can cause death
Artemisia absinthium	Wormwood, madderwort, absinthium, mugwort	Severe mental and nervous system impairment; contains a narcotic poison
Atropa belladonna	Deadly nightshade	Produces anticholinergic symptoms
Conium maculatum	Hemlock, spotted parsley, St. Bennett's herb	Toxic plant
Lobelia inflata	Indian tobacco, asthma weed, emetic weed	Severe vomiting, pain, paralysis; can result in death
Vinca major; vinca minor	Periwinkle, vinca	Liver, kidney, and neurological damage

periwinkle plant, are common antineoplastic agents frequently used in the treatment of Hodgkin's disease, leukemia, and breast and testicular cancer. Reserpine (*Sepasil*), made from rauwolfia derivatives, comes from a shrub grown in India and the tropics and is used to treat high blood pressure.

REPRESENTATIVE DRUGS FOR VITAMIN AND MINERAL DEFICIENCIES

CATEGORY, NAME[a], AND ROUTE	USES AND DISEASES	ACTIONS	USUAL DOSE[b] AND SPECIAL INSTRUCTIONS	SIDE EFFECTS AND ADVERSE REACTIONS
Fat-Soluble Vitamins				
Vitamin D Oral, IM	Rickets; hypocalcemia; malabsorption	Promotes absorption and utilization of calcium	Initially, 12,000 IU PO or IM daily; increased up to 500,000 IU daily	Rare; seen only with vitamin D toxicity
Vitamin K (aqua mephyton) PO, SC, IM	Hypoprothrombinemia	Formation of pro-thrombin	25 to 100 mg PO, SC, or IM daily	Rare; flushing, taste alterations, redness at injection site
Water-Soluble Vitamins				
Thiamine hydrochlo-ride (vitamin B$_1$) Oral, IM, IV	Beriberi; malabsorption syndrome; anemia; polyneuritis	Combines with ATP enzyme necessary for carbohydrate metabolism	Beriberi: 10 to 500 mg IM tid for 2 weeks, followed by 5 to 100 mg for 1 month Anemia and polyneuritis: 100 mg PO daily Crisis state: 500 mg to 1 g IV	Rare; skin rash, itching, wheezing after IV administration
Riboflavin (vitamin B$_2$) Oral	Malnutrition, malabsorption	Converted into 2 coenzymes necessary for normal tissue respiration	50 mg PO daily	Rare; bright yellow urine with high doses
Cyanocobalamin (vitamin B$_{12}$) Oral, SC, IM	Malabsorption, pernicious anemia, strict vegetarianism	Necessary for red blood cells, protein, fat, and carbohydrate metabolism	30–100 mcg SC or IM daily for 5 to 10 days; monthly maintenance dose 100 mcg to 200 mcg IM	Rare; itching
Vitamin C (ascorbic acid) SC, IM, IV	Poor nutritional habits; delayed wound healing	Promotes tissue repair and wound healing	200 to 500 mg	Rare
Macrominerals				
Calcium carbonate (*Oscal, Caltrate, Titralac, Tums, Tums Ex*) Oral	Hypocalcemia; osteoporosis	Replaces and maintains calcium	250 to 650 mg PO daily	Constipation; cardiac changes if calcium level goes too high
Potassium (*K-Dur, Micro-K*) Oral	Hypokalemia; diuretic use; vomiting; diarrhea; starvation diet	Replaces and maintains potassium	40 to 100 mg PO TID or QID	Cardiac changes if potassium level goes too high
Microminerals				
Iron (*FeSol, Imferon*) Oral, IM	Iron deficiency anemia	Formation of red blood cells	325 mg PO TID or QID, 50 to 100 mg IM daily	Constipation; black stools; nausea

[a]Trade names given in parentheses are examples only. Check current drug references for a complete listing of available products.
[b]Average adult doses are given. However, dosages are determined by a physician and vary with the purpose of the therapy and the particular patient. The doses presented in this text are for general information only.

Match the medical terms to their definitions.

_____ 1. Inorganic elements essential to the body   a. homeostasis

_____ 2. Condition resulting from a diet lacking in vitamins   b. vitamins

_____ 3. Organic substances essential for normal metabolism   c. ion

_____ 4. State of fluid balance within the body   d. minerals

_____ 5. Particle that carries an electrical charge   e. hypovitaminosis

Complete the following statements by filling in the blanks.

6. The level of intake for essential nutrients considered to be adequate to meet the nutritional needs of healthy individuals is called _____.

7. Another name for microminerals is _____.

8. A food guide pyramid was developed by the _____ to assist in the buying and preparation of food.

Answer the following questions in the spaces provided.

9. Name the water-soluble vitamins. _____

_____

_____

_____

_____

_____

10. List at least five food sources for fat-soluble vitamins. _____

_____

_____

_____

_____

_____

11. Name the fat-soluble vitamins. _____

_____

12. Both a deficiency and excess of which mineral causes cardiac abnormalities? _____

_____

_____

_____

Continued

Match each vitamin to its function.

_____ 13. Nerve conduction

_____ 14. Formation of collagen

_____ 15. Maintenance of healthy bones and teeth

_____ 16. Formation of prothrombin for blood clotting

a. vitamin K

b. vitamin D

c. vitamin C

d. vitamin B_1

Match each mineral to its function.

_____ 17. Formation of hemoglobin

_____ 18. Development of the thyroid gland

_____ 19. Controls fluid balance in the body

_____ 20. Formation of bones and teeth

a. iodine

b. calcium

c. iron

d. sodium

■ CASE STUDIES FOR CRITICAL THINKING

From this list, choose the vitamin or mineral you would give to each patient described below, and explain why.

Vitamin C   Calcium   Vitamin B_1 Vitamin A   Iodine

21. Mrs. Smith is admitted to the hospital with tingling and numbness of the extremities.

_____

22. Mr. Jones is diagnosed with scurvy and is experiencing bleeding gums, bruising, and a wound that does not heal.

_____

23. Mr. Gerber comes to the physician's office complaining of rough, dry skin and night blindness.

_____

24. Mrs. Peterson is shrinking in height, and sustained a broken hip without having fallen.

_____

25. Mrs. Scott has been diagnosed with decreased thyroid function.

_____

■ APPLICATIONS

Obtain a current copy of a drug reference book or PDR® and use it to answer the following questions.

26. Look up potassium chloride and list all its trade names. _____

_____

_____

27. From the dosage section, summarize the information referring to child and adult dosages for potassium chloride. _____

_____

_____

The use of herbs for the treatment of common illnesses and disorders is becoming increasingly popular. To learn more about the use of herbs in medicine, check out the Herb Research Foundation at http://www.herbs.org. This site will take you to resources and scientific articles. The site also gives information on the common uses of herbs and plants in medicine.

CHAPTER

6 Antibiotics and Antifungals

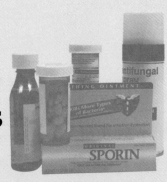

In this chapter you will learn how an infection develops. You will learn how infection affects the body and how drugs are used to treat it. You will also learn how health care workers can stop the spread of infection.

OBJECTIVES

After studying this chapter, you should be able to

- differentiate between the external and internal immune systems.
- explain why infection is more dangerous in a hospital or long-term care unit than elsewhere.
- state the two main actions of antibiotics and microorganisms.
- explain why drug resistance, drug sensitivity, and superinfection are important concerns in antibiotic drug therapy.
- name at least two problems that may arise in giving penicillin.
- list the most common uses of sulfonamides and aminoglycosides.
- outline the importance of patient education with each of the various types of antibiotics (penicillins, cephalosporins, tetracyclines, macrolides, aminoglycosides, sulfonamides, and quinolones).
- describe the correct procedure for hand washing before and after giving medications.
- describe the correct procedure for administering a medication to a patient in isolation.
- state three primary ways a health care worker can be exposed to hepatitis B virus and human immunodeficiency virus.
- explain standard, airborne, droplet, and contact precautions.

KEY TERMS

aerobic: bacteria that can survive only in the presence of oxygen

AIDS: acquired immune deficiency syndrome

anaerobic: bacteria that can survive without oxygen

anaphylaxis: severe, possibly fatal, systemic hypersensitivity reaction to a sensitizing agent—that is, a drug, food, or chemical

antibiotic: antimicrobial agent, either natural or synthetic, that kills or stops the growth of other organisms

antibody: a proteinlike substance produced in the body to fight microorganisms

antifungal: drug that kills or prevents the growth of fungi

aseptic: free of pathogens

autoclave: machine that sterilizes with steam under pressure, usually at 250°F, for a designated time

bactericide: an agent that is destructive to bacteria

bacteriostatic: an agent that inhibits the growth or multiplication of bacteria

broad-spectrum antibiotics: antibiotics that are effective against a wide variety of pathogens

culture and sensitivity test: laboratory technique for finding out which, if any,

microbes are present, and which antibiotic will be effective against a specific pathogen

disinfectant: chemical capable of killing bacteria; used in sterilization process

fungi: plantlike parasitic microorganisms

Gram stain: laboratory test for identifying microbes

HBV: hepatitis B virus

HIV: human immunodeficiency virus

hypersensitivity: an exaggerated response to a drug or other foreign agent

immune: able to resist damage from pathogens

immunization: a way of stimulating production of antibodies by exposing the body to weakened or killed germs

infection: an invasion by pathogens that reproduce, multiply, and cause disease

infectious disease: disease caused by direct or indirect spread of pathogens from one person to another

inoculation: immunizing by administration of a vaccine

isolation: keeping a patient in an environment where pathogens cannot spread from patient to health care worker and/or vice versa

leukocytes: white blood cells that defend the body against bacteria

microorganisms: tiny, one-celled plants and animals; some are pathogenic/

disease-producing and others are non-pathogenic; also called *microbes*

mycoses: infections caused by fungi

narrow-spectrum antibiotics: antibiotics that are effective against specific pathogens

nosocomial: refers to an infection that occurs in a hospital or long-term care facility

pathogens: disease-producing microorganisms

penicillinase: enzyme produced by microbes that makes them resistant to penicillin

photosensitivity: sensitivity to light, often a side effect of certain drugs; can cause rash

resistance: the ability of a particular microorganism to resist the effects of a specific antibiotic

Standard Precautions: primary strategies for prevention of infection transmitted through blood, body fluid, nonintact skin, and mucous membranes

superinfection: secondary infection that occurs while the antibiotic is destroying the first infection

Universal Precautions: safety measures that consider all patients potentially infectious with blood-borne pathogens

vaccination: introduction of an infectious agent for the purpose of establishing resistance to an infectious disease

INFECTION AND IMMUNITY

We are literally surrounded by tiny, one-celled plants and animals—called germs or, more properly, **microorganisms** or microbes. They are in the air we breathe, on the food we eat, and on the things we touch. Many of them are harmless. Some are even beneficial; for example, certain bacteria that live in the intestine help create important vitamins out of the waste products of digestion. But some microorganisms produce infection and disease. These harmful microorganisms—known as **pathogens**—include bacteria, fungi, protozoa, rickettsiae, and viruses (Figure 6.1 on page 108).

Infection is an invasion by pathogens that reproduce, multiply, and cause disease. For an infection to develop, certain conditions must be present in the environment:

• food
• oxygen (presence or absence)
• moisture
• heat
• pH of 5 to 8 (slightly alkaline)
• darkness

Microorganisms require some type of nutrition. Some thrive on organic matter, such as *Clostridium perfringens,* which causes gangrene. Others, such as *E. Coli,* receive nourishment from undigested food in the colon. **Aerobic** bacteria grow in the presence of oxygen, whereas **anaerobic** bacteria can survive without oxygen. For example, an infection deep within the body, such as in a joint, grows without oxygen. Moisture is necessary for most pathogens to survive. A few pathogens, such as botulism and tetanus, can survive without water. There are even some pathogens that can survive exposure to extreme temperatures. Pathogens also require an alkaline and dark environment to flourish.

Infectious diseases—those caused by direct or indirect spread of pathogens from one person to another—have distinct sets of symptoms that help in diagnosis. Fever, chills, headache, nausea, vomiting, diarrhea, and pus formation at the infection site are some of the signs that may indicate an infection.

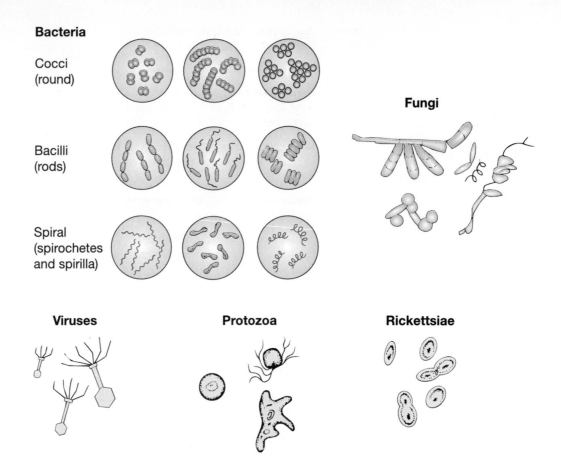

Bacteria

Cocci (round)

Bacilli (rods)

Spiral (spirochetes and spirilla)

Fungi

Viruses

Protozoa

Rickettsiae

Figure 6.1
Pathogens produce infection and disease.

THE IMMUNE SYSTEM

The immune system has two parts: external and internal.

External Immune System. The external immune system protects against infection because of normally functioning defenses. The most important of these is the skin. It provides a tough physical barrier to microorganisms. When the skin barrier is damaged, as when cut or burned, microorganisms can enter the body and cause infection.

Internal Immune System. The internal immune system is made up of microscopic substances whose specialized function is to fight infection. Certain cells, called neutrophils, surround and digest the microorganisms. **Leukocytes,** also called white blood cells, produce antibodies, which are proteins that help destroy microorganisms as they enter the body.

Antibodies. **Antibodies** are proteins that either destroy or stop the growth of certain types of microorganisms. Antibodies are carried in the bloodstream and can readily move to the site of entry.

Specific antibodies act against specific microorganisms. When an unfamiliar microorganism enters the body, proteins in the blood are stimulated to produce a special antibody to act against it. The next time that same microorganism enters the body, the antibody "remembers" it and proceeds to destroy it. Antibodies make the body **immune** to a great many infections.

Immunity can be either temporary or permanent, depending on the type of antibody. People who, for some reason, cannot form antibodies are at risk because they cannot defend themselves against the microorganisms to which we are all constantly exposed.

Sometimes, despite all these defenses, microorganisms can multiply and spread in the body, and the result is infection. The infection can be local, such as in a cut or a surgical wound, or it can be systemic and affect the whole body, as in measles.

IMMUNIZATION

Because of the pioneering work of Edward Jenner, Jonas Salk, and others, we are able to prevent many deadly or debilitating infectious diseases that in the past affected many lives. Through **immunization,** we are able to stimulate the body to produce antibodies against disease-producing microorganisms. Antibodies are produced by placing a small amount of dead or weak disease germs into the body, a process called **inoculation** or **vaccination.** Because the microorganisms are not at full strength, they do not cause full-blown disease, but they provide enough material to stimulate the body to manufacture the necessary antibodies. Thus, when living microorganisms come along, the antibodies are already there to fight them off. Immunization has been so successful that diseases that used to kill thousands of people during sweeping epidemics, such as polio and yellow fever, are now rare.

PATIENTS AT RISK

Most individuals can fight off infection successfully. If they are in good health, their natural defenses prevent the spread of microorganisms, so that there are few disease symptoms. Even when a disease develops, generally healthy people are able to survive while the infection runs its course. It is the people who are *not* healthy who are at greatest risk. Age, nutritional status, stress, medical condition, or an actual medical treatment may predispose an individual to infection.

Patients with surgical wounds or with lowered resistance because of other conditions, such as **AIDS** (acquired immune deficiency syndrome), are especially prone to infections. Weakened patients have a harder time shaking off infections and avoiding complications. Very young and very old people also have less resistance to infection.

CAUTION: Risk Factors for Infection in the Geriatric Patient

- Thin, less elastic skin
- Decreased sensitivity
- Decreased saliva production
- Less ability to perform oral hygiene
- Decreased secretion of stomach acid
- Decreased cough reflex
- Decreased hormone production
- Weakened muscular structures
- Poor nutrition
- Use of corticosteroids or cytotoxin drugs
- Residency in a long-term care facility

Hospitals and other health care facilities have large numbers of at-risk patients located in one place. A **nosocomial** infection is an infection that occurs in a hospital or long-term care facility. Once started, an infection can spread rapidly through such settings. For this reason, medical personnel must be especially concerned with avoiding the spread of pathogens. They are trained in **aseptic** or pathogen-free techniques of caring for patients. Medical personnel also learn to wash their hands before and after caring for each patient. They learn to sterilize equipment, change bed linens frequently, and wear protective clothing when handling certain infected patients.

Staph (staphylococcal) infections are a common danger for hospitalized patients. People who develop such infections must be kept in **isolation.** No one may enter or leave these patients' rooms without special precautions against spreading staph pathogens. Practice Procedure 6.1 at the end of this chapter shows you how to prepare to administer medications to a patient in isolation.

Standard Precautions are the primary strategies for prevention of infections. The term applies to infections caused by blood, body fluids, nonintact skin, and mucous membranes. Standard Precautions combine the major features of the previous categories—Universal Precautions and body substance isolation. They provide protection for the health care worker as directed by the Occupational Safety and Health Administration (OSHA) and the Centers for Disease Control (CDC). Standard Precautions apply in the care of all patients in hospitals regardless of their diagnosis or presumed infection status. They reduce the transmission of microorganisms in both recognized and unrecognized infections in patients. The CDC developed new guidelines in 1995 for isolation precautions, both Standard Precautions and Transmission-based Precautions. Transmission-based Precautions are used for patients who are known to be infected or suspected to be infected with a pathogen that is epidemiologically significant and can be transmitted by air or droplet or by contact with contaminated surfaces.

ANTIBIOTIC DRUGS

The discovery of so-called miracle drugs—the antibiotics—changed the practice of medicine radically. **Antibiotics** are drugs that destroy microorganisms. The major classifications of antibiotics are penicillins, cephalosporins, tetracyclines, macrolides, aminoglycosides, sulfonamides, and quinolones. (See Table 6.1.)

TABLE 6.1: Antibiotics and Antivirals

Antibiotics

Penicillins
  Penicillin BK (*Pentids*)
  Ampicillin (*Amcill*)
  Amoxicillin (*Amoxin*)
  Ampicillin/sulbactam (*Unasyn*)
  Amoxicillin/clavulanate (*Augmentin*)
  Nafcillin (*Unipen*)
  Oxacillin (*Bactrocill*)
  Dicloxacillin (*Dynapen*)
  Carbencillin (*Geocillin*)
  Ticarcillin (*Ticar*)
  Ticarcillin/clavulanate (*Timentin*)
  Azlocillin (*Azlin*)
  Mezlocillin (*Mezlin*)
  Methicillin (*Staphcillin*)
  Piperacillin (*Pipracil*)
  Piperacillin/tazobactam (*Zosyn*)
Quinolones
  Norfloxacin (*Noroxin*)
  Ciprofloxacin (*Cipro*)
  Ofloxacin (*Floxin*)
  Enoxacin (*Penetrex*)
Cephalosporins
  Cefazolin (*Ancef, Kefzol*)
  Cephalexin (*Keflex*)
  Cephradine (*Velosef, Anspor*)
  Cephalothin (*Keflin*)
  Cephadroxil (*Duricef*)
  Cefonicid (*Monocid*)
  Cefamandole (*Mandol*)

Cefuroxime (*Zinacef, Kefurox*)
Cefaclor (*Ceclor*)
Cefuroxime axemil (*Ceftin*)
Cefoxin (*Mefoxin*)
Cefmetazole (*Zefazone*)
Cefotetan (*Cefotan*)
Cefotaxime (*Claforan*)
Ceftizoxime (*Cefizox*)
Ceftriaxone (*Rocephin*)
Cefixime (*Suprax*)
Cefoperazone (*Cefobid*)
Cefrazidime (*Fortaz, Tazicef*)
Sulfonamides
  Sulfadiazine (*Microsulphan*)
  Sulfasoxazole (*Gantrisin*)
  Sulfamethoxazole/trimethoprim
    (*Bactrim, Septra*)
Aminoglycosides
  Gentamicin (*Garamycin*)
  Tobramycin (*Tobrex, Nebcin*)
  Amikacin (*Amikin*)
  Netilmicin (*Netromycin*)
  Streptomycin
  Kanamycin (*Kantrex*)
  Neomycin
Macrolides
  Erythromycin (eryc), *E-mycin,*
  Ilosone, EES
  Azithromycin (*Zithromax*)
  Derivatives
  Clarithromycin (*Biaxin*)

Tetracyclines
  Tetracycline hydrochloride
    (*Achromycin V, Stecil*)
  Doxycycline (*Vibramycin*)
  Oxytetracycline (*Terramycin*)
  Minocycline (*Minocin*)
Miscellaneous Antibiotics
  Aztreonam (*Azacram*)
  Chloramphenical (*Chloromycetin*)
  Imipenen/cilastatin (*Primaxin*)
  Metronidazole (*Flagyl*)
  Spectinomycin (*Trobicin*)
Antifungals
  Amphotericin B (*Fungizone*)
  Flucanazole (*Diflucan*)
  Flucytosine (*Anocobon*)
  Griseofulvin (*Grisactin*)
  Ketoconazole (*Nizoral*)
  Miconazole (*Monistat*)
  Mistatin (*Mycostatin*)

Antivirals
  Acyclovir (*Zovirax*)
  Ganciclovir (*Cytovene*)
  Foscarnet (*Foscarir*)
  Zidovudine (AZT) (*Retrovir*)
  Didanosine (ddl) (*Videx*)
  Dideoxyctidine (ddC) (*Hivid*)
  Ribavirin (*Virazole*)
  Amantadine (*Symmetrel*)

Antibiotics kill microorganisms either directly (indicated by the suffix *-cidal*, as in *bacteriocidal*) or keep them from growing (suffix *-static*, as in *bacteriostatic*). Some interfere with cell wall production in the microorganisms. Others inhibit protein synthesis. Still others mix up the chemical messages for producing nucleic acid, a major substance in cell growth. Some act better on rapidly multiplying pathogens, whereas others are more effective with slowly growing organisms.

ADMINISTRATION CONSIDERATIONS

Before prescribing antibiotics for specific ailments, a physician must consider three points.

- *Condition of the patient's defense system.* The physician must note whether the patient's immune system is functioning properly. Some antibiotics kill microorganisms directly and others slow the growth or reproduction of microorganisms. Both types depend on the body's natural defenses (leukocytes and antibodies) for help in eliminating an infection.
- *Type of infection and its cause.* What organism is causing the infection is important. Some infectious diseases have distinct symptoms, but many have similar symptoms. When in doubt, an attempt must be made to identify the bacteria. The identity of the pathogen determines the choice of a specific antibiotic. Specific identification of bacteria requires a **Gram stain** and culture with chemical testing.

    When placed on a microscope slide along with a stain, some microbes turn blue and others turn red. The blue-staining microbes are called gram-positive microbes and the red-staining ones gram-negative. The shape of the microbes changes into either rods (slender straight bar) or cocci (spherical or ovoid). These changes, along with the color changes, help identify the correct antibiotic to use. For example, vancomycin is effective against most gram-positive microbes, and tobramycin is effective against most gram-negative microbes.
- *Type of drug and its effects.* The physician must consider the type of antibiotic because these drugs have varying degrees of effectiveness and varying side effects. Although the initial antibiotic selection may be made by the physician's examination of the patient and the Gram stain, the antibiotic may be changed following a **culture and sensitivity test.** A sample of fluid (e.g., pus obtained from a throat scraping) is taken from an infected person and used to start a culture of bacteria in the laboratory. Then pieces of paper saturated with samples of different antibiotics are placed on the culture. The results show which drugs kill the bacteria, and which drugs are resistant to the bacteria. The physician chooses one of the drugs that is sensitive to the bacteria and has the fewest side effects for the particular patient (Figure 6.2).

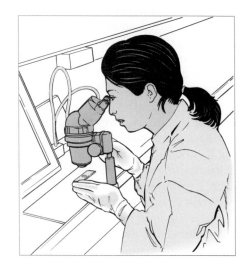

Figure 6.2
Physicians try to choose the antibiotic that is most effective against a particular bacterium and that causes the fewest side effects for the patient.

Sometimes it is hard to isolate the microorganism that is causing an ailment. In these situations a physician may prescribe a **broad-spectrum antibiotic.** This type of antibiotic destroys a great variety of microorganisms. The cephalosporins are one group of broad-spectrum antibiotics. In contrast, **narrow-spectrum antibiotics** are effective against only a few types of pathogens.

If the disease-producing organism can be identified, a narrow-spectrum drug is usually a better choice than a broad-spectrum drug. Pathogens are able to develop **resistance** to antibiotics. After exposure to a certain antibiotic for a while, a particular pathogen may no longer be sensitive to its action. Once this happens, it is useless to continue giving that antibiotic to the patient. (Note that the *bacteria,* not an individual, becomes resistant to an antibiotic.) Use of broad-spectrum antibiotics gives more types of organisms a chance to develop resistance. Because of resistance, the overuse of antibiotics is now recognized as an important public health problem. The results of overuse are seen in hospitals where certain strains of resistant bacteria have appeared, causing hospital-acquired or nosocomial infections.

Another problem a doctor considers in prescribing antibiotics is drug **hypersensitivity.** Hypersensitivity can occur in reaction to all antibiotics. It is an altered state of reactivity in which the body reacts with an exaggerated immune response. Some antibiotics may cause a minor rash, which the patient may easily tolerate. Other antibiotics can cause an anaphylactic reaction, which is a serious medical emergency.

The physician weighs the benefits of the drug against the dangers of not giving the drug. Usually the physician has several drugs to choose among, with a varying range of side effects. A more dangerous drug is chosen only when a less dangerous one has failed to stop an infection, when the patient has become hypersensitive to the drug, or when the bacteria has become resistant to it.

Superinfection is a secondary infection that occurs while an antibiotic is destroying the first infection. Most antibiotics decrease or destroy normal flora in the GI tract. Approximately 2 percent of patients contract superinfections. Patients are at higher risk of developing superinfections if they are taking more than one antibiotic or a broad-spectrum antibiotic. When a superinfection occurs, the drug should be changed to another drug to which the organism is sensitive.

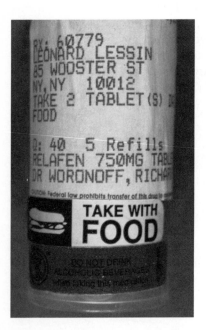

SCHEDULES

Timing is important in antibiotic therapy. Pathogens may be present long after symptoms disappear. The physician must order the antimicrobial drug in the appropriate dose and for a long period. It is important for patients to take the drug until they have finished all the doses. An antimicrobial drug often fails because the dose is too small or the drug is taken too briefly. Antimicrobial drugs should not be discontinued until the patient has been fever-free and feeling well for 48 to 72 hours. Follow-up cultures should be done to determine if the drug was effective.

Time of day is also important, because doses of antimicrobials must be scheduled around mealtimes. Oral antimicrobials can cause gastric irritation. Giving them on a full stomach or with milk can help soothe irritation. On the other hand, some are made less effective when food or milk is present in the stomach. It is important to find out if oral antimicrobials should be given with food or milk or on an empty stomach. Instructions to "give between meals" mean that drug is to be given at least 1 hour before or 2 hours after meals, when the stomach is assumed to be empty.

ANTIBIOTICS

An antibiotic is a substance with the ability to destroy life. It is produced by a microorganism and has **bactericidal** activity or **bacteriostatic** activity on other microorganisms.

Penicillins. The penicillins are a large group of antibiotics that are the most effective and least toxic of all antimicrobials. They come in many forms, to be given by different routes according to the therapeutic aim.

Natural penicillins are made from a mold that grows on bread and fruit. Penicillin G potassium (*Pentids*) and penicillin V (*Pen-Vee, V-Cillin K*) are the most common natural penicillins. They are commonly used to treat syphilis and strep throat. Amoxicillin, a type of penicillin, may be given preventively to patients with heart disease and rheumatic fever. Infections considered susceptible to penicillins include gonorrhea, syphilis, pneumonia, meningitis, diphtheria, osteomyelitis, and otitis media. Penicillins are also effective against infections caused by staphylococci, streptococci, Escherichia coli, and salmonella bacteria.

Unfortunately, some pathogens fight back when attacked by penicillin. They secrete a substance called **penicillinase.** The pathogens are then resistant in the ongoing battle against these penicillinase-producing bacteria. Protection can be provided, though, by adding a penicillin decoy. When the penicillinase attacks the decoy, it leaves the penicillin able to kill the bacteria. Examples of this penicillin and decoy strategy are amoxicillin + clavulanate (*Augmentin*), ticarcillin + clavulanate (*Timentin*), ampicillin + sulbactam (*Unasyn*), and, most recently, piperacillin + tazobactam (*Zosyn*), put on the market in 1994.

Although penicillins are usually safe and well tolerated, patient education is essential. There is the danger of penicillin allergy. Severe rashes can occur as a result of penicillin allergy. Other reactions can be life-threatening. A person can go into **anaphylaxis,** which is signaled by difficulty in breathing, swelling of the throat so as to cause suffocation, and shock symptoms. Persons who have penicillin allergies should wear a medical ID to alert the medical staff in case emergency treatment is needed.

 PATIENT EDUCATION

Penicillins

- Take the full course of medication even after feeling better and being symptom-free.
- Take doses at the prescribed times to maintain therapeutic blood levels.
- Never take an antibiotic prescribed for someone else, because it may be for a different type of infection.
- Generally the medication should be taken on an empty stomach, but there are some exceptions.

- Penicillins affect the effectiveness of estrogen-containing contraceptives.
- Patients with diabetes mellitus should use Clinistix or Ketodiastix urine glucose tests instead of the Clinitest, because of the likelihood of false-positive results.
- The most common side effects are mild diarrhea, nausea, and vomiting.
- Notify the physician if rash, fever, or chills occur, because they may indicate an allergic reaction.

Cephalosporins. Cephalosporins are broad-spectrum, semisynthetic drugs that are chemical modifications of the penicillin structure. They are classified into three generations. Each generation is used for specific pathogens. It wasn't until the third generation that cephalosporins were prescribed for serious infections. Initially, they were considered advantageous over penicillin because of their resistance to the enzymatic activity of penicillinase. However, drug resistance has since been demonstrated in all three generations. Cephalosporins are often prescribed for patients who are allergic to penicillin. Generally, only about 6 percent to 18 percent of patients who are allergic to penicillin are also allergic to cephalosporins. Examples are cephalexin (*Keflex*) and cephalothin (*Keflin*). Patient education is important for patients taking cephalosporins.

 PATIENT EDUCATION

Cephalosporins

- Take all doses of the medication even after being symptom-free and feeling better.
- Take doses at the prescribed times to maintain therapeutic blood levels.
- Take the medicine with food if gastrointestinal upset occurs.
- Patients with diabetes mellitus should use Clinistix or Ketodiastix urine glucose tests instead of the Clinitest, because of the likelihood of false-positive results.

- Avoid alcohol or alcohol-containing medications because they interact with cephalosporins to produce abdominal pains, nausea, vomiting, decreased blood pressure, rapid pulse, and sweating.
- Read labels, such as on cough syrup, for alcohol-containing ingredients.
- Tell the physician of any history of bleeding tendencies.
- The physician may order liver and renal blood tests to monitor the drug in patients with liver or renal impairment.

Tetracyclines. The tetracyclines were the first broad-spectrum antibiotics. They are used to treat many infections. Tetracyclines pose a greater risk of superinfection than other microbials, so patients must be monitored for symptoms of secondary infections. As with all antibiotics, their effectiveness depends on the patient's compliance with treatment. Examples of this drug group are tetracycline hydrochloride (*Achromycin V*) and doxycycline (*Vibramycin*).

 PATIENT EDUCATION

Tetracyclines

- Take all doses of the medication at the prescribed times until the medication is gone.
- Perform good oral and perineal hygiene to prevent Candida superinfection.
- Except for doxycycline (*Vibramycin*) and minocycline (*Minocin*), take the medication on an empty stomach (1 hour before or 2 hours after meals).
- Take the medication with a full glass of water to prevent gastrointestinal irritation.

- Avoid taking antacids, iron products, and laxatives containing aluminum, calcium, or magnesium, because they decrease absorption of the tetracyclines.
- Avoid milk and milk products for 1 hour before or 2 hours after tetracycline administration.
- Avoid direct ultraviolet and sunlight (tetracyclines can cause a rash due to **photosensitivity**).
- Notify the physician if discoloration of teeth appears.

Macrolides. There are four macrolide antibiotics: azithromycin (*Zithromax*), clarithromycin (*Biaxin*), erythromycin, and troleandomycin (*Tao*). They are both bacteriostatic and bactericidal. *Zithromax* and *Biaxin* are the two newest macrolide antibiotics. Although both drugs cause gastrointestinal side effects, they have a lower incidence than erythromycin and *Tao*. Patients receiving erythromycin should be monitored closely if also receiving theophylline (a bronchodilator), because there is a potential for increasing the serum levels of theophylline. Caution is also necessary if the patient is taking astemizole (*Hismanal*) because it causes heart problems. Educating the patient about the medication is an important part of treatment success.

PATIENT EDUCATION

Macrolides

- Take all the medicine at prescribed times until the medicine is gone.
- Usual course of treatment is 10 days.

- Take the medicine on an empty stomach (1 hour before or 2 hours after meals) with a full glass of water, because food decreases absorption.
- Patients may be monitored closely if there is a diagnosis of liver impairment.

Aminoglycosides. Aminoglycosides are potent bactericidal antibiotics that are generally used to treat only serious or life-threatening infections. These drugs must be used with extreme caution because of their high incidence of toxic effects on several body systems. Patients receiving muscle relaxants or who have myesthenia gravis or Parkinson's disease experience greater weakness. Extreme caution must be used with elderly patients because they are susceptible to hearing loss and to toxic effects on the kidney. Patient education is essential with these drugs to decrease the incidence of toxic side effects. Examples of aminoglycosides are amikacin (*Amikin*), gentamicin (*Garamycin*), and tobramycin (*Tobrex, Nebcin*). They are also available as one ingredient in creams and ointments for topical use (e.g., *Neosporin, Cortisporin Otic*) and in oral forms for a local antibacterial effect.

PATIENT EDUCATION

Aminoglycosides

- Take the full course of medication as prescribed.
- Take medication with a full glass of water to decrease the risk of toxic effects on the kidneys.
- Report any ringing or buzzing in the ears that may indicate hearing loss.

- Report any change in urinary pattern or blood in the urine, which indicate a toxic effect on the kidney.
- Report any dizziness, numbness, tingling, or twitching, which indicate vestibular or nervous system toxicity.

Sulfonamides. Sulfonamides, or sulfa drugs, are useful for many different types of infection (see page 116). They are primarily bacteriostatic rather than bactericidal. They are frequently used for urinary tract infections. The combination of a sulfonamide, sulfamethoxazole, with trimethoprim makes a very powerful antibiotic regimen. It is so useful, in fact, that this combination has been given the name "cotrimoxazole," which is the active ingredient in the drugs *Bactrim* and *Septra*.

Side effects from sulfonamides are frequent. Common side effects are fever, rash, nausea, vomiting, and diarrhea. Low blood counts can also result from taking this medicine. Sulfonamides may cause crystals to form in the urine. This can cause urinary complications. For this reason, patient education is important.

PATIENT EDUCATION

Sulfonamides

- Take the full course of medication even after feeling better.
- Take the medication on an empty stomach and with a full glass of water to enhance absorption.
- If the common side effects of nausea and vomiting occur, medication may be taken with food.
- Avoid taking the medication with antacids because they decrease absorption of the sulfonamide.

- Drink at least 3 quarts of fluids per day.
- Avoid acidic juices, such as orange juice, and vitamin C (ascorbic acid), because they cause the urine to be acidic.
- Report any skin reactions, such as a rash or itching.
- Fever and joint pain may occur after 7 days, and must be reported immediately to the physician.
- Avoid direct sunlight.

Quinolones. Quinolones are newer, broad-spectrum, synthetic antibiotics that are bactericidal. They are used in the treatment of respiratory, gastrointestinal, bone, skin, and urinary infections. Two commonly used quinolones are ciprofloxacin (*Cipro*) and ofloxacin (*Floxin*). Because they have a wide range of gastrointestinal and central nervous system side effects, they are to be used with caution in the elderly. They are not to be used with infants or children. Patient education is important to enhance the effectiveness of these drugs.

PATIENT EDUCATION

Quinolones

- Take all doses of the medication at prescribed times.
- Report dizziness, lightheadedness, blurred vision, or depression immediately to the physician; they may indicate central nervous system toxicity.

- Avoid taking with antacids.
- Avoid direct sunlight.
- Avoid activities that require coordination and alertness because of the possibility of central nervous system symptoms.

MISCELLANEOUS ANTIBIOTICS

Aztreonam (Azactam). *Azactam* is the first drug in a new class of antibiotics known as *monobactams.* It is a synthetic bactericidal antibiotic that is effective in the treatment of respiratory, urinary, intra-abdominal, gynecological, and skin infections. The most frequent side effects are rash and itching.

Chloramphenicol (Chloromycetin). *Chloromycetin* is a potent inhibitor of protein synthesis that is generally bacteriostatic. However, in high doses, with certain susceptible organisms, it may be bactericidal. *Chloromycetin* is very toxic to the bone marrow and is reserved for use in infections for which other antibiotics have been ineffective. As a result of its bone marrow toxicity, patients should be monitored closely for bleeding tendencies.

ANTIFUNGAL DRUGS

Infections caused by **fungi,** plantlike parasitic microorganisms, are called **mycoses.** These are treated with **antifungal** drugs. Mycoses can range from superficial to severe and life-threatening. The fungi can be inhaled, orally ingested, or implanted under the skin after an injury. *Candida albicans* is a species of fungi that is usually part of the normal flora of the mouth, skin, intestines, and vagina. Systemic infection and overgrowth of *Candida albicans* (candidiasis) can result from certain drug therapies such as antibiotics, corticosteroids, and antineoplastics. Oral candidiasis, also called *thrush,* is common in newborns and in immunocompromised patients such as those with cancer and AIDS. Vaginal candidiasis frequently occurs in women who are taking oral contraceptives, are pregnant, or who have diabetes mellitus.

ANTIVIRAL DRUGS

Antiviral drugs are synthetic and developed to fight specific viruses. Examples of viral diseases are herpes zoster, herpes simplex (shingles), influenza, acquired immune deficiency syndrome (AIDS), and the common cold. The development of antiviral drugs has been much more difficult than the development of antibacterials. The reason is that the virus often reaches its peak before clinical symptoms actually appear. For an antiviral to be effective, the drug must be given before the disease begins.

Table 6.2 lists the various categories of infectious diseases.

TABLE 6.2: Infectious Diseases

Bacterial Infections	Fungus Infections (mycoses)	Spirochetal Infections
Anthrax	Actinomycosis	Lyme disease
Bacillary dysentery	Candidiasis (moniliasis)	Syphilis
Bacterial endocarditis	Coccidioidomycosis	**Virus Infections**
Blood poisoning	Histoplasmosis	AIDS
Boils	**Parasitic Infections**	Chickenpox
Botulism	Flukes	Cold sores (herpes simplex)
Brucellosis (undulant fever)	Hookworm	Common cold
Cholera	Pinworm	Encephalitis
Diphtheria	Roundworm	Genital herpes
Gastroenteritis (food poisoning)	Schistosomiasis	Influenza (flu, grippe)
Gonorrhea	Tapeworm	Lymphogranuloma
Meningitis	Trichinosis	Measles
Osteomyelitis	**Protozoan Infections**	Mononucleosis
Plague	Amebic dysentery (amebiasis)	Mumps
Pneumonia	Malaria	Poliomyelitis
Strep throat	Toxoplasmosis	Psittacosis (parrot fever)
Tetanus	Trypanosomiasis (sleeping sickness)	Rabies
Trench mouth	**Rickettsial Infections**	Shingles (herpes zoster)
Tularemia	Rocky Mountain spotted fever	Viral hepatitis
Typhoid fever	Typhus	Yellow fever
Chlamydial Infections		

ISOLATION PROCEDURES

There are two basic situations in which isolation procedures may be used:

- when a patient must be protected from any microorganisms that you carry.
- when you must be protected from any microorganism the patient is carrying.

Depending on the specific disease or microorganism danger, there are special types of isolation requiring different precautions. The CDC's isolation guidelines are outlined in Table 6.3.

TABLE 6.3: CDC Isolation Guidelines

TYPE OF PRECAUTION	CRITERIA FOR USE	BARRIER PROTECTION
Standard precaution	Any contact with all body fluids, secretions, excretions (except sweat), nonintact skin, mucous membranes	• Wash hands between patient contact • Gloves • Masks, eye protection or face shield only if splash with body fluids or blood is possible • Gowns only if soiling with body fluids or blood is possible • Patient care items must be properly cleaned • Contaminated linen is placed in leak-proof bag and labeled • All sharp instruments and needles are disposed of in puncture-resistant container (never recap needles after use) • Private room only if the patient's hygienic practices are careless and pose a risk to other patients
Airborne precautions	Droplet nuclei smaller than 5 microns; chickenpox, measles, tuberculosis	• Private room • Close patient room door to control direction of air flow • Mask or high filtration respirator • Wash hands between patient contact • Gowns and gloves only if risk of exposure with body fluids or blood • Patient should wear mask when ambulating or being transported outside of their room
Droplet precautions	Droplets larger than 5 microns; pharyngeal diphtheria, rubella, pneumonia, streptococcal pharyngitis, pertussis, mumps	• Private room • Mask or filtration respirator • Wash hands between patient contact
Contact precautions	Direct patient or environmental contact, infection with drug resistant organism; major wound infections, herpes simplex, scabies varicella zoster, shigella and other enteric pathogens	• Private room • Gloves • Gowns, hand washing

STRICT ISOLATION

The patient is kept in a separate room, or shares a room with a patient who has the same disease, with the door closed. All involved staff wear protective gowns, masks, and gloves. Hands must be washed upon entering and leaving the room. All equipment for drug administration must be discarded in special containers after use or must be disinfected and sterilized.

This type of isolation is ordered for hospital staph infections and serious infectious diseases that can be spread by touch and by air. It protects the medical staff (and other patients) from microorganisms the patient is carrying.

RESPIRATORY ISOLATION

The patient is kept in a separate room, with the door closed. Staff members wear protective masks only. Hands must be washed upon entering and leaving the room. Gloves are not necessary, but any object that is contaminated with fluids from the patient's nose and lungs must be disinfected so that the patient's microorganisms are not spread to others. Meningitis, measles, mumps, and tuberculosis are diseases requiring respiratory isolation.

REVERSE ISOLATION (PROTECTIVE ISOLATION)

The patient is kept in a separate room, with the door closed. Gown, mask, and gloves must be worn by the staff. Hands must be washed upon entering and leaving the room. This type of isolation protects patients who have no immunity or who have weakened immunity because of leukemia or cancer chemotherapy; the patient is being protected from microorganisms you are carrying.

SPECIAL CONSIDERATIONS WHEN CARING FOR INFECTIOUS PATIENTS

Special procedures are also followed when handling patients with burns and skin infections (wound and skin precautions), and open sores, blood infections, and draining wounds (discharge precautions). These do not require a separate room for the patient, but aseptic procedures must be followed to avoid causing or spreading infection. When a patient has a disease that is spread by direct or indirect contact with feces, enteric precautions are implemented. Generally, a private room is used, especially if the patient's hygiene is poor.

Before administering drugs to an isolation patient, you should review isolation procedures in your agency's procedure manual or in a good nursing manual. The steps are specific and should be followed. There are usually instructions for putting on and taking off gowns, masks, and gloves and for disposing of materials and equipment. Personal protective equipment is shown in Figure 6.3.

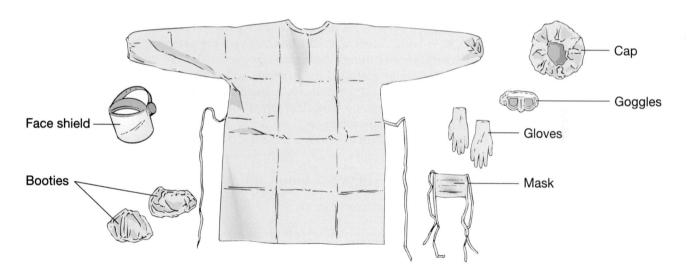

Face shield

Booties

Cap

Goggles

Gloves

Mask

Figure 6.3
Personal protective equipment acts as a barrier between the health care worker and patients who may be carrying infectious diseases.

The procedure you will use most often, whether working with an isolation patient or not, is washing your hands. You will wash your hands both before and after administering a medication. Practice Procedure 6.1 on page 122 will refresh your skill in the proper hand-washing technique.

When administering medications to an isolation patient, you may wonder which items are considered contaminated. The answer is everything that has been in direct or indirect contact with the patient. An example of indirect contact would be your touching a glass that has remained near a coughing patient, even if the patient had never actually touched the glass. Your gown and mask protect you (or the patient) from indirect contact. Your gloves protect you from direct contact. For additional protection, you may ask patients to take their own medications and dispose of supplies while you watch, as long as they are able to do this.

When working with a patient who has an infectious disease, it is helpful to know the main places where infection can be picked up. Infection may leave the body of a diseased person in the secretions of the nose and mouth; in material coughed up from the lungs; in the feces or anything touched by feces (bedclothes, toilet, etc.); in the urine; in the vaginal area; in drainage from infected wounds; and in the blood (as in the case of hepatitis).

You may take advantage of disposable materials to avoid carrying infection from one place to another. Where disposable materials are not available or not practical (as with permanent pieces of equipment), contaminated items must be washed and sterilized by using a special machine. Machines can kill infectious organisms by subjecting them to extreme heat, searing them with steam, or by means of sound waves or ultraviolet rays. A common sterilizing machine is the **autoclave,** which uses steam. A variety of chemicals called **disinfectants** kill infectious organisms and are also available for sterilizing surgical tools and other pieces of equipment.

Disposal procedures are also important when you work with infected patients. Equipment and disposable materials must be specially wrapped and often labeled before being discarded or sent to the facility's sterilization unit. Agencies usually have their own disposal procedures described in a procedure manual.

UNIVERSAL BLOOD AND BODY FLUID PRECAUTIONS

Universal Precautions mean that all patients are considered potentially infectious with blood-borne pathogens. Examples are hepatitis B virus (**HBV**) and human immunodeficiency virus (**HIV**), the virus that causes AIDS. Health care workers are exposed to these pathogens primarily through mucous membranes, nonintact skin, and needlesticks.

Blood is the most important vehicle for transmission of these pathogens. Other body fluids that can be involved are cerebrospinal (CSF), synovial (joint), pleural (lung), peritoneal (abdominal), and amniotic fluids; semen; vaginal secretions; and human breast milk. Gloves and other protective clothing should be used routinely in handling contaminated needles and other sharp instruments. The Universal Blood and Body Fluid Precaution Guidelines are frequently revised, so be sure your facility has the current, up-to-date guidelines in use (see Table 6.4).

TABLE 6.4: Universal Blood and Body Fluid Precautions

Employer: Protect Health Care Worker
- Explain activities that expose workers to blood-borne pathogens.
- Develop standard operating procedures to prevent worker exposure.
- Provide initial and ongoing education on universal precautions.
- Follow up worker compliance with guidelines.
- Redesign the workplace and modify the workplace environment.

Health Care Worker: Use Appropriate Barrier Precautions
- Wear gloves to reduce blood contamination to skin surface.
- Wash hands/skin immediately when exposed.
- Change and discard punctured or torn gloves.
- Change gloves between patients.
- Wear mask, gowns, and eye/face shields during procedures that are likely to generate splashes of blood or body fluids.
- Do not work if you have exudative lesions.
- If pregnant, do not risk exposing the fetus to blood-borne pathogens by lack of precautions.

Health Care Worker: Prevent Needlestick Injuries
- Do not break, bend, or remove needles by hand from syringes.
- Do not recap needles if avoidable.
- Place disposable needles in puncture-resistant containers.
- Place these containers as close to the work area as possible.
- Place nondisposable needles and equipment in puncture-resistant containers and transport them to the processing area.
- Transport contaminated equipment to the appropriate area.

REPRESENTATIVE ANTIMICROBIALS

CATEGORY, NAME[a], AND ROUTE	USES AND DISEASES	ACTIONS	USUAL DOSE[b] AND SPECIAL INSTRUCTIONS	SIDE EFFECTS AND ADVERSE REACTIONS
Antibiotics				
Amoxicillin clavulante (*Augmentin*) PO	Lower respiratory infection, otitis media, urinary tract infection, skin infections	Inhibits bacterial cell wall synthesis	250 mg PO q 8 hrs; 500 mg 1 8 hrs (severe infection); watch patient closely for allergic reaction	Nausea, vomiting, diarrhea, hypersensitivity reactions such as rash, chills, shortness of breath
Erythromycin PO, IV	Acute pelvic inflammatory disease, endocarditis prophylaxis for dental work, respiratory infection	Inhibits protein synthesis	250–550 mg PO q 6 hrs	Nausea, vomiting, diarrhea, abdominal pain
Gentamicin (*Garamycin*) IV, IM	Bloodstream infections, serious infections, meningitis, endocarditis prophylaxis for GI or GU surgery	Inhibits protein synthesis	3 mg/Kg daily in divided doses; IM or IV infusion q 8 hrs	Kidney damage, hearing loss, upset of balance; drug levels must be closely monitored
Sulfamethoxazole/trimethoprim (*Septra, Bactrim*) IV, PO	Bronchitis, urinary tract infections, otitis media	Blocks folate metabolism pathway	One double-strength tablet PO q12h; encourage fluids	Nausea, vomiting, diarrhea, rash, allergic reaction to sulfa
Ciprofloxacin (*Cipro*) PO	Pneumonia, bone infection, urinary tract infection, skin infection	Inhibits DNA gyrase	500 mg PO q12hr; do not take with antacids	Headache, nausea, diarrhea, rash
Antifungals				
Amphotericin B (*Fungizone*) IV, PO	Systemic fungal infections	Damages fungal cell wall	100 mg PO QID for 7 to 10 days	Fever, chills, nausea, weight loss, anorexia, kidney damage, vein irritation
Antivirals				
Acyclovir (*Zovirax*) IV, PO, top	Herpes simplex, chickenpox, genital herpes	Stops viral replication	200 mg PO 1 4 hr	Kidney damage, headache, confusion, irritability, nausea, vomiting

---

[a]Trade names given in parentheses are examples only. Check current drug references for a complete listing of available products.

[b]Average adult doses are given. However, dosages are determined by a physician and vary with the purpose of the therapy and the particular patient. The doses presented here are for general information only.

PRACTICE PROCEDURE 6.1

Administering Medication to an Isolation Patient

You may wish to practice the procedure several times using a different type of isolation each time.

■ EQUIPMENT

Medication order for an oral medication to be taken with water

Kardex, medication record, patient chart

Oral medication

Medication tray and disposable medication cup

Gown, mask, and gloves

Instructions for basic isolation procedures in your facility's procedure manual

Water pitcher and glass (next to patient's bed)

■ PROCEDURE

1. Assemble equipment. Use disposable equipment, if possible.

2. Read medication order and set up medication. Check to see that you have the RIGHT DOSE of the RIGHT MEDICATION for the RIGHT PATIENT by the RIGHT ROUTE at the RIGHT TIME.

3. Check to see what kind of isolation the patient is under—respiratory, strict, reverse, or special precautions (enteric, skin wounds, discharge, etc.). A sign on the door of the patient's room or on the Kardex should tell the type of isolation.

4. Review isolation procedures for the specific type of isolation and decide what clothing you must wear—gown, mask, and/or gloves. Here is a brief reminder:

   For reverse isolation. Wear gown, mask, and gloves. This provides protection for the patient.

   For respiratory isolation. Wear a mask only. This protects you from airborne bacteria that may be inhaled into the lungs.

   For strict isolation. Wear gown, mask, and gloves. This provides protection for you, since you must not touch anything contaminated. But remember to wash your hands before you put on the protective clothing.

5. Wash your hands, using antiseptic liquid soap and warm water to make a lather and then scrub each finger and the front and back of each hand with a circular motion. Rinse, keeping hands lower than elbows so that water flows from the cleaner area toward the dirtier area. The washing process should last for at least 1 to 2 minutes. Dry hands with a paper towel, from the fingers (cleanest area) to wrists (least clean area).

6. Now put on your gown, mask, and/or gloves, following the proper procedure.

7. Carry the medication into the patient's room in a disposable medication cup. Leave the drug cart or tray outside the door.

8. Identify the patient, following agency procedure. Explain what you are going to do (e.g., give the patient an antibiotic to help heal or fight an infection). If necessary, assist the patient into a comfortable position for taking the medication.

9. Administer the medication. Have the patient pour a glass of water from the bedside pitcher and then take the medication from the medication cup and swallow it with water while you watch.

10. Give any special instructions regarding the medication; for example, describe mild side effects that may be expected. Make the patient comfortable before leaving the room.

Continued

11. Remove gown, mask, and/or gloves and discard according to the rules of your agency. Wash your hands, following standard nursing practice. Use a paper towel to turn off the water faucet, unless there is a foot or knee pedal.

12. Chart the medication, noting the time, dose, and anything unusual that you may have noticed or that the patient may have mentioned.

Demonstrate this procedure for your instructor or the nurse in charge.

Define each term.

1. Antibody   _____

2. Immunization   _____

3. Pathogen   _____

4. Bacteriostatic   _____

5. Bactericidal   _____

6. Hypersensitivity   _____

7. Penicillinase   _____

Answer the following questions in the spaces provided.

8. List two ways in which antibiotic drugs fight infection. _____
   _____
   _____

9. Which parts of the body may be damaged by aminoglycosides? _____
   _____
   _____

10. What is another name for erythromycin? _____
    _____

11. Why might a physician order a Gram stain? _____
    _____

12. Why are isolation procedures used? _____
    _____

13. List the three main types of isolation (in which patients are kept in separate rooms). _____
    _____
    _____
    _____

Match these antibiotics to their descriptions.

_____ 14. Semisynthetic forms of penicillin

_____ 15. Broad-spectrum antibiotics that should not be taken
with antacids or milk

_____ 16. Semisynthetic drugs that can substitute for penicillin
when germs have developed resistance

_____ 17. Broad-spectrum antibiotics that can cause nerve damage

_____ 18. Synthetic drugs used mostly for urinary tract infections

a. tetracyclines

b. cephalosporins

c. sulfonamides

d. ampicillin, amoxicillin

e. kanamycin, gentamicin

_____ 19. Blood protein containing antibodies, given to protect the body from infection   f. macrolides

_____ 20. Substitute for penicillin   g. gamma globulin

Match these terms to their descriptions.

_____ 21. Laboratory test to identify pathogens   a. narrow spectrum

_____ 22. Laboratory test to determine which drug will kill a specific pathogen   b. resistance

c. Gram stain

_____ 23. Drugs that affect many pathogens

d. broad spectrum

_____ 24. Drugs that affect only a few pathogens

e. hypersensitivity

_____ 25. A germ's immunity to the effects of pathogen-killing drugs

f. culture and sensitivity test

_____ 26. Allergiclike reaction to a drug after taking several doses

■ CASE STUDIES FOR CRITICAL THINKING

Answer the following questions in the spaces provided.

27. Why are staph and other infections a special problem in hospitals and long-term care units? Give at least three reasons. _____

_____

_____

_____

_____

_____

28. List three ways in which a health care worker can be exposed to HBV and HIV. _____

_____

_____

_____

29. List at least three possible problems associated with the use of penicillin. _____

_____

_____

_____

30. You have just administered penicillin to Mrs. Mosley. Within minutes she goes into shock, has difficulty breathing, and shows signs of swelling in the throat. What is probably the matter, and what should you do?_____

_____

_____

_____

Continued

31. Why should oral tetracyclines not be given to a patient who is using antacids or dairy products?

_____

_____

_____

32. List at least three ways in which microorganisms leave an infected person's body. _____

_____

_____

_____

■ APPLICATIONS

Obtain a current copy of a drug reference book or the PDR.® Use it to answer the following questions in a notebook or on index cards.

33. Choose one of the drugs from the Representative Antimicrobials table on page 121 and differentiate between the generic and trade names. _____

_____

_____

_____

_____

34. For the drug chosen in #33, outline the action, uses, adult dose, adverse reactions, and nursing considerations. _____

_____

_____

_____

_____

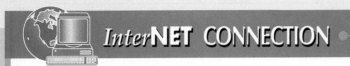 *Inter*NET CONNECTION

To learn more about the use of antibiotics and the efforts being made to curb resistance to antibiotics, go to http://www.heathsci.tufts.edu/apua. This is the site for the Alliance for the Prudent Use of Antibiotics. Click on Patient. This gives a listing of common antibiotics, facts on antibiotic resistance, and other Web sources.

Drugs for the Eye and Ear

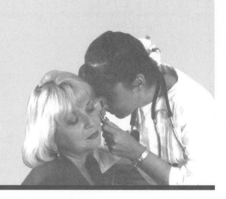

In this chapter you will learn the functions of the various parts of the eye and ear and how sight and hearing occur. You will learn about the disorders of the eye and ear and how drugs are used to control them. You will learn how to administer eyedrops, eye ointments, and ear drops.

OBJECTIVES

After studying this chapter, you should be able to

• identify the external parts of the eye and ear.

• describe the major disorders of the eye and ear for which medications are given.

• describe the actions and give examples of the following drug groups: miotics, carbonic anhydrase inhibitors, beta-adrenergic blocking agents, eye antibiotics, mydriatics, and ear antibiotics.

• follow general instructions for administering eye and ear medications.

• follow proper procedures for instilling eyedrops, eye ointments, and ear drops.

KEY TERMS

acoustic: pertaining to hearing or sound

air conduction: middle and external ear function to conduct and amplify sound waves from the environment

blepharitis: bacterial infection of the eyelid that causes crusting, redness, and irritation

canthus: angle at either end of the slit between the eyelids

central hearing loss: difficulty understanding the meaning of words heard; inability to understand the meaning of incoming sounds or words; caused by problems of the central nervous system from the auditory nucleus to the cortex

cerumen: earwax

cochlea: part of the inner ear; the primary organ of hearing

conductive hearing loss: alteration in the perception of or sensitivity to sounds; occurs with problems in the external and middle ear

conjunctiva: a thin, mucous membrane lining the eye sockets and eyelids

conjunctivitis: an inflammation of the mucous membrane that lines the back of the eyelids and the front of the eye except the cornea

diplopia: double vision

eardrum: round disk that vibrates and transmits sound from the outer ear to the middle ear; also called *tympanic membrane*

external auditory meatus: part of the external ear; the ear canal

external otitis: an inflammation and infection of the epithelium of the auricle and ear canal

floater: nontransparent specks that are small pieces of cells floating across the visual field

glaucoma: condition characterized by increased pressure within the eye caused by failure of the aqueous humor to drain

hordeolum: a hard cyst on the eyelid resulting from a blocked sebaceous duct; also called a sty

lacrimal gland: gland that produces tears

optic: pertaining to the eyes or sight

otic: pertaining to the ear

photophobia: abnormal intolerance to light

presbycusis: decreased ability to hear high-pitched sounds

presbyopia: farsightedness brought about by decreased accommodation of the eye as a result of the aging process

sclera: fibers meshed together to form opaque structure referred to as the "white" of the eye

sensorineural hearing loss: alteration in the perception of or sensitivity to high-pitched sounds; occurs with problems in the inner ear

tinnitus: ringing in the ears

tragus: small cartilage projection in front of entrance (exterior meatus) to the ear

vertigo: dizziness; inability to maintain balance in either a sitting or standing position

The eye is a group of tissues that are specialized to permit vision. It is housed in a bony eye socket and is surrounded by fatty tissue and muscles that serve to protect and to move the eye. The eyelids, lashes, tears, and blinking also protect the eye. The eyelid covers the outer eye and quickly closes (blinks) to prevent a foreign body from entering the eye. Lashes on the eyelid help to keep dust and dirt from entering the eye. At the edge of the eyelid is a **lacrimal gland,** which produces tears to keep the eye moist and to wash away dust particles. Tears are drained off through the tear ducts into the nose. The eyelids and sclera are lined with mucous membranes called the **conjunctiva.**

The eye itself is made up of three layers: the external protective layer (cornea and sclera); the middle layer (choroid, iris, and ciliary body); and the retina, which is sensitive to light. Within these layers are the many parts that work together to produce sight (Figure 7.1).

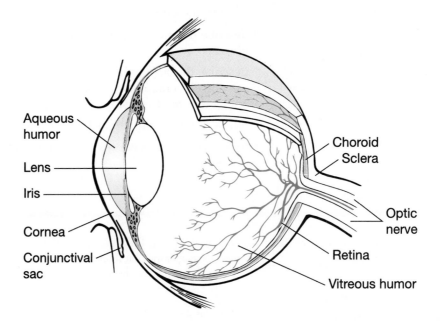

Figure 7.1
Structure of the eye.

The cornea is the transparent anterior portion of the eye. Continuous with the cornea is the **sclera,** which is nontransparent and is commonly referred to as the "white" of the eye. Within the middle layer is the choroid, which is the highly vascular structure that provides nourishment to the ciliary body; the iris; and the outer part of the retina. The iris gives the eye its color. The ciliary body is the vascular section of the eye that lies between the base of the iris and the anterior portion of the choroid. The lens is transparent, lies behind the iris, and serves to ensure that a received image falls in sharp focus on the retina.

For light to reach the retina, it must pass through the cornea, aqueous humor, lens, and vitreous humor. The aqueous humor is a clear, watery fluid that fills both the anterior and posterior chambers of the anterior cavity of the eye. It bathes and nourishes the lens, iris, and the posterior side of the cornea. The aqueous humor is the substance that usually leaks out when the eye is injured. The vitreous humor is a soft, gelatin substance in the posterior cavity of the eye. It helps maintain sufficient intraocular pressure to prevent the eyeball from collapsing.

The **optic** nerves (one from each eye) carry information back to the brain. The brain then codes the information into visual images.

EFFECTS OF AGING ON THE VISUAL STRUCTURES

As an individual ages, changes occur to every structure of the visual system. **Presbyopia** is farsightedness that normally occurs between the ages of 40 and 45. The eye loses its ability to accommodate, and the individual experiences eye fatigue and blurred vision. Bifocal lenses are prescribed to correct vision.

Many of the changes of aging are relatively insignificant, but some may result in a decrease in vision (Table 7.1). Someone who loses part or all of the ability to see must make a major psychological adjustment.

TABLE 7.1: Effects of Aging on Visual Structures

VISUAL STRUCTURE	EFFECTS OF AGING
Eyebrows and eyelashes	Loss of pigmentation (brows and lashes turn grey)
Eyelids	Loss of orbital fat; weakened muscles; sensitivity to touch
Conjunctiva	Formation of small yellow spots
Sclera	Yellowing
Cornea	Yellow ring around cornea; decreased corneal sensitivity and luster; blurred vision
Lacrimal ducts	Decreased tear production; dry, irritated eyes
Iris	Decreased pupil size; slower dilatation after exposure to light; decreased near vision and accommodation
Lens	Cataracts; opacity resulting in glare; yellowing
Retina	Change in color perception; decreased sharpness of vision; loss of central vision; vascular changes resulting from arteriosclerosis and hypertension
Vitreous humor	Floaters (specks)

EYE DISORDERS

GLAUCOMA

Glaucoma is an eye disorder characterized by increased intraocular pressure. The increased pressure damages the optic nerve. Usually the patient has no symptoms until the loss of vision is significant. If it goes unnoticed and untreated, glaucoma can cause blindness. Glaucoma is the second leading cause of blindness in the United States. There are three types of glaucoma—primary, secondary, and congenital. All three are treatable. Primary glaucoma is either narrow-angle or wide-angle glaucoma. Drugs are needed to control narrow-angle glaucoma prior to surgery. Wide-angle glaucoma must be controlled by permanent drug therapy. Secondary glaucoma results from previous eye disease or following removal of a cataract and is also dependent on drug therapy. Congenital glaucoma is treated by surgery. The drug therapy of choice for treating glaucoma is miotics, carbonic anhydrase inhibitors, and beta-adrenergic blocking agents. The side effects of these drugs include **diplopia,** or double vision.

EYE INFECTIONS

The treatment of eye infections is generally determined only after a laboratory test is performed to determine the infective organism. Eye infections can also cause an increase in **floaters,** which are cells in the form of nontransparent specks that float across the visual field. **Conjunctivitis** is an inflammation of the mucous membrane that lines the back of the eyelids and the front of the eye except the cornea. Conjunctivitis, referred to as "pink eye," is a common eye disorder and highly contagious among children. Symptoms include redness, itching, excessive tearing, and, occasionally, **photophobia,** extreme sensitivity to light. **Blepharitis** is a bacterial infection of the eyelids that causes crusting, redness, and irritation of the eyelids. Infection of the sebaceous glands, **hordeolum,** commonly referred to as a sty, creates a hard cyst on the eyelid as a result of a blocked sebaceous duct.

STRUCTURE AND FUNCTION OF THE EAR

The ear is a complex organ designed for hearing. It also plays a part in the body's sense of balance. It has three basic parts: the external ear, the middle ear, and the inner ear (Figure 7.2). The external ear consists of an auricle or pinna and the **external auditory meatus,** or ear canal. Ceruminous glands in the external ear produce wax, or **cerumen.** Small hairs in the canal move this wax toward the outer opening. The wax protects the ear by trapping foreign materials and dust. The function of the external ear is **acoustic,** pertaining to sound. It collects and transmits sound waves to the tympanic membrane, or **eardrum.**

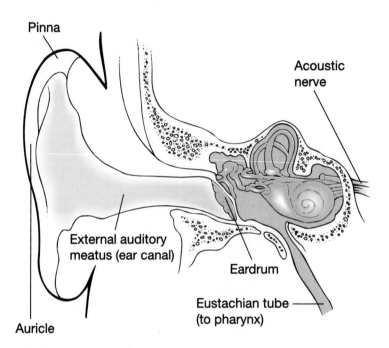

Figure 7.2
Structure of the ear.

The eustachian (auditory) tube connects the middle ear to the nasopharynx. The eustachian tube is usually collapsed, except during swallowing, chewing, yawning, or when moving the jaw. This tube equalizes air pressure on both sides of the eardrum, preventing it from rupturing. The external and middle ear function to conduct and amplify sound waves from the environment. This is called **air conduction.** Problems with either the external or middle ear cause a **conductive hearing loss,** an alteration in the patient's perception of or sensitivity to sounds. The vibrations of the eardrum are picked up by three tiny bones in the middle ear—the malleus, incus, and stapes bones. These three bones transmit vibrations to specialized hearing cells in the inner ear.

The inner ear is also called the labyrinth, because of its complicated shape. It is made up of the bony labyrinth that contains the vestibule, cochlea, and semicircular canals, and the membranous labyrinth. The vestibule is necessary to maintain equilibrium. The **cochlea** is the primary organ of hearing. When disease or injury occurs in the inner ear, a **sensorineural hearing loss** results, and the patient experiences an alteration in the perception of or sensitivity to high-pitched tones. Problems with the central auditory system cause a **central hearing loss,** which results in difficulty understanding the meanings of words heard or the inability to understand the meaning of incoming sounds and words. This condition results from damage to the central nervous system from the auditory nucleus to the cortex.

EFFECTS OF AGING ON THE AUDITORY STRUCTURES

Changes that occur to the structures of the auditory system as a result of aging can result in impaired hearing (Table 7.2). **Presbycusis** is a lessened ability to hear high-pitched sounds. **Tinnitus,** ringing in the ears, may accompany hearing loss. Loud noises, such as highly amplified music or noisy equipment, may cause hearing loss. Whenever a hearing loss occurs, especially later in life, severe depression and isolation may occur. The older individual may withdraw from social contacts and neglect personal hygiene. As a result of people's living longer, the incidence of hearing loss is increasing. In your role as a member of the health care team, helping with early identification of problems with auditory structures can contribute to patients' living more active and happier lives into their seventies and eighties.

TABLE 7.2: Effects of Aging on Auditory Structures

AUDITORY STRUCTURE	EFFECTS OF AGING
External ear	Increase in cerumen; drier cerumen; increase in hair
Middle ear	Conductive hearing loss
Inner ear	Decrease in ability to hear high-pitched sounds; tinnitus; alteration in balance

EAR DISORDERS

EXTERNAL OTITIS

External otitis is an inflammation and infection of the epithelium of the auricle and ear canal. It is more common in the summer and is associated with swimming in contaminated water. It is called "swimmer's ear." It can be caused by either bacteria or fungi. The ear promotes the growth of microorganisms because it is a warm and dark environment. After a culture and sensitivity test is performed to identify the causative organism, topical antibiotics may be administered.

CERUMEN

Cerumen, or earwax, can decrease hearing when it collects in the ear canal. Cerumen becomes a greater problem with age because the earwax becomes drier, harder, and cannot be easily removed. Treatment of cerumen may be irrigation of the ear canal or lubricating drops placed in the canal to soften the earwax.

DRUG THERAPY FOR EAR DISORDERS

TOPICAL ANTIBIOTICS

Topical antibiotics for external ear disorders include polymyxin B, colistin, neomycin, and chloromycetin. Nystatin is used for fungal infections. Corticosteroids may be used for infections except those that are fungal. After the ear canal is cleansed, a medication-soaked wick of cotton is placed in the canal to assist in the delivery of the antibiotic ear drops. Side effects of topical antibiotics such as chloramphenicol (*Chloramycetin Otic*) are ear itching and irritation.

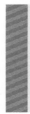

CAUTION: Ear Wicks

Be cautious about placing a cotton wick in the ear of a very young, a confused, a psychotic, or an elderly patient, because they may push the wick further into the ear.

Otic (ear) drops should be administered at room temperature, because cold drops can cause dizziness. Avoid touching the tip of the dropper to the auricle because that contaminates the remainder of the solution in the bottle. Administering antibiotics in the ear canal is an excellent opportunity to teach the patient how to prevent future ear infections or hearing problems.

PATIENT EDUCATION

Preventing Hearing Problems

- Do not put objects in the ears.
- Avoid environmental noise, such as loud music, equipment, and airplanes.
- Get all childhood and adult immunizations, particularly mumps, measles, and rubella.
- Congenital deafness can occur if a pregnant woman is exposed to rubella during the first 16 weeks of gestation.
- When taking medications, report any hearing loss, **vertigo** (dizziness), nausea, vomiting, or a spinning sensation in the head while sitting.

- Chronic mouth breathing may result from enlarged adenoids, which may block the eustachian tubes and predispose one to infection.
- Always take the full course of an antibiotic, even if a condition improves before the medicine is gone.
- Report any symptoms that may indicate hearing loss, such as asking others to speak up, answering questions inappropriately, and increased sensitivity to even slight changes in noise level.
- Avoid self-medicating.

REPRESENTATIVE DRUGS FOR THE EYE AND EAR

CATEGORY, NAME[a], AND ROUTE	USES AND DISEASES	ACTIONS	USUAL DOSE[b] AND SPECIAL INSTRUCTIONS	SIDE EFFECTS AND ADVERSE REACTIONS
Eye Medications				
Polymyxin B, bacitracin, neomycin (*Neosporin Ophthalmic, Mycitracin*) Topical	Superficial eye infections	Bactericidal effect against gram-positive and gram-negative organisms	1-cm (⅜″) strip every 3–4 hours	Stinging, itching, swelling, redness
Pilocarpine HCl (*Isopto Carpine*) Topical	Glaucoma	Miotic agent that causes pupil constriction, reduces intraocular pressure by increasing aqueous humor outflow	1 drop every 4–8 hours; gently press tear duct for 1–2 minutes to prevent systemic absorption	Blurred vision, brow pain, eye irritation, myopia

REPRESENTATIVE DRUGS FOR THE EYE AND EAR

CATEGORY, NAME[a], AND ROUTE	USES AND DISEASES	ACTIONS	USUAL DOSE[b] AND SPECIAL INSTRUCTIONS	SIDE EFFECTS AND ADVERSE REACTIONS
Eye Medications				
Betaxolol (*Betoptic*) Topical	Glaucoma	Beta-adrenergic blocking agent that decreases production of aqueous humor	1 drop of 5% solution or 1–2 drops of 0.25% suspension BID.	Eye stinging at time of instillation, photophobia, tearing
Acetazolamide (*Diamox*) PO	Glaucoma	Carbonic anhydrase inhibitor that decreases production of aqueous humor	250 mg PO q 4 hrs	Transient myopia; paresthesia, especially tingling in extremities; drowsiness; nausea; vomiting
Atropine sulfate (*Isopto Atropine*) Topical	Iritis, uveitis, refraction during eye exam	Mydriatic and cycloplegia agent that dilates pupil and causes paralysis of muscles	1 drop of 1% solution or ½ inch ointment daily for iritis and uveitis; 1 to 2 drops of 1% solution before refraction examination	Blurred vision, photophobia
Ear Medications				
Polymyxin B, neomycin, hydrocortisone (*Cortisporin otic*) Topical	Bacterial infection of outer ear, postsurgical ear infection	Bactericidal, suppresses inflammation and itching	3 or 4 drops TID or QID	Superinfection, hypersensitivity
Chloramphenicol (*Chloromycetin otic*) Topical	Infections of the ear canal	Bacteriostatic or bactericidal	2–3 drops into ear canal TID.	Ear itching and irritation
Triethanolamine polypeptid oleate-condensate (*Cermenex*) Topical	Cerumen	Softens ear wax	Fill ear canal with solution and insert cotton ball	Ear redness and itching

[a]Trade names given in parentheses are examples only. Check current drug references for a complete listing of available products.
[b]Average adult doses are given. However, dosages are determined by a physician and vary with the purpose of the therapy and the particular patient. The doses presented in this text are for general information only.

PRACTICE PROCEDURE 7.1

Instilling Eyedrops and Eye Ointment

■ EQUIPMENT

Physician's orders for eyedrops and eye ointment

Kardex, medicine cards, medication record, patient chart

Medication tray or cart

Bottle of eyedrops and sterile eyedropper

Tube of ophthalmic ointment

Sterile cotton balls or gauze

Continued

Tissues to wipe up spills

Disposable gloves

■ PROCEDURE

1. Set up medications on tray or cart. Check for the "five rights."

2. Wash your hands.

3. Don gloves.

4. Identify the patient and explain the procedure.

5. Gently wash eyelid margins or inner **canthus** (angle or corner of the eye) if crusting or drainage is present. If dry, cleanse with damp cloth. Wash from inner to outer canthus.

6. Instill eyedrops:

   • Position the patient lying down or sitting back in a chair with head slightly hyperextended.
   • In your nondominant hand, gently resting on the patient's cheekbone, hold the cotton ball or tissue. With the dominant hand resting on the patient's forehead, hold dropper ½ to ¾ inch above conjunctival sac (Figure 7.3).

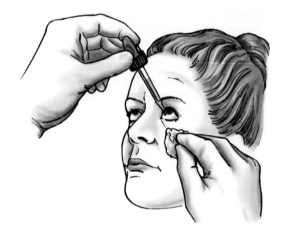

Figure 7.3
Instilling eye-
drops.

   • Drop prescribed number of drops into the conjunctival sac.
   • If patient blinks or if drop lands on outer eyelid, repeat.
   • Wipe up any liquid overflow with cotton or tissue.

7. If administering a drug that causes systemic effect, cover your finger with tissue and press gently against the inner corner of the eye and the nose bone. This keeps the medication from entering the tear ducts and the nose. Do this for 30 to 60 seconds.

8. Instill eye ointment:

   • Instruct patient to look up.
   • Holding ointment applicator above lower lid, apply small layer of ointment evenly along inner edge of lower lid margins on inner conjunctiva from inner canthus to outer canthus (Figure 7.4).
   • Instruct the patient to close the eye and rub the eyelid in a circular motion with cottonball to spread the ointment over the eye.
   • Wipe up excess ointment with tissue or cotton.

9. Help the patient back into a comfortable position.

10. Remove gloves and wash your hands.

Continued

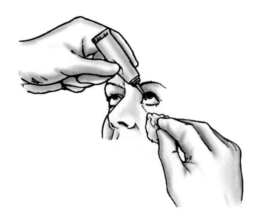

Figure 7.4
Instilling eye
ointment.

11. Chart the procedure, including drug name, concentration, number of drops, time, and which eye received the medication.

12. Application of eye ointment may result in temporary blurred vision.

Demonstrate this procedure for your instructor.

PRACTICE PROCEDURE 7.2

Instilling Ear Drops

■ **EQUIPMENT**

Medication order for ear medication

Medication record, medicine cards, and chart

Ear medication in bottle with dropper (marked with drops or milliliters)

Medication tray or cart

Tissue

Cotton-tipped applicator

Cotton ball (optional)

Disposable gloves

■ **PROCEDURE**

1. Set up medication. Make sure it is at room temperature or warmed to body temperature, according to instructions. Check for the "five rights."

2. Wash your hands.

3. Don gloves.

4. Identify the patient, explain the procedure, and position the patient lying on the back with the head turned to the side.

5. Gently wipe out outermost portion of ear canal with cotton-tipped applicator if cerumen or drainage is blocking it.

6. Instill ear drops.

- Grasp the outer ear and pull gently to straighten the ear canal. In children, pull the auricle down and back; in adults, pull the auricle upward and outward (Figure 7.5).

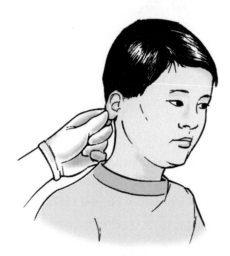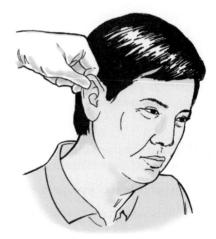

Figure 7.5
Positioning the patient's ear for instilling drops. To straighten a child's ear canal (left), pull the auricle down and back; to straighten an adult's ear canal (right), pull upward and outward.

- Instill prescribed drops, holding dropper ½ inch above ear canal.
- Instruct patient to remain in side-lying position for 2 to 3 minutes.
- Gently apply pressure or massage the **tragus** (small cartilage projection in front of entrance) of the ear with finger to help move medication inward.

7. Wipe up any spills with tissue.

8. If ordered, place a cotton ball in the outermost portion of the ear canal to prevent the medication from leaking out. Remove cotton in 15 minutes.

9. Remove gloves and wash your hands.

10. Chart the procedure. Be sure to record the number of drops instilled and which ear was treated.

Demonstrate this procedure for your instructor.

Match the terms to their definitions.

_____ 1. Referred to as the "white" of the eye   a. cochlea

_____ 2. Mucous linings of the eye socket and eyelid   b. conjunctiva

_____ 3. Ear canal   c. external auditory meatus

_____ 4. Earwax   d. cerumen

_____ 5. Primary organ of hearing   e. sclera

_____ 6. Gland that produces tears   f. lacrimal

Define each of the terms listed below.

7. Acoustic _____

_____

_____

8. Vertigo _____

_____

_____

9. Otic _____

_____

_____

10. Optic _____

_____

_____

11. Tinnitus _____

_____

_____

12. Diplopia _____

_____

_____

Fill in the blank with the word or phrase that best completes the statement.

13. The tiny bones in the middle ear that receive the vibrations of the eardrum are the
    _____, _____, and _____.

14. The covering of the outer eye that closes quickly to prevent a foreign body from entering the eye
    is the _____.

15. The _____ tube connects the middle ear to the nasopharynx and is usually
    collapsed except when one is chewing, yawning, or moving the jaw.

Define the purpose of the following drug categories.

16. Miotics _____

_____

_____

17. Mydriatics _____

_____

_____

Match drug names to their use.

_____ 18. *Betoptic, Diamox, Timoptic*   a. cerumen

_____ 19. *Isopto, Atropine*   b. glaucoma

_____ 20. *Chloramphenicol*   c. superficial eye infections

_____ 21. *Neosporin Ophthalmic*   d. infections of the ear canal

_____ 22. *Cerumenex*   e. iritis, ureitis, refraction during eye exam

Fill in the blanks with the word or phrase that best completes the statement.

23. Eye ointment may cause _____ for a while after application.

24. Before instilling ear medications, the ear canal must be _____.

25. For patient comfort, ear drops should be _____ in the hand or in warm water.

26. Never administer a topical medication to the eyes unless it is labeled _____.

Answer the following questions in the spaces provided.

27. List at least three things you can teach a patient about the prevention of hearing loss. _____

_____

_____

_____

28. List at least five effects of aging on the visual structures. _____

_____

_____

_____

_____

_____

_____

Continued

■ CASE STUDIES FOR CRITICAL THINKING

Select the disorder that best matches the patient description. Write the name of the disorder in the blank.

Cerumen	External otitis	Glaucoma	Conjunctivitis

29. Jackie Palmer went swimming last week in a polluted stream and developed an infection in his right ear. _____

30. Mr. Brown comes to the physician's office complaining of a "hollow sensation" and decreased hearing. _____

31. Mr. Crane is having an operation to relieve increased intraocular pressure inside his eye. Without this surgery, he may become blind. _____

32. Danny, who is five years old, has an inflammation of the mucous membranes that line the back of the eyelids and the front of the eye except the cornea, referred to as "pink eye." _____

■ APPLICATIONS

Obtain a current copy of the PDR®. Use it to answer the following questions in a notebook or on file cards.

33. In Section 4 of the *PDR®*, Generic and Chemical Index, find another trade name for each of the drugs in the Representative Drugs table.

34. In Section 2 of the *PDR®*, Product Name Index, identify the pages that provide detailed information about one of the drugs you listed in item 33. Read about this drug in Section 6, Product Information Section.

If you have trouble finding a particular drug in the *PDR®*, look in the back of the *PDR®* under Discontinued Products to see if it has been discontinued.

 Inter*NET* CONNECTION •

Ear infections and conjunctivitis are common among young children. To learn more about these conditions, go to the American Medical Association Web site at http://www.ama-assn.org. Point to the Health and Fitness Information box and click on Kids Health. Click on Childhood Infections. This will take you to a listing, which includes conjunctivitis and ear infections. When you click on any of the listings, you will get detailed information on causes and treatments of these common infections.

CHAPTER 8

Drugs for the Skin

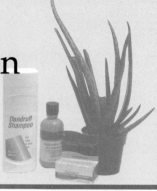

In this chapter you will learn about the structure of the skin and its functions. You will study major skin disorders, the medical terms for their symptoms, and the drugs used to treat them. You will learn to administer topical drugs to the skin with a proper understanding of their uses and action.

OBJECTIVES

After studying this chapter, you should be able to

- name the two layers of skin tissue and describe the structure of each.
- list the main functions of the integumentary system.
- name the secretions of the sebaceous and sudoriferous glands.
- state the normal body temperature.
- explain the process of inflammation.
- list and define the common symptoms of skin disorders.
- describe the major skin disorders.
- state the actions and give examples of the following topical medication categories: keratolytics, protectives, astringents, antipruritics, topical corticosteroids, vasoconstrictor/venous insufficiency treatments, antiseptics, topical anesthetics, miticides, and transdermal patches.
- list five ways of increasing absorption of drugs into the skin layers.
- follow general instructions for administering topical medications to the skin (psychological support, preparing the patient, applying bandages, etc.).
- follow the correct procedures for applying topical creams, lotions, liniments, ointments, and aerosol sprays.

KEY TERMS

acne: inflammatory condition of sebaceous glands

antihistaminic: drug that works against the effects of histamine

anti-inflammatory: drug that suppresses inflammation

antipruritic: drug that relieves itching

antiseptic: agent that inhibits the growth of microorganisms

comedo: blackhead

contact dermatitis: reaction to an irritating substance that has touched the skin

corticosteroids: drugs used on the skin because they suppress inflammation, tighten blood vessels, and relieve itching

dandruff: scaling of the dead tissue of the scalp

dermatitis: inflammation of the skin causing redness, irritation, and skin lesions; also called eczema

dermis: inner layer of skin that contains blood, lymph, nerves, glands, and hair follicles

disinfectant: chemical capable of killing bacteria

ecchymosis: discoloration of the skin or bruising caused by leakage of blood into the subcutaneous tissue

eczema: dermatitis

edema: swelling

epidermis: outer skin layer

erythema: reddening of the skin caused by dilation of superficial capillaries

hair follicle: a structure of the skin from which hair grows

histamine: substance normally present in the body; actively released in response to tissue injury

hives: lesions of the skin caused by exposure to an allergen, or by various other factors, such as fatigue and emotions

inflammation: protective response of body tissues to irritation and injury; a process that results in swelling, reddening, heat, and pain

integumentary system: skin and its appendages—hair, nails, and sweat and sebaceous glands

keratin: hard protein contained in cells of the epidermis, nails, and hair that is both waterproof and acts as a barrier to pathogens and chemicals

keratolytic: drug that loosens and facilitates the shedding of the outer layer of skin

keratosis: overgrowth and thickening of keratin in the skin

lesion: area of pathological tissue

macerate: soften a solid, such as the skin, by moistening, causing increased absorption through the skin

miticides: drugs that kill parasites on the skin

occlusive dressing: dressing that seals in drugs, body heat, and moisture

parasite: organism that lives on or in another organism (e.g., lice, mites, tapeworms) and obtains nourishment from it

pediculicide: drug that kills lice

pediculosis: infection caused by lice

petechiae: tiny, purplish-red spots on the skin resulting from small hemorrhages

photodermatitis: irritation caused by skin sensitivity to light

pressure ulcer: bedsore, pressure sore, decubitus ulcer

protective: soothing, cooling preparation that forms a film on the skin

pruritus: itching

psoriasis: chronic skin disease of unknown cause; characterized by itching, red macules, papules, or plaques covered with silvery scales

scabicide: drug that kills mites

scabies: infestation caused by mites

scaling: an excess of keratin in the epidermis

sebaceous glands: glands in the skin that produce sebum or oil

seborrheic dermatitis: inflammatory irritation of the scalp, face, or groin producing greasy scales

sebum: oil that lubricates the skin, produced by the sebaceous glands

sense receptor: structure that picks up sensations of hot, cold, touch, pain, or pressure in the skin

subcutaneous tissue: loose connective tissue that attaches skin to underlying muscle and bone

sudoriferous glands: glands that produce sweat

transdermal patch: patch containing medication that is absorbed continually through the skin and acts systemically

transdermal/transcutaneous: passing, entering, or penetrating the skin

ulceration: open sore

vasoconstrictive/venous insufficiency treatment drugs: drugs that tighten blood vessels in an area of inflammation and reduce swelling

INTEGUMENTARY SYSTEM

The **integumentary system** consists of the skin (the integument), along with the hairs, nails, and glands that are embedded in it. The skin is the largest organ of the body in terms of its function in homeostasis. It forms a waterproof, protective covering for the entire body. It protects the internal organs and acts as a barrier to microorganisms.

The skin also senses temperature changes in the environment and helps to regulate body temperature. The body's normal temperature is about 98.6°F (37°C). This is the temperature at which the cells maintain their normal functioning. When body temperature goes up, the blood vessels in the dermis dilate, causing perspiration. When body temperature goes down, blood flow decreases, causing the skin to constrict to conserve heat.

The skin is also an organ of sensation. Sensations such as heat, cold, pressure, and pain are perceived through nerve endings. Other functions of the skin include secretion and excretion of fluid and electrolytes. The skin is also important to body image. For example, conditions such as acne can have a negative impact on an adolescent's self-esteem.

The skin is made up of two distinct layers: the epidermis and the dermis (Figure 8.1 on page 142).

EPIDERMIS

The outermost avascular (without blood) layer, the **epidermis,** is made up of two types of cells, melanocytes and keratinocytes. The melanocytes contain melanin, a skin-color pigment that gives a person's skin its characteristic color. The more melanin an individual has, the darker the skin.

Keratinocytes produce a hard protein, **keratin,** which is both waterproof and acts as a protective barrier to pathogens and chemicals.

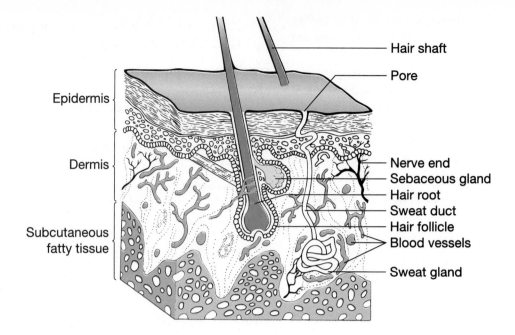

Figure 8.1
Cross section of skin showing the epidermis and dermis and the subcutaneous layer that attaches skin to muscle and bone.

Labels in figure:
- Hair shaft
- Pore
- Epidermis
- Dermis
- Nerve end
- Sebaceous gland
- Hair root
- Sweat duct
- Hair follicle
- Blood vessels
- Subcutaneous fatty tissue
- Sweat gland

Any break in the epidermis, such as a puncture or a cut, lets in bacteria that may attack the deeper tissues. For this reason, all skin wounds must be kept clean until they heal.

DERMIS

Just beneath the epidermis lies a second layer, the **dermis.** The dermis is made up primarily of collagen, blood vessels, nerves, lymphatic tissue, and connective tissue. It also contains several other structures:

- **Hair follicles,** from which grow the tiny hairs that cover the body.
- **Sebaceous glands,** or oil glands, that lubricate the hairs with oil or **sebum.**
- **Sudoriferous glands,** or sweat glands, that help regulate body temperature.
- **Sense receptors,** which send messages to the brain when they feel pain, pressure, heat, cold, and touch.

SUBCUTANEOUS LAYER

The **subcutaneous** layer is not actually part of the skin, but is generally discussed with the skin because it attaches the skin to muscle and bone. The nerves and blood vessels that supply the skin are also found in the subcutaneous layer. The subcutaneous layer provides support, insulation, nutrition, and cushioning or padding.

SKIN DISORDERS

The skin reflects the changes inside the body caused by infectious diseases, such as measles and chickenpox, and by irritating substances that have been touched, swallowed, or inhaled. The skin is also a mirror of human emotions, which reveal themselves through blushing, paleness, and rashes.

Disorders that are confined mainly to the skin area itself produce symptoms that are similar to those of systemic diseases. Symptoms of local irritation are the result of the body's natural response to injury: **inflammation.**

Inflammation is a process that occurs wherever and whenever there is cell damage. The capillaries around the damaged area expand to bring in white blood cells (leukocytes), which fight to destroy microorganisms, and cell repair is begun. Localized response to inflammation is characterized by redness, swelling, heat, and pain. Someone experiencing this reaction may be very uncomfortable, but the inflammatory process establishes an environment suitable for healing and repair.

SYMPTOMS OF SKIN DISORDERS

The following symptoms are common to many skin disorders.

- **Pruritus** (itching)—caused by the release of histamine from the skin cells during allergic reactions.
- **Erythema** (reddening)—caused by an expansion of the capillaries close to the skin surface.
- **Edema** (swelling)—caused by a buildup of fluid in the tissues.
- **Scaling**—an excess of a protein, keratin, in the epidermis. When a layer of dead cells builds up and becomes hard, the resulting condition is called **keratosis.**
- **Lesions**—circumscribed areas of pathological tissue that are classified as primary or secondary. Primary lesions include macules, papules, plaques, nodules, pustules, and wheals. Secondary lesions occur as a result of primary lesions and include scales, scars, erosions, ulcers, fissures, atrophy, and crusts.
- **Ulcerations**—open lesions that are the result of tissue damage that starts below the skin and then erupts onto the skin surface.
- **Hives** or welts (urticaria)—raised, irregularly shaped skin eruptions that have red margins and pale centers. Hives can appear on parts of the body or cover the whole body. They are caused by sensitivity to some substance in the environment, or by various other factors, such as fatigue and emotions.

MAJOR SKIN DISEASES

Many diseases and conditions cause the symptoms of inflammation. You should be familiar with a few of the most common conditions.

Contact Dermatitis. **Contact dermatitis** is an inflammation resulting from direct contact with a substance to which the skin is sensitive (Figure 8.2 on page 144). Most commonly, these substances are metal compounds, rubber compounds, poison oak, poison ivy, poison sumac, cosmetics, soaps, and some dyes. The main symptoms are red, hivelike papules, itching, pain, and oozing, scaly lesions usually seen on the face, neck, hands, forearms, and genitalia. The treatment is to avoid causa-tive agents. Other treatment includes a protective astringent lotion to prevent itching, dry up oozing, and guard against infections. For serious cases, an oral antihistamine may be given to counteract the allergic reaction and itching.

Eczema (Dermatitis). **Eczema,** or **dermatitis,** is an inflammation with eruptions of pimplelike bumps, blisters, scales, or scabs. The lesions may be dry or "weepy" (having a watery discharge).

Eczema is a set of symptoms rather than a disease in itself. It is characterized by redness, swelling, itching, and a feeling of warmth to the touch. Eczema can be a reaction to a drug or a common substance. Creams, lotions, and ointments containing corticosteroids help suppress the inflammation of eczema. Oral antihistamines may be given instead, as eczema patients often develop sensitivity to the topical preparations.

Psoriasis. **Psoriasis** is a chronic (long-term) dermatitis identified by its red, raised lesions covered with dry, silvery scales. The cause is unknown, but there is a family predisposition. It appears mainly on the knees, palms, soles, elbows, lower back, and scalp. The fingernails may become thick and irregular.

The aim of treatment is to retard the growth of epidermal cells. There is no cure, and psoriasis is difficult to medicate. Topical corticosteroids may be used. Corticosteroids may be injected into the lesions of chronically affected areas.

Acne. **Acne** lesions develop in adolescence when growth hormones speed up the secretions of the oil (sebaceous) glands. The open pores of the skin become plugged with oil (sebum) and dead cells. This produces

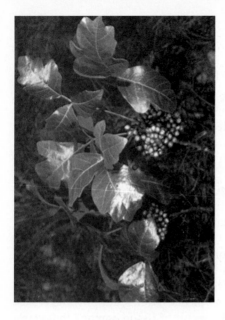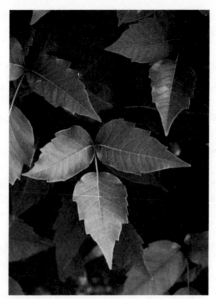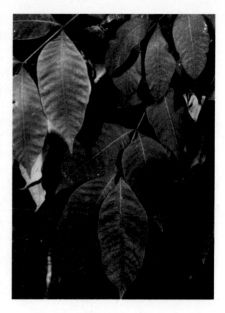

Figure 8.2
Poison oak, poison ivy, and poison sumac are common plants that can cause contact dermatitis.

noninflammatory lesions, such as a **comedo** (blackhead). Treatment consists of topical application of benzoyl peroxide, tretinoin (retinoic acid), topical or systemic long-term antibiotic therapy, and isotretonin (*Accutane*) for long-term remission.

Seborrheic Dermatitis. **Seborrheic dermatitis** is an inflammatory skin disorder of unknown cause that begins on the scalp. It is characterized by yellow or brownish-grey greasy scales. Treatment includes frequent shampooing and mild **keratolytic** agents.

Dandruff. **Dandruff** is a scaling of the scalp that produces dry, white flakes. It may sometimes be due to seborrhea. Treatment consists of regular shampooing with medicated shampoo.

Burns. Burns are classified according to type and extent of injury. The types of burns include thermal, chemical, smoke and inhalation, and electrical burns. Thermal burns are caused by heat, such as a flame, scalding, or contact with a hot object. Chemical burns are the result of contact with a caustic agent such as acid. Smoke and inhalation burns occur from inhaling hot air or noxious chemicals. Electrical burns are the result of coming into contact with some kind of electrical current.

Burns are also classified as first-, second-, or third-degree burns. First-degree burns involve only the epidermis. The burn is painful, red, blanches (whitens) on pressure, and has mild swelling without blistering. Second-degree burns involve the epidermis and dermis to various depths. These burns are red, fluid-filled blisters causing pain as a result of nerve involvement. The most severe type of burn is the third-degree burn. It involves complete destruction of the epidermis and the dermis and produces a dry, white, leathery-appearing skin without pain (because of nerve destruction). The Rule of Nines is used to calculate the percentage of body surface affected by burns. The body is divided into areas that are multiples of nine percent. It is used for calculating the size of burn injury in an adult patient whose weight is in normal proportion to his or her height. See Figure 8.3.

Silver sulfadiazine (*Silvadene*) is the preferred anti-infective agent used in most burn centers. Gentamicin sulfate (*Garamycin*) has been replaced for the most part because of the development of bacterial resistance, especially to Pseudomonas organisms. Mafenide (*Sulfamylon*) is one of the most common agents used in treating second- and third-degree burns.

Extended exposure to the sun can cause sunburn, premature aging of the skin, and a predisposition to cancer. Skin preparations may be applied to absorb or reflect the sun's harmful rays. Absorbing agents include aminobenzoic acid (formerly known as Para-aminobenzoic acid, or PABA),

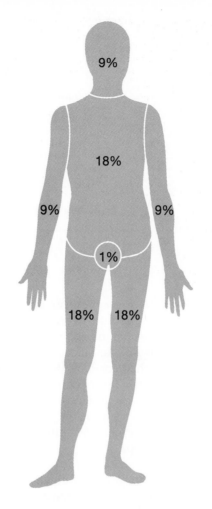
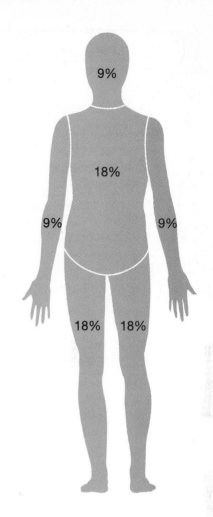

9%

9%

18%

18%

9%

9%

9%

9%

1%

18% 18%

18% 18%

Figure 8.3
The Rule of Nines is used to calculate the percentage of body surface affected by burns. A child's body proportions are not the same as an adult's, so the percentage is different.

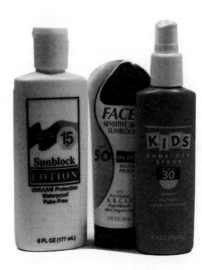

Figure 8.4
The general recommendation for sun blocks and sun screens is a sun protection factor (SPF) of 15 or higher.

cinamates, benzophenones, and anthranilates. PABA was removed from products because it causes dermatitis and stains clothing. Agents that reflect rays are titanium dioxide and zinc oxide. Because they come as a thick paste and must be heavily applied, most people don't like to use them. The Food and Drug Administration has classified sun products according to their sun protection factor (SPF). The general recommendation is a minimum of SPF 15. See Figure 8.4.

Because burns are a common occurrence, especially among the elderly, patient education for preventing burns is essential.

PATIENT EDUCATION

- Never smoke in bed
- Install smoke detectors in kitchens and near bedrooms
- Keep a fire extinguisher in an easily accessible place
- Avoid cooking when wearing loose-fitting clothing
- Avoid setting the water heater too high to prevent scalding
- Use a microwave oven appropriately
- Identify fire exits when in public places

Pressure Ulcers. **Pressure ulcer,** pressure sore, decubitus ulcer, and bedsore are all terms used to describe impaired skin integrity caused by prolonged pressure that damages skin and underlying tissue. The most appropriate term is pressure ulcer. This condition occurs in patients who lie in bed or sit in a chair for long periods of time without moving. Pressure ulcers develop where a bony prominence is in contact with the bed or chair (e.g., at the elbows, heels, and hips). Unrelieved pressure on the skin squeezes small blood vessels that supply the skin with oxygen and nutrients. When the skin is deprived of oxygen and nutrients for too long, the tissue dies and a pressure ulcer develops.

Prevention is the best cure for pressure ulcers. Once the tissues begin to break down, it becomes very difficult for the area to heal. Lotions may be rubbed into pressure spots to stimulate blood flow. The skin must be kept dry at all times.

Pressure ulcers that have begun to break down should be rinsed with saline. Do not use antiseptics, such as hydrogen peroxide or iodine, because they damage sensitive tissue and prevent healing.

Infections. Skin infections are caused by microbes invading the skin tissues. They may enter through a break in the skin. Or they may attack when the skin's natural protective chemistry is unbalanced. The signs of infection are the same as those of inflammation: reddening, swelling, warmth to the touch, and pain. In bacterial skin infections there is usually also pus, a thick, yellowish fluid made of dead white blood cells and debris. Impetigo and boils are examples of bacterial infections.

Scabies and Pediculosis. **Scabies** is a parasitic infestation caused by the itch mite. (**Parasites** are organisms that live on or in another organism.) Mites burrow under the skin, and about a month later, the patient begins to develop symptoms such as watery blisters between the fingers and severe itching. The infestation spreads quickly. Special topical insecticides called **scabicides** are used to destroy the mites. The drug of choice is the scabicide crotamiton (*Eurax*). There is no easy or fast treatment for scabies because the mites are difficult to eliminate. Bedding and clothing must be treated to help destroy the mites.

Pediculosis is caused by lice. These are insect parasites that lay eggs at the base of the hair of the head or in the pubic area. Pediculosis was once attributed to crowded housing and poor hygiene, but this theory has proven false. The lice are transmitted by close contact with infested individuals, clothing, combs, and bedding. Drugs called **pediculicides,** such as pediculicide lindane (gamma-benzene hexachloride), are available to kill the lice. Clothing, combs, and bedding must never be shared. To avoid repeated infection, patients must practice good hygiene.

MAJOR CATEGORIES

Each skin disorder has its own best treatment and drugs, although many of the drugs share characteristics. They belong to certain general categories or drug groups. If you learn these categories, you will understand how many drugs operate. For instance, suppose you know that a particular drug is in the category "anti-infective." You then know that it works something like other anti-infectives you studied in Chapter 6. Memorize the technical terms for these drug categories, which will be a help when you are looking up drugs in drug reference books.

Oral drugs such as sedatives, antihistamines, and analgesics are sometimes ordered to make patients with skin diseases more comfortable. These oral drugs are described in other chapters.

Most topical drugs for the skin fall into one or more of the following drug groups.

Keratolytics. Keratolytic drugs soften and destroy the outer layer of skin so that it is sloughed off (shed). Strong keratolytics are effective for removing warts and corns. Milder preparations are used to promote the shedding of scales and crusts in eczema, psoriasis, and acne. Very weak keratolytics irritate inflamed skin, which speeds up healing. Common keratolytics are salicylic acid and resorcinol.

Protectives and Astringents. These drugs work by covering, cooling, drying, or soothing inflamed skin. **Protectives** do not penetrate the skin or soften it, but instead form a long-lasting film. This film protects the skin from air, light, and dust. Nonabsorbable powders such as zinc stearate, zinc oxide, bismuth preparations, and talcum powder are listed as protectives, although they are not especially useful because they stick to wet surfaces. Collodion is a 5 percent solution of pyroxylin in a mixture of ether and alcohol. When applied, the ether and alcohol evaporate and leave a film on the skin. Astringents shrink the blood vessels locally, dry up secretions from weepy lesions, and lessen skin sensitivity. Styptic collodion contains 20 percent tannic acid, so it is both a protective and an astringent.

Antipruritics. **Antipruritics** relieve itching caused by inflammation. Calamine lotion, cornstarch, and oatmeal baths may help relieve itching. **Corticosteroid** drugs relieve itching by suppressing the inflammation itself. **Antihistaminic drugs,** such as diphenhydramine (*Benadryl*) and hydroxyzine (*Atarax*), lessen the effects of **histamine**, the cause of the itching.

Anti-Inflammatory Drugs (Topical Corticosteroids). The corticosteroids have three actions that relieve symptoms of skin disorders:

- **Antipruritic**—relieves itching.
- **Anti-inflammatory**—suppresses the body's natural reactions to irritation.
- **Vasoconstrictive/venous insufficiency treatment**—tightens the blood vessels in the area of the inflammation. This reduces the swelling due to edema.

Most of the top-selling prescription drugs for the skin are corticosteroids. Examples are hydrocortisone, betamethasone (*Valisone, Diprosone*), triamcinolone (*Aristocort, Kenalog*), fluocinonide (*Lidex*), fluocinolone acetate (*Synalar*), and flurandrenolide (*Cordran*). Vasoconstrictors or venous insufficiency treatment drugs are *Debrisan* beads or paste and *DuoDERM*/Hydroactive paste. The actions of corticosteroids are further described in Chapter 14.

Antiseptics. **Antiseptics,** such as alcohol, benzalkonium chloride (*Zephiran*), thimerosal (*Merthiolate*), mercurochrome, and povidone-iodine (*Betadine*), inhibit the growth of microorganisms on skin surfaces. They are used only topically, never orally. Antiseptics prevent infections in cuts, scratches, and surgical wounds. **Disinfectants** are bactericidal drugs used only on nonliving objects such as surgical tools. Fungi, viruses, and spores that live on these surgical tools may, however, be resistant to destruction.

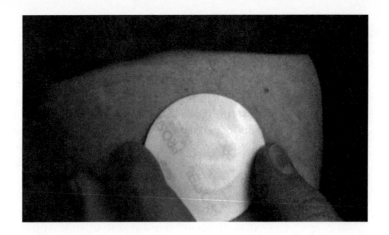

Figure 8.5
A transdermal patch can deliver medication into the bloodstream through absorption into the skin.

Topical Anesthetics. For pain on skin surfaces or in mucous membranes, such as wounds, hemorrhoids, and sunburns, the physician may order a topical anesthetic. These relieve pain and itching by numbing the skin layers and mucous membranes. They are applied directly to the painful areas by means of sprays, creams, and suppositories. Examples are benzocaine (*Solarcaine*) and dibucaine (*Nupercainal*).

Miticides. **Miticides** are drugs that kill insect parasites that infest the skin. Scabicides kill the mites that cause scabies. Pediculicides kill the lice that cause pediculosis. A miticide that is effective against both scabies and lice is lindane (*Kwell*).

Transdermal Delivery System. Many prescription drugs that were always taken orally are now available in **transdermal patch** form to be absorbed into the bloodstream through the skin. The patch is an easy and convenient way to take medicine. For example, patients with high blood pressure may use a clonidine patch (*Catapres-TTS*). Other patches or **transdermal** (penetrating the skin) delivery system drugs include nitroglycerin (*Nitro-Dur, Transderm-Nitro*) and estrogen. People who are trying to stop smoking cigarettes may be prescribed nicotine patches (*Nicoderm, Habitrol*) (Figure 8.5).

An important part of applying drug patches is to mark the date and time the patch is applied to the patient's skin. When applying a new patch, remove the old patch first. Leaving more than one drug patch on a patient can cause a possible overdose. Wear disposable gloves or cover the old patch with a tissue to prevent any of the remaining medication on the patch from absorbing into your skin.

Table 8.1 lists some skin preparations that are available without a prescription. You will handle these over-the-counter drugs regularly. The table of Representative Drugs at the end of this chapter lists some drugs for treating skin disorders. The table lists the drug category to which each drug belongs, its uses, actions, hints for application, and side effects. You will administer these drugs frequently. Be sure to consult drug references and package inserts when you have questions or need additional information.

ABSORPTION OF DRUGS INTO THE SKIN LAYERS

Drugs for the skin are prepared in the form of powders, lotions, gels, creams, ointments, beads, pastes, and plasters. The form that is chosen for a topically administered drug depends on the desired therapeutic effect.

The form affects the absorption of a drug into the deeper skin layers. Few drugs used on the skin are intended to be absorbed into the bloodstream unless they are delivered via the transdermal delivery system. Some, like protectives and antiseptics, are supposed to remain only on the skin surface. Others are designed to sink into the dermal and subcutaneous layers to provide anti-inflammatory or soothing actions. The physician must carefully choose the type of drug, its form, and the treatment that goes with it to achieve the proper effect.

When absorption into the underlying skin layers is desired, the following measures increase absorption:

TABLE 8.1: Selected OTC Drugs for the Skin

CONDITION	PRODUCTS	ACTION
Acne	*Cuticura Medicated, Clearasil, Stri-Dex Medicated Pads*	Keratolytic
Dandruff	*Selsun Blue, Head and Shoulders*	Keratolytic/cytostatic
Diaper rash, prickly heat	*A & D Ointment, Desitin, Vaseline, Baby Magic, Johnson's Medicated Powder,* zinc oxide	Protective/antimicrobial
Dry skin	*Keri, Corn Huskers*	Emollient
Eczema, psoriasis	*Tegrin, Psorex, Zetar*	Keratolytic/antipruritic
Insect bites and stings	*Dermoplast, Nupercainal*	Anesthetic/antipruritic
Minor burns	*Medi-Quick, Solarcaine, Unguentine, Noxema*	Anesthetic/antimicrobial
Minor wounds	*Betadine, Zephiran Chloride, Baciguent, Neosporin, Neo-Polycin, Mycitracin*	Antiseptic/antibiotic
Poison ivy, poison oak	*Calamine, Caladryl, Ivy Dry Cream, Ziradryl*	Antipruritic/antihistaminic

- *Apply wet dressings.* Wet dressings soften or **macerate** the skin. This permits the drug to pass through the epidermis, which is normally "waterproof." These dressings are frequently used to treat wounds that require debridement, or removing dead tissue from the wound.
- *Use a fat- or lipid-soluble drug.* Fat- and lipid-soluble drugs are absorbed better than a water-soluble drug.
- *Rub the preparation into the skin.* Do this only when the skin is not covered with lesions that could be damaged by rubbing. Rub creams in gently; rub liniments in vigorously. Hard rubbing also stimulates the skin, which increases circulation to the area.
- *Keep medicine in contact with skin for an extended period of time.* One way to achieve extended contact is to cover the area with a dressing that prevents the drug from being rubbed off by sheets or clothing. Another way is to reapply the medication as soon as it seems to have worn off and recover it.
- *Apply an occlusive dressing if ordered by the physician.* An **occlusive dressing** does not permit air to enter under the dressing. An example of an air-occlusive dressing is a plastic wrap. Petroleum jelly is an occlusive ointment. They both trap and prevent water loss (sweat) from the skin.
- *Use a stronger concentration of the drug.* A preparation that has more of the drug in it has more drug available to be absorbed.

CAUTION: Treating Mucous Membranes

When administering medications, mucous membranes are treated differently than skin. These membranes make up the linings of body orifices such as the mouth, the eyes, the rectum, and the vagina. Unlike the skin, mucous membranes do not have a tough outer layer of dead cells to protect the underlying tissues. Instead, their surfaces are moist and easily penetrated. Therefore, drug absorption through the mucous membranes is rapid. Topical preparations for the skin are formulated differently from those for mucous membranes. Never apply skin medications to mucous membranes, accidentally or otherwise; this invites the risk of overmedicating the patient.

Absorption into the skin is most complete when several techniques are used together—for example, a strong preparation held against the skin for a long period under an occlusive dressing. Absorption is also greater in young children and elderly patients because both groups have thinner layers of skin.

Drugs applied to the skin are rarely intended to be absorbed into the bloodstream. However, if the skin is cut, scratched, or scraped, or if there are many open sores, the drug may readily enter the bloodstream. This is usually undesirable and can be dangerous. Safe and effective absorption of each topical drug depends on many factors. It is important that you understand and follow instructions when applying any topical medication.

GENERAL INSTRUCTIONS FOR MEDICATING THE SKIN

PSYCHOLOGICAL SUPPORT

People who have skin conditions need psychological support. Living with constant itching or pain is stressful. Patients may lose sleep because they are uncomfortable. They may become depressed about their condition, especially if it lasts for a long time. Depression may affect appetite and intake of fluids.

Because of the psychological problems associated with skin diseases, doctors sometimes prescribe sedatives and tranquilizers. Patients with conditions like psoriasis, for which there is no permanent cure, may need counseling to help them live with the disease. Acne can be especially traumatic for adolescents, when body image is so important.

Show your support for these patients by accepting their feelings and responding to their needs with patience and understanding.

PATIENT CONSIDERATIONS

If a skin condition is painful, the doctor may order an analgesic drug prior to administration of a topical medication. It is best to apply topical medications approximately 30 minutes after a dose of an analgesic, especially with burn patients.

Before giving the medication, explain to the patient what you are going to do. Inform him or her of any unusual sensations the drug may cause. For example, some gels produce warmth or a burning sensation on the skin.

Find a position that is comfortable for the patient and that lets you easily reach the skin area you need to work on. Place protective pads under the affected area to keep the bed and the patient's clothing clean. (Some skin medications cause stains.) If possible, position the affected area so that the patient cannot see it while you are applying the medication. Afterward, be sure to help the patient back into a comfortable position.

WOUND PREPARATION

As lesions heal, the fluids that are produced dry out, and crusting may appear on the skin surface. If ordered, cleanse the wound with the prescribed antiseptic solution or normal saline. Use a separate swab for each cleansing stroke. Clean from the least contaminated to the most contaminated area.

Apply medications only on the affected area. In the case of irritating substances, such as corn and wart removers, healthy skin surrounding the lesions needs to be protected. A film of petroleum jelly provides good protection against absorption and irritation.

Some drugs must be diluted (mixed with water or some other liquid) before being applied. Follow instructions carefully to prepare the drug. Check with the pharmacy if you do not understand the directions. A drug that is improperly diluted could cause irritation or poisoning or be ineffective.

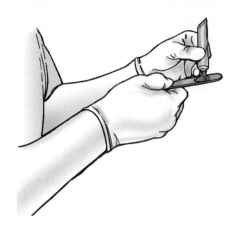

Figure 8.6
Apply ointments with a wooden tongue blade or a cotton swab.

APPLYING THE MEDICATION

Apply drugs as directed. In general, rub in creams and liniments by hand. Pat lotions onto the skin with pieces of cotton. Apply ointments with a wooden tongue blade or cotton swab (Figure 8.6). Use a glove to protect your skin. When infection or an open wound is present, use a sterile glove.

When opening the medication container, place the cap upside down on the medicine tray or cart. Use a sterile tongue blade or cotton swab to dip out a quantity of medication from the container. Do not dip in and out with the same applicator you are using on the patient! Then apply the medication according to instructions (the physician's or those in the package insert). Administer medication from the center outward, never going back over skin. (See Practice Procedure 8.1 on page 154.)

A few skin drugs are administered by means of a medicated bath (e.g., coal tar for a psoriasis patient), a special soap or shampoo (e.g., acne soaps, pediculicides), or an injection directly into a lesion.

The instruction "Apply as needed" is given only for drugs that carry no danger of overdose. Reapply the medication whenever symptoms flare up, or when the thin film of drug has worn off or has been absorbed into the skin. A nurse or physician is frequently responsible for deciding when to reapply medication. Others may do so if they have the permission of the physician or nurse.

DRESSINGS

Because they hold in body heat and increase absorption, dressings should be used only when ordered by the physician. Some lesions must be covered to protect them from clothing and scratching. Others must be covered to keep the medication in constant contact with the affected skin. A dressing can, however, be irritating rather than helpful. Many lesions heal more quickly when left exposed to air.

Infected lesions that are actively producing pus are usually covered with a dressing to soak up the drainage. The dressing must be changed frequently. Usually the physician orders the frequency for changing a dressing.

Be careful when removing the dressing from a wound so as to avoid pulling away the scab. A dressing that is sticking to a lesion may be softened by moistening it with normal saline. To avoid removing and reapplying tape each time you change a dressing, you may use butterfly tape strips.

FOLLOW-UP

Charting Observations. Each time you prepare to apply a topical medication, note the appearance of the skin. Has there been a change for better or for worse since you last saw it? If there is no change, perhaps the medication is not working. Are there signs of irritation? Chart your observations to help in evaluating the patient's progress and pinpointing problems.

Side Effects. Observe for signs of irritation that do not seem to come from the disease itself. Many people are sensitive to certain drugs. They may develop rashes, dryness, redness, tiny purplish-red spots, and ruptures of surface blood vessels **(petechiae, ecchymosis)**, sensitivity to light **(photodermatitis)**, and/or itching in the area where you applied the medication. Chart these signs and report them to the nurse in charge. The strength of the drug may be changed or another drug or treatment may be ordered.

Patient Education. Instruct patients in how to apply skin medications properly. If theirs is a long-lasting condition, they will be responsible for their own skin care. A drug reference book, the PDR®, or the package insert are good places to look for information that will be useful to the patient.

REPRESENTATIVE DRUGS FOR THE SKIN

CATEGORY, NAME[a], AND ROUTE	USES AND DISEASES	ACTIONS	USUAL DOSE[b] AND SPECIAL INSTRUCTIONS	SIDE EFFECTS AND ADVERSE REACTIONS
Keratolytics				
Salicylic acid Topical	Seborrheic dermatitis, psoriasis, warts, corns, calluses	Swells and softens excess keratin for easy removal or shedding	Dosage depends on form and strength of preparation. Soaking skin before use assists drug action. Apply dressing as ordered. Do not put drug in contact with eyes, mucous membranes, or normal skin	Irritation, burning
Astringents				
Calamine and diphen-hydramine (*Caladryl*) Lotion	Itching from poison ivy or poison oak, insect bites, or other skin irritations; mild sunburn	Relief of itching; soothes mild sunburns; drying action	Apply topically 3 or 4 times daily. Clean and dry area before applying	Burning or itching
Antipruritics				
Trimeprazine tartrate (*Temaril*) Oral	Urticaria, contact dermatitis, drug rash	Relief of itching; both antihistamine and antipruritic; has drying effect and sedative effect	2.5 mg 4 times daily	*Short-term therapy:* drowsiness, hypotension, bradycardia, faintness, and very rarely, anorexia, nausea, and vomiting, dry mouth *Long-term therapy:* skin pigmentation, extrapyramidal reactions (dyskinesia)
Anti-Inflammatory Drugs (Topical Corticosteroids)				
Betamethasone valerate (*Valisone*) Topical	Contact dermatitis, psoriasis	Suppresses inflammation, relieves itching and swelling	Dosage depends on form and strength of preparation. Apply sparingly. Massage gently into affected area. Do not apply in or near eyes. Available as aerosol; do not inhale spray. Check skin regularly for signs of irritation. Use occlusive dressing as ordered	Irritation, burning, itching, dryness, redness

REPRESENTATIVE DRUGS FOR THE SKIN

CATEGORY, NAME[a], AND ROUTE	USES AND DISEASES	ACTIONS	USUAL DOSE[b] AND SPECIAL INSTRUCTIONS	SIDE EFFECTS AND ADVERSE REACTIONS
Anti-Inflammatory Drugs (Topical Corticosteroids) continued				
Triamcinolone (*Aristocort*) Topical	Contact dermatitis, oral lesions	Suppresses inflammation, relieves itching and swelling	Apply TID and HS	Irritation, burning, itching, dryness, redness
Hydrocortisone *OTC: Hytone* 0.5% ointment *Delacort* 0.5% lotion *Bactine* 0.5% cream *Aeroseb* HC 0.5% spray *Cortef* Rectal Itch 0.5% ointment	*OTC:* Temporary relief of many minor skin, genital, anal itching, rashes; anorectal products for severe inflammation and swelling have other ingredients such as belladonna, benzocaine	Anti-inflammatory, antipruritic, and vasoconstrictive actions	Use sparingly and rub in lightly. Cover *only as directed* with occlusive dressing. Protect patient's face from aerosols; avoid inhalation	Burning and itching sensations, irritation, dryness, skin maceration, especially with occlusive dressings. Systemic effects may occur with excessive or prolonged use
Prescription: Dermacort 1.0% lotion *Synacort* 2.5% cream *Sensacort* 0.5% spray *Nutracort* 1.0% gel *Cort-Dome* 15 mg suppositories *Proctofoam* 1.0% aerosol	*Prescription:* Relief of inflammatory and pruritic manifestations of corticosteroid-responsive dermatosis			
Anti-Infectives, Antibacterials, Antifungals				
Mafenide acetate (*Sulfamylon*) Topical	Second- and third-degree burns	Broad spectrum sulfonamide, bactericidal for many organisms	Cleanse area of debris before application. Apply with sterile tongue blade or gloved hand to a thickness of ⅟₁₆th inch. Keep area covered with medication at all times. Apply dressing as ordered	Pain, burning, stinging, allergic reactions, fungal superinfection
1% silver sulfadiazine (*Silvadene*) Topical cream	Adjunct for prevention and treatment of wound sepsis (poisoning) in second- and third-degree burns	Bactericidal and antimicrobial activity	Cleanse and debride; cover with drug at all times. Reapply 1 or 2 times daily using sterile technique to a thickness of ⅟₁₆th inch	Itching, burning, or rash; pain
Vasoconstrictors/Venous Insufficiency Treatments				
Debrisan Topical paste and beads	Adjunct treatment of wet ulcer (e.g., decubitus ulcers)	Reduces swelling and edema; increases venous flow	Dosage depends on strength of beads or paste. Packets are 25–60 g each; paste available in 10-g foil packets	Pain, transitory bleeding, blistering, erythema
DuoDERM hydroactive Granules/beads, paste	Dermal exudating ulcers; dermal ulcers	Local management of ulcer by forming gel-like substance of moisture in ulcers or wounds	Sterile 30-g tube; avoid use when muscle, bone, or tendon is involved; do not use on pressure sores, ulcers from tuberculosis, or deep fungal infection	Infection; odor or change in color due to infection; fever, cellulitis

(continued)

REPRESENTATIVE DRUGS FOR THE SKIN (continued)

CATEGORY, NAME[a], AND ROUTE	USES AND DISEASES	ACTIONS	USUAL DOSE[b] AND SPECIAL INSTRUCTIONS	SIDE EFFECTS AND ADVERSE REACTIONS
Antiseptics				
Povidone-iodine (*Betadine*) Topical	Surface infections, burns, minor wounds, vaginitis	Kills germs	Apply as ordered; avoid contact with eyes	Irritation, redness, swelling
Anesthetics				
Benzocaine (*Solarcaine*) Topical	Pruritus, minor burns; oral, nasal, and gingival mucous membranes	Inhibits conduction of nerve impulses from sensory nerves	Give smallest effective dose according to age	Sensitization

[a] Trade names given in parentheses are examples only. Check current drug references for a complete listing of available products.
[b] Average adult doses are given. However, dosages are determined by a physician and vary with the purpose of the therapy and the particular patient. The doses presented in this text are for general information only.

PRACTICE PROCEDURE 8.1

Applying Topical Medication to the Skin

■ EQUIPMENT

Disposable gloves; sterile gloves when changing sterile dressing

Sterile dressings and coverings

Sterile applicators: tongue blades, gauze, cotton balls, or swabs

Medication (lotion, ointment, cream, liniment, or aerosol spray)

Bag for disposal

Medication record, Kardex, medicine card, or the form used by your agency

■ PROCEDURE

1. Assemble equipment, medications, and patients' records.

2. Read the Kardex, medication record, or medicine card. Check this information against the medication label. Be sure you have the RIGHT DRUG and the RIGHT DOSE for the RIGHT PATIENT at the RIGHT TIME by the RIGHT ROUTE.

3. Read the application instructions on the package insert.

4. Identify the patient and explain the procedure. Check the patient's wrist ID or follow agency policy for identifying patients.

5. Administer a systemic analgesic (if ordered) approximately 30 minutes prior to administering topical medication.

6. Position the patient and the affected area comfortably. Protect clothing and bed linen with pads, if necessary.

7. Wash your hands and don gloves.

8. Remove old, soiled dressings. Discard them in a disposal bag. Be careful not to pull the scab from a newly healed area. If the dressing sticks to the wound, apply normal saline. Let it soak for 5 to 10 minutes.

9. Change gloves (use disposable or sterile gloves as appropriate). Open the dressings, applicators, and medication. Place the lid of the medication container upside down on the table or tray to avoid contaminating the medication.

10. Cleanse and remove dead tissue or crusts from lesions if ordered. Use a cleansing liquid ordered by the physician. Remove crusts with cotton swabs.

11. Reread the label to make sure you have the right drug.

12. Take medication from its container using a sterile applicator (tongue blade or swab). Try to dip out the entire amount you will need for one application.

13. Apply the medication using the correct procedure.

   - Creams: rub in gently.
   - Lotions: pat or dab on skin.
   - Liniments: rub in vigorously.
   - Ointments: apply with wooden blade or cotton swab.
   - Aerosol sprays: hold can upright and spray area from a distance of 3 to 6 inches; spray a second and a third time.
   - Foam medication: hold can inverted next to the skin and spray.
   - Beads: mix with suitable substance (e.g., glycerin) and apply directly to wound with sterile wooden spatula.
   - Paste: puncture tube by inverting cap back into tube; squeeze paste onto the wound.

14. Apply a thin or thick amount (one-fourth the thickness for paste or beads) as ordered by the physician or as stated on the package directions. Systematically cover the affected area.

15. Cover the area with wet or dry dressings, if ordered. (See doctor's orders, package insert, or procedure manual for instructions.) Secure dressings with adhesive tape or butterfly tape strips.

16. Instruct the patient in further care of the skin. See package directions or the doctor's orders. Remove your gloves.

17. Make the patient comfortable before leaving. Fluff pillows, return the patient to a comfortable position, secure call button, and so forth.

18. Remove, clean, and/or discard equipment and supplies. Put away medications, rereading the labels as you do so. Dispose of used supplies in the appropriate area. Wash your hands.

19. Record the application of medication. Note:

   - Condition of the skin or skin lesions (on nurses' notes).
   - Reactions of the patient (on nurses' notes).
   - Date, time, medication, and dosage (on medication record).

Demonstrate this procedure for your instructor.

Match these skin structures to the function they perform.

_____ 1. Hair follicles   a. grows tiny hairs covering the body

_____ 2. Epidermis   b. secretes oil

_____ 3. Subcutaneous tissue   c. secretes sweat

_____ 4. Sebaceous gland   d. feels pressure or pain

_____ 5. Sense receptor   e. provides padding

_____ 6. Sudoriferous gland   f. acts as waterproof covering

Define these medical terms.

7. Pruritus   _____

8. Erythema   _____

9. Edema   _____

10. Keratin   _____

11. Parasite   _____

12. Acne   _____

13. Antiseptic   _____

14. Sebum   _____

Describe the purpose of the following types of drugs.

15. Antipruritics   _____

16. Keratolytics   _____

17. Protectives   _____

Match drug names to drug categories.

_____ 18. *Aristocort, Valisone, Cordran*   a. topical corticosteroids

_____ 19. *Tinactin, Mycostatin, Lotrimin*   b. miticides

_____ 20. *Kwell*   c. topical anesthetics

_____ 21. *Neosporin, Sulfamylon*   d. oral antipruritics

_____ 22. Zinc oxide, calamine   e. topical antibacterials

_____ 23. *Temaril, Atarax*   f. topical antifungals

_____ 24. *Betadine*, alcohol, *Merthiolate*   g. antiseptics

_____ 25. *Benzocaine*   h. protectives and astringents

_____ 26. *Zithromax*, clarithromycin   i. oral antibacterial

■ CASE STUDIES FOR CRITICAL THINKING

Select the skin disorder that best matches each patient's description.

   Decubitus   Pediculosis   Seborrheic dermatitis   Eczema (dermatitis)   Psoriasis

27. Mr. Yee has applied *Kwell* cream on his body to combat scabies. After a few hours his skin becomes dry and scaly. It is red, swollen, itchy, and warm to the touch.

   _____

   _____

28. Miss Barnett has suffered from dry scales on the backs of her hands for many years. The symptoms are kept under control with *Celestone*.

   _____

   _____

29. Fred Entler is annoyed to find dry, white, greasy scales on his scalp.

   _____

   _____

30. Fran Graham is bedridden with a muscle disease. A sore is developing where her tailbone touches the sheets.

   _____

   _____

31. While washing her children's hair, Mrs. Johnson discovers tiny eggs in their scalps at the base of the hairs.

   _____

   _____

■ APPLICATIONS

Obtain a current copy of a drug reference book or the PDR®. Use it to answer the following questions in a notebook or on file cards.

32. In Section 4 of the *PDR®*, Generic and Chemical Name Index, find another product name for each of the categories of drugs listed on the chart Representative Drugs for the Skin on pages 152–154 of this text.

33. In Section 3 of the *PDR®*, Product Category Index, find Psoriasis Agents (under Dermatologicals). List all the agents found there.

If you have difficulty finding a drug in the *PDR®*, turn to the back and look under Discontinued Products to see if it has been discontinued.

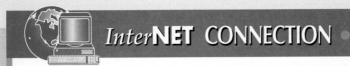

InterNET CONNECTION

To obtain information about common skin disorders such as acne, go to the Web site of the American Academy of Dermatology at http://www.aad.org. Click on AcneNet and then click on Table of Contents. If you click on Acne Treatments, you will find information on both prescription and non-prescription medications.

Drugs for the Cardiovascular System

In this chapter you will learn about the organs and functions of the cardiovascular system and what goes wrong with them during common cardiovascular disorders. You will study the types of drugs used to treat each disorder and learn to classify common generic and trade name drugs according to their drug categories. You will also practice step-by-step procedures for administering oral, buccal, and sublingual medications.

OBJECTIVES

After studying this chapter, you should be able to

- name the parts of the cardiovascular system and state their functions.
- state the names of instruments used to measure blood pressure and to record the heartbeat.
- state the average blood pressure and pulse rate.
- list the main components of blood.
- state the functions of the lymphatic system.
- identify the proper medical terms for common symptoms of cardiovascular disorders.
- explain the major disorders for which cardiovascular drugs are given.
- describe the actions and give examples of the following drug groups: vasopressors, vasodilators, diuretics, antihypertensives, calcium channel blockers, antilipemics, cardiac glycosides, antidysrhythmics, anticoagulants, thrombolytics, hemostatics, and hematinics.
- state the difference between an initial and a maintenance dose.
- follow the proper procedure for administering oral and sublingual medications to patients with cardiovascular disorders.
- state the special procedures for administering vasopressors (vasoconstrictors), vasodilators, antihypertensives, digitalis, antidysrhythmics, anticoagulants, hemostatics, and hematinics.

KEY TERMS

ACE: angiotensin converting enzyme

anemia: any condition in which the oxygen-carrying capacity of the blood is reduced

angina pectoris: chest pain resulting from lack of oxygen in the heart tissue

anticoagulant: drug that inhibits or delays blood from clotting

antihypertensive: drug that lowers high blood pressure

antilipemic: drug that lowers the level of lipids in the blood

apical pulse: heart rate measured with the bell or diaphragm of a stethoscope placed on the apex of the heart

arteriosclerosis: thickening of the walls of the arterioles with a loss of elasticity and ability to contract

artery: blood vessel that carries blood away from the heart

atherosclerosis: accumulation of cholesterol and lipids on the walls of the arteries

blood pressure: force of the blood against vessel walls

bradycardia: slow heartbeat (fewer than 60 beats per minute)

capillaries: microscopic vessels that carry blood from the smallest arteries to the smallest veins

cardiac: pertaining to the heart

cardiac arrest: sudden cessation of breathing and of sufficient circulation of blood by the heart

cardiac glycoside: drug that strengthens the force of the myocardial contraction, slows the heart, and improves the tone of the myocardium coronary: pertaining to the heart vessels

cyanosis: bluish color of the skin due to lack of oxygen

diastolic pressure: force of the blood when the heart is at rest between contractions; lowest point at which sounds are heard when taking a blood pressure

diuretic: drug that reduces fluid volume in the body by stimulating urine flow

dyspnea: labored or difficult breathing

dysrhythmia: any deviation from the normal rhythm of the heartbeat; also referred to as arrythmia

edema: abnormal accumulation of fluids in the interstitial tissues

electrocardiogram (ECG): graphic record showing the spread of electrical excitation to different parts of the heart

embolus: small amount of fat or air or a blood clot that circulates in the blood until it lodges in a blood vessel

endocardium: innermost layer of the heart

fibrillate: to quiver or contract spontaneously, causing ineffective contractions of the heart

hematinic: drug that increases the hemoglobin content in the blood; also called antianemic

hematoma: a collection of blood in an organ or tissue caused by a break in a blood vessel

hemoglobin: iron-containing substance that carries oxygen from the lungs and to the tissues

hemoptysis: coughing up blood

hemostatic: drug used to help in the formation of blood clots

hypertension: high blood pressure; two or more systolic readings above 140mm Hg

hypotension: low blood pressure; the systolic reading falls to 90mm Hg or below

interstitial fluid: fluid that fills most of the cells of the body and provides a large portion of the liquid environment of the body

leukemia: general term to describe a group of malignant conditions affecting the blood-forming tissues of the bone marrow, lymph system, and spleen

lymph: clear, watery-appearing fluid found in lymphatic vessels which carry fluid from the interstitial spaces to the blood

myocardial infarction: "heart attack" or death of a part of the heart muscle due to lack of oxygen

myocardium: the heart muscle; the middle layer of the heart wall

orthostatic hypotension: a condition of low blood pressure that occurs when a person rises from a sitting or lying position

palpitations: rapid and throbbing heartbeats that can be felt by the patient

pericardium: sac that encases the heart

phlebitis: inflammation of a vein

plasma: the liquid part of blood and lymph

platelets: aid in blood clotting

point of maximum impulse (PMI): heartbeat felt at fifth intercostal space, about two inches left of midline

pulmonary: referring to the lungs

pulse rate: the number of heartbeats that can be felt by touching the radial, carotid, femoral, or pedal arteries

sphygmomanometer: device for measuring blood pressure

spleen: organ of the lymphatic system that works in the body's defenses, produces red blood cells, stores platelets, and serves as a reservoir for blood

systolic pressure: force of blood pushing against the artery walls when the ventricles contract; the first tap-like sound heard when measuring blood pressure

tachycardia: rapid heartbeat (more than 100 beats per minute)

thrombolytic: drug that is capable of dissolving blood clots

thrombophlebitis: inflammation of a vein blocked by a thrombus

thrombosis: condition in which a blood clot, or thrombus, is formed within a blood vessel

thrombus: a blood clot formed in a blood vessel

vasodilator: drug that expands blood vessels; used to treat angina pectoris and hypertension

vasopressor: drug that causes narrowing of blood vessels, or vasoconstriction

vein: vessel that carries blood toward the heart

CARDIOVASCULAR SYSTEM

The cardiovascular system consists of the heart, the blood vessels, and the blood. It transports vital substances throughout the body. These substances include nutrients, waste products, oxygen, carbon dioxide, minerals, hormones, drugs, and body heat. The blood plays an important role in the body's defense against disease (see Chapter 6).

BLOOD VESSELS

The three main types of vessels are the arteries, veins, and capillaries. **Arteries** carry blood away from the heart. Except for the pulmonary artery, the arteries carry oxygenated blood. As arteries get farther away from the heart, they branch into increasingly smaller arteries called arterioles. **Veins** travel toward the heart and, except for the pulmonary vein, carry deoxygenated blood. The smallest veins are called venules.

The arterioles and venules are connected by thin-walled vessels called **capillaries.** The capillaries serve the important function of carrying oxygen and other nutrients to the tissues and taking away the waste products.

THE HEART

The heart is a hollow, muscular, four-chambered organ approximately the size of the fist that lies within the thorax and between the lungs. The heart can be felt beating at the fifth intercostal space, about two inches left of the midline. This area is called the **point of maximum impulse (PMI)** and is an important landmark when taking the **apical pulse** before administering certain cardiac drugs.

The wall of the heart is made up of three layers. The **endocardium** is the innermost layer. The **myocardium** is the middle layer, and the most important structure of the heart. The **pericardium** or pericardial sac encases the heart. The four chambers of the heart are divided into two chambers on the right side and two chambers on the left side. The upper chambers are called the atria and the lower chambers are the ventricles (Figure 9.1).

Cardiac drugs are designed to affect specific parts of the heart.

- *Myocardium* (cardiac muscle)—Certain cardiac drugs affect the force of myocardial contractions. Cardiac glycosides such as digoxin (*Lanoxin*) increase cardiac output.
- *Coronary arteries*—The **coronary** arteries are the arteries that supply the myocardium and heart with blood. If these arteries are narrowed, chest pain or angina pectoris occurs. If the blood flow in one or more of the coronary arteries is interrupted, that part of the heart muscle supplied may not get sufficient oxygen. Antianginal drugs such as nitroglycerin, or calcium channel blockers such as nifedipine (*Procardia*), produce coronary dilation and increase the oxygen to the heart, thereby reducing the workload on the heart.
- *Electrical conduction system*—The heartbeat is controlled by "pacemaker" cells that stimulate the heart muscle when it is supposed to contract. Each

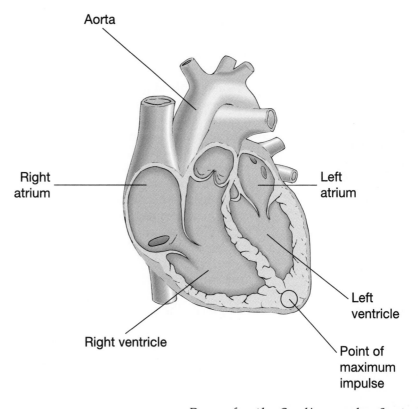

Figure 9.1
Anatomy of the heart.

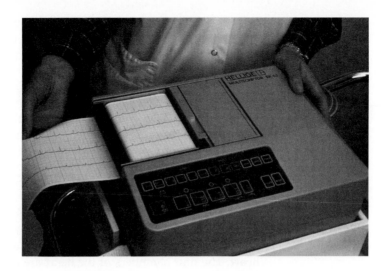

Figure 9.2
An electrocardiograph records the heart's electrical signals.

heartbeat is caused by a wave of electricity that passes from the pacemaker cells to the heart muscle. The electrical signals can be picked up by a machine called an electrocardiograph. The electrocardiograph records these signals on a chart called an **electrocardiogram** (ECG). The electrocardiograph records the signals so they can be used in diagnosing heart problems (Figure 9.2). The heart alternately contracts and then relaxes about 72 times a minute (the normal range at rest is approximately 60 to 80 beats per minute). The heartbeat you hear is the sound of the heart valves opening and closing during these contractions.

Antidysrhythmic drugs such as propranolol hydrochloride (*Inderal*) are given in the treatment of cardiac arrythmias to decrease cardiac excitability.

After the blood has transported oxygen through the arteries, capillaries, and veins and has picked up waste products, it must go through the lungs. There it picks up new oxygen and gets rid of carbon dioxide wastes (see Figure 9.1). In this way, the cardiovascular system is linked to the respiratory system, described in Chapter 10. The cardiovascular system is closely linked to all the other body systems, because blood is essential in all body functions.

BLOOD PRESSURE AND PULSE

One way to tell if the heart and vessels are working properly is by measuring a patient's **blood pressure.** This is the force of the blood against the walls of the blood vessels. One's blood pressure results from a combination of two factors: the force of the heartbeat and the condition of the vessels.

The walls of normal blood vessels are elastic and able to expand. If vessels lose elasticity because of disease, such as arteriosclerosis, the heart must pump against stiff, narrow vessel walls. The heart must also pump harder if vessels are partially blocked by deposits of fat, as in atherosclerosis. Either situation results in a higher blood pressure reading.

To measure blood pressure, you will use a **sphygmomanometer** that consists of a pressure manometer, an occlusive (closing) cuff enclosing an inflatable rubber bladder, and a pressure bulb with a release valve to inflate the cuff (Figure 9.3). When the cuff is inflated, it tightens around the patient's arm, and you will listen for two types of sounds:

- *systolic*—the peak pressure exerted against the arteries when the heart contracts
- *diastolic*—the minimal pressure when the heart is at rest between contractions

Blood pressure is recorded as two numbers: systolic pressure over diastolic pressure. The numbers represent the amount of mercury (Hg) that is

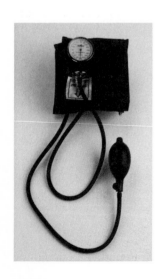

Figure 9.3
Blood pressure is measured by means of a sphygmomanometer.

displaced on the sphygmomanometer, measured in millimeters. The average blood pressure measures about 120/80 mm Hg ("120 over 80"). Generally, readings of 90/60 to 140/90 are variations used when giving medications. High blood pressure, **hypertension,** is not determined with one reading. A diagnosis of hypertension is made after two readings greater than 140/90 on two separate occasions. Hypertension is never considered normal and must be taken seriously. Report an elevated blood pressure reading immediately to your supervisor. Low blood pressure, **hypotension,** is a systolic blood pressure reading of less than 90mm Hg. Unlike hypertension, it does not always indicate illness. There are some individuals who normally have low blood pressure. When it does indicate disease, the individual may be pale, have clammy skin, be confused, have an increased pulse rate, and have decreased urine output. This is the case with shock, such as after a blood loss.

The **pulse rate** is another way to tell how well the cardiovascular system is working. Pulse rate is most commonly measured by taking the radial pulse. Place the tips of your first two fingers along the thumb side of the patient's wrist and lightly compress so you can feel the pulse (Figure 9.4). If the pulse is regular, count for 30 seconds and multiply by 2. If the pulse is irregular, count for one full minute. A normal pulse is strong and full and about 60 to 80 beats per minute.

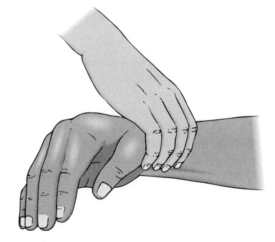

Figure 9.4
You will usually take a patient's pulse at the wrist, along the radial artery.

If the heart or blood vessels are diseased, or if there is too little blood in the system, the pulse may be weak and irregular. A weak pulse taken at the wrist but a strong one taken elsewhere (foot or neck) may mean that vessels in the wrist are narrowed or blocked.

You will often be required to take your patient's pulse and/or blood pressure before administering a cardiac drug. Review the procedures in your agency's procedure manual to be sure you know how to do these tasks. You must chart the results each time. Unless there is a special form for this, pulse and blood pressure (abbreviated P and B/P) are usually charted on the nurses' notes.

BLOOD

Blood has two component parts: fluid called **plasma,** and solid elements called cells. Plasma is about 90 percent water and 10 percent solutes. Approximately 80 percent of these solutes are proteins. The remaining 20 percent is made up of glucose, amino acids, lipids, urea, creatinine, oxygen, carbon dioxide, hormones, and certain enzymes.

There are three main kinds of blood cells:

- *Red blood cells (erythrocytes)* carry oxygen. The major component of erythrocytes is **hemoglobin.** It is made up of iron and protein and gives blood its red appearance. The function of hemoglobin is to carry oxygen.

- *White blood cells (leukocytes)* are made up of granulocytes, monocytes, and lymphocytes. The granulocytes and monocytes consume bacteria and other foreign matter that enter the body. The lymphocytes play an important role in the development of immunity.
- *Platelets* (thrombocytes) are critical in clotting. When a blood vessel is cut or punctured, the platelets release a substance that causes fibers to form over the wound. These fibers eventually harden into a scab.

Table 9.1 summarizes the primary characteristics of blood carried by arteries and veins.

TABLE 9.1: Characteristics of Blood

	COLOR	OXYGEN LEVEL	ROUTE
Arterial Blood	Bright red	Highly oxygenated	Travels from heart to capillaries
Venous Blood	Dark red	Mostly carbon dioxide and wastes; low oxygen	Travels from capillaries to heart

LYMPHATIC SYSTEM

The lymphatic system is actually part of the circulatory system, because it consists of moving fluid that goes throughout the body. The lymphatic system consists of lymphatic capillaries, ducts, and lymph nodes and carries fluid from the interstitial spaces to the blood. This **interstitial fluid** that fills most of the cells of the body is called **lymph.** The system carries away waste products that the blood cannot carry, such as dead cells and debris. These wastes are removed at the lymph nodes, which act like small filtration stations. They are located mainly in the groin, the armpits, and the neck. After being filtered, the lymph is poured back into the veins near where they enter the heart.

Unlike the blood, lymph is not pumped, but merely collected from the various body parts through open-ended lymph vessels. As the body moves, the lymph is pushed through its vessels.

Another part of the circulatory system is the **spleen.** The spleen, a soft, purplish organ in the upper left side of the abdomen, has four functions. It plays a vital part in the body's resistance against microorganisms. It serves as a filter, removing old and defective red blood cells from the bloodstream. The spleen also has an immune function, and stores approximately 30 percent of the body's platelets.

EFFECTS OF AGING

Heart disease is a major problem that increases with age. Most deaths from cardiovascular disease occur in the aged population. High blood pressure, coronary artery disease, heart attacks, and congestive heart failure occur much more frequently in the over-60 age group. Certain changes in the heart are associated with aging. The heart usually becomes larger because it loses its elasticity, and it has a deeper color because there is less oxygen in the heart tissue. The endocardium becomes thicker and sclerotic (hardened), and the aorta and the arteries are less elastic. The valves thicken and are more rigid. These changes lead to problems in filling and emptying the heart, which result in decreased oxygen intake and output. Even with these changes, the heart is able to meet most demands. Under stress, however, declining heart function is apparent.

Anything that interferes with the functioning of the heart and vessels deprives the body of the vital nutrients that circulate in the blood. Any change in the rate, rhythm, and force of the heartbeat or in the force and quantity of blood running through the vessels thus endangers the entire body.

SYMPTOMS

The presence of cardiovascular disorders is indicated by a number of symptoms.

Dyspnea is labored or difficult breathing that occurs because of fluid accumulation in the interstitial tissues and lungs. The patient becomes short of breath, with rapid and shallow respirations. Dyspnea can occur at rest or while exercising. Knowing when the dyspnea began (e.g., when the patient was lying down, sitting, or performing a strenuous physical activity) gives clues to the type of heart problem.

Angina pectoris, chest pain, is a symptom of some types of heart disease. It can be caused by a lack of blood in the heart muscle, by inflammation of the heart, or by anxiety.

Edema is an abnormal accumulation of fluid in the interstitial tissues. It occurs in cardiovascular disorders when the blood is not being pumped quickly or strongly enough. Some of the blood fluid "backs up" in the tissues, and swelling results. Edema is a common sign of congestive heart failure. It can occur in the legs, liver, abdominal cavity, or lungs.

Dysrhythmias are irregular heartbeats or palpitations that may indicate a heart problem. Patients may complain that their heart is pounding or jumping or missing a beat. Disturbances of the heartbeat are **tachycardia** (very rapid heartbeat—pulse above 100 beats per minute) and **bradycardia** (very slow heartbeat—pulse below 60 beats per minute).

Hemoptysis (coughing up blood) may indicate serious cardiovascular disease in which blood is leaking into the lungs. A patient in congestive heart failure may cough up frothy, blood-tinged sputum.

Fainting and fatigue can be symptoms that the heart or vessels are not functioning at their best. When tissues do not receive all the oxygen they need, the patient may experience pain. When oxygen content in the blood is low, the skin may turn bluish, a condition called **cyanosis.**

Cardiac arrest is a sudden and unexpected stopping of the heart and circulation. It can be brought on by myocardial infarction, electric shock, severe allergic reactions, drug overdose, or surgery. Unless immediate steps are taken to restore the heartbeat, cardiac arrest is fatal. Circulation and respiration must be restored immediately. Irreversible damage occurs when the brain is deprived of oxygen for 10 minutes.

CONGESTIVE HEART FAILURE

Congestive heart failure (CHF) results from the inability of the heart to pump adequately enough to meet the body's metabolic needs. Congestive heart failure is not a disease, but a syndrome caused by some other disease. Regardless of the cause, the ventricles of the heart are not able to contract and pump properly. The patient exhibits signs of fatigue, dyspnea, tachycardia, chest pain, and edema.

CHF is treated by giving digoxin (*Lanoxin*), a cardiac glycoside. It increases the force of and strengthens the heartbeat. Diuretic drugs are also given to help the kidneys eliminate excess fluids.

Angiotensin converting enzyme (**ACE**) inhibitors are the vasodilators of choice for CHF. Amrinone (*Inocor*) is another drug given for its vasodilating effect. It is used in patients who do not respond to the usual therapy of

Lanoxin, diuretics, and vasodilators. Common causes of congestive heart failure are

- Coronary artery disease
- Myocardial infarction (heart attack)
- Cardiomyopathy (enlarged heart)
- Dysrhythmias (abnormal cardiac rhythms)
- Hypertensive heart disease
- Anemia

DYSRHYTHMIAS

Dysrhythmia is any deviation from the normal rhythm of the heartbeat. These disturbances in cardiac rhythm result from an abnormality in the electrical conduction of the heart muscle. Dysrhythmias frequently occur within 4 to 72 hours after a heart attack. They can also occur in coronary artery disease or after cardiac surgery. Dysrhythmias may appear if parts of the heart vibrate **(fibrillate),** skip contractions, or beat very rapidly (tachycardia). These irregularities endanger the body because they affect the heart's ability to pump blood efficiently. Antidysrhythmic drugs are given to stabilize the heart's electrical impulses. *Quinidine, Pronestyl, Norpace,* and *Inderal* are examples of antidysrhythmic drugs.

CORONARY ARTERY DISEASE

Coronary artery disease (CAD) is a disorder of the blood vessels that falls under the general category of **atherosclerosis,** accumulation of cholesterol and lipids in the walls of the arteries. CAD takes many years to develop. The three main manifestations of CAD are angina pectoris, myocardial infarction, and sudden cardiac death. Myocardial infarctions remain the leading cause of all cardiovascular deaths and of deaths in general.

Angina pectoris is a clutching pain in the chest caused by oxygen starvation resulting from narrowed coronary arteries. It usually lasts only 3 to 5 minutes and subsides when the contributing factor, such as exertion, is removed. It should not last longer than 20 to 30 minutes after giving nitroglycerin under the tongue (sublingually). Chest pain that lasts for more than 20 to 30 minutes may be a sign of "heart attack" or **myocardial infarction** (MI). Myocardial infarction means that a part of the heart muscle dies because its supplying artery is completely blocked. This event severely weakens the heart. The most common complication after an MI is dysrhythmia. Dysrhythmias are present in approximately 80 percent of MI patients. Thrombolytic therapy is the standard treatment after an MI. This involves the administration of an agent such as tissue plasminogen activator, streptokinase, or urokinase to dissolve an arterial clot. Sudden cardiac death is an unanticipated collapse and cardiopulmonary arrest of a person within one hour after the onset of symptoms.

BLOOD VESSEL DISEASES

Thrombophlebitis. **Thrombophlebitis** involves the formation of a blood clot **(thrombus)** in a blood vessel associated with inflammation **(phlebitis).** Thrombophlebitis may be caused by pooling of blood in the veins. Pooling is associated with immobility, obesity, pregnancy, CHF, and steroid therapy. Other causes include long-term IV therapy and the administration of high-dose antibiotics, cancer drugs, potassium, and other drugs that are irritating to the veins. **Thrombosis** (thrombus formation) also occurs in certain blood disorders and in patients taking oral contraceptives. The thrombus blocks the flow of blood to the part of the body served by the particular vessel. The body part becomes pale and cold and sometimes bluish (cyanotic). If a vein is partially blocked by a blood clot, the thrombus may break off into the blood vessel and circulate back to the heart and into the **pulmonary** (pertaining to the lungs) circulation. It is then called an **embolus** (the blocking of a blood vessel is called an embolism). An embolus can also be an air bubble or any kind of particle that can block a vessel. It may travel to another part of the body and cut off blood circulation to a vital area. For example, an embolus to the brain can cause a stroke, while an embolus to the coronary arteries can cause a heart attack.

A patient with thrombophlebitis may exhibit warm, red skin, edema, elevated temperature, and pain upon dorsiflexing, or flexing the foot back toward the body, when the leg is raised. Treatment consists of anticoagulant therapy and bed rest for 5 to 7 days with the affected leg elevated.

Arteriosclerosis. **Arteriosclerosis** is the most common arterial disorder, characterized by thickening, loss of elasticity, and calcification of arterial walls. Atherosclerosis is a form of arteriosclerosis in which fat and fibrin (white, tough, elastic, fibrous protein formed when blood clots) are deposited in the arteries. Together, these disorders are called peripheral vascular disease. Most of the symptoms occur in the lower extremities, such as pain on walking. Many patients with arteriosclerosis and atherosclerosis also have coronary artery disease and take vasodilators and beta-blockers (drugs that decrease the heart rate and force of contraction by blocking adrenergic stimulation). Analgesics are also given for pain control.

Hypertension. High blood pressure is a chronic (long-term) disease with no single cause but many risk factors. Over time, hypertension can weaken the heart and affect vital organs such as the kidneys and eyes. Hypertension is also the leading cause of strokes. Because hypertension is called the "silent killer" and may go without symptoms for a long time, it is important to teach patients about the risk factors, which include the following:

- Men in young adulthood and early middle age
- Women after the age of 55
- African-Americans
- Family history of hypertension
- Obesity
- Cigarette smoking
- Sedentary lifestyle
- Elevated blood cholesterol levels
- High-sodium diet
- Excessive alcohol consumption
- Continued stress
- Diabetes mellitus

Hypertension can be controlled by weight reduction, decreased sodium and alcohol intake, increased physical activity, stress management, and antihypertensive drugs.

SHOCK

Shock occurs as a result of decreased blood flow to the body's tissues that causes organs to fail. Shock has many causes. It is important not to define shock solely in terms of hypotension, because shock can occur without hypotension.

Shock can be brought on by severe blood loss, surgery, severe infections, allergic reactions, or heart failure. Signs of shock may be low blood pressure; high pulse rate; pale, clammy skin; and mental confusion. Shock requires emergency treatment. Because patients can die rapidly from shock, the goal of treatment is to improve circulation so enough oxygen is available to the tissues. Drugs called vasopressors cause vasoconstriction which elevates blood pressure. Epinephrine and norepinephrine are two vasopressors frequently used to treat shock. Blood transfusions or intravenous fluids are also given to restore the proper volume of blood in the system.

DISEASES OF THE BLOOD AND LYMPH

Blood and lymph diseases involve abnormal blood clotting processes, excessive bleeding, or disturbances in the production of blood cells.

Anemia. **Anemia** is a decrease in the number of erythrocytes, the quality of hemoglobin, and the volume of hematocrit, which reflects the ratio of red blood cells to plasma. The body needs a good supply of hemoglobin because this is the substance that transports oxygen to all tissues of the body. The entire body is affected by fatigue and other symptoms when too little oxygen is delivered to body tissues. Anemia can be caused by lack of iron or cyanocobalamin (vitamin B_{12}) in the diet, by severe bleeding, by diseases in which red blood cells are destroyed (hemolytic diseases), or by failure to produce red blood cells. Treatment varies with the cause, but usually iron supplements, an iron-rich diet, treatment of underlying diseases, vitamin B_{12}, and folic acid are given, and transfusions, if necessary.

Leukemia. **Leukemia** is a general term used to describe a group of malignant disorders that affect the blood-forming tissues in the bone marrow, spleen, and lymph system. There is an elevated number of white blood cells, because they do not go through the normal cell life cycle. The symptoms of leukemia vary depending on the type, but may include fatigue, pallor, weakness, weight loss, anemia, and increased bleeding tendencies. The drugs used to treat leukemia interfere with the abnormal production of white blood cells (see Chapter 18).

Hodgkin's Disease. Hodgkin's disease is a malignant disorder characterized by the growth of abnormal giant, multinucleated cells called Reed-Sternberg cells, which are located in the lymph nodes. Hodgkin's disease makes up 15 percent of all lymphomas (malignant tumors of the lymphatic tissue). The cause is unknown. Symptoms include enlargement of lymph nodes, fever, weight loss, and night sweats. Treatment is with chemotherapeutic drugs.

Non-Hodgkin's Lymphoma. Non-Hodgkin's lymphoma is a malignant disorder of the immune system. It involves the lymphocytes and can originate outside of the lymph nodes. Its method of spread is unpredictable and generally advanced at the time of diagnosis. The most common symptom is painless lymph node enlargement. Other symptoms may include fever, night sweats, and weight loss. Treatment consists of chemotherapy drugs and radiation.

DRUGS FOR CARDIOVASCULAR AND BLOOD DISORDERS

VASOPRESSORS

Vasopressors (also known as vasoconstrictors) raise blood pressure by causing the blood vessels to contract. They are used in the treatment of shock, heart block (failure of electrical impulses to stimulate the heartbeat), and adverse reactions to medications. Vasoconstrictors are powerful drugs. Many are used in the intensive care unit, where the patient must have close monitoring of heart rate, blood pressure, kidney, and pulmonary function. Patients must be watched carefully to make sure they are not getting too strong a reaction—in other words, hypertension. The blood pressure must be checked regularly and often.

Norepinephrine (*Levophed*) is a vasoconstrictor used in hospital emergency treatment. Metaraminol (*Aramine*) is a less powerful vasoconstrictor. Both are given parenterally with great care. An IV line with two large-gauge catheters must be established as soon as possible. Other vasoconstrictors are mephentermine (*Wyamine*), methoxamine (*Vasoxyl*), phenylephrine (*Neo-Synephrine*), dopamine (*Intropin*), and dobutamine (*Dobutrex*).

VASODILATORS (NITRATES)

Vasodilators relax or dilate the walls of the arteries, so that less force is needed to push the blood through them. The classic vasodilators are nitrates. They are used especially in the control of angina pectoris. Nitrates dilate the arteries so that the heart receives more blood and more oxygen. Sublingual nitroglycerin (*Nitrostat*) is the most common vasodilator. Taken at the beginning of an angina attack, it takes effect within about 2 minutes. Isosorbide (*Isordil*) is another vasodilator used to treat angina.

Sublingual nitroglycerin may be left at the patient's bedside to be taken whenever the patient feels an angina attack coming on. If this is done, you must keep track of how many tablets are left each time you check on the patient—and chart the number taken. If there is no improvement or relief of chest pain (angina), the nurse in charge should be notified.

Time-release tablets, capsules, and topical preparations of nitroglycerin are available for longer-lasting effects. If applying nitroglycerin ointment, you will usually squeeze out 1 to 2 inches and apply it every 8 hours and at bedtime. Avoid touching the ointment with your fingers, because you will experience the vasodilating effects. Wash off the last application. Rotate sites, which include the chest, abdomen, anterior aspect of the thigh, and the forearm. Cover the new application with a transparent wrap and tape it. Sites must also be rotated for transdermal patches. Side effects of nitroglycerin include dizziness, headaches, nausea, vomiting, facial flushing, and increased pulse rate. Patient education is important to effective nitrate therapy.

PATIENT EDUCATION

Nitrates

- Avoid alcoholic beverages
- Identify situations that precipitate attacks requiring use
- Take a dose 5 or 10 minutes before an activity known to cause an attack
- Side effects include dizziness, lightheadedness, and mild headache
- Report severe headache, dry mouth, and blurred vision to the physician; they are symptoms of overdose

- Air, heat, and moisture inactivate nitrates
- Discard unused tablets after 6 months
- Prevent tolerance by removing paste or patch for 12 hours—a "no nitrate" time
- If pain occurs during the day, use the nitrate during the day and remove it at night
- If pain occurs during the night, use the nitrate during the night

DIURETICS

Diuretics are drugs that help the body eliminate excess fluids through urinary excretion (see Chapter 12). In so doing, they reduce the amount of blood that the heart has to pump. This effect is helpful for people with CHF. Because some also help to dilate the blood vessels, certain diuretics are often given along with antihypertensive drugs in the treatment of high blood pressure. Commonly used diuretics are the thiazides, potassium-sparing diuretics, and "loop" diuretics.

The thiazides are chlorothiazide (*Diuril*) and hydrochlorothiazide (*HydroDiuril, Esidrix*). The potassium-sparing diuretics are spironolactone (*Aldactone*), triamterene (*Dyrenium*), and amiloride. "Loop" diuretics are furosemide (*Lasix*), metolazone (*Zaroxolyn*), ethacrynic acid (*Edecrin*), and bumetanide (*Bumex*).

Loop, or high-dose thiazide, diuretics can cause severe potassium loss in the urine. There are three ways of preventing this:

- Have the patient eat potassium-rich foods, such as bananas and potatoes.
- Give potassium supplements (such as *K-Dur, Micro-K, K-Lor, Slow-K, K-lyte*, etc.).
- Combine a potassium-losing diuretic with one that is potassium-sparing, such as hydrochlorothiazide/triamterene (*Maxzide, Dyazide*), HCTZ/amiloride (*Morduretic*), or HCTZ/spironolactone (*Aldactazide*).

ANTIHYPERTENSIVES

There are several types of drug strategies to lower blood pressure. Some drugs work by relaxing the vessel walls. Others interfere with the nerves that cause the vessel walls to become tense. Hydralazine (*Apresoline*), captopril (*Capoten*), propranolol (*Inderal*), methyldopa (*Aldomet*), and metoprolol (*Lopressor*) are some of the major **antihypertensive** drugs used to control high blood pressure.

Antihypertensive therapy is done by starting with a less potent drug and then moving up to a more potent drug or adding additional drugs, depending on the patient's response.

Because they act on the nervous system, which controls muscle tension, most antihypertensives have some unwanted side effects such as headache, dizziness, fainting, mental depression, and inability to achieve an erection. Each antihypertensive has its own set of side effects, which you should check in a drug reference. A sign to watch for with most of them, however, is extreme low blood pressure when the patient stands up quickly, or **orthostatic hypotension**. This may indicate that the dose is too high. Caution your patient to rise slowly from a sitting or lying position to avoid dizziness or fainting. Hot showers and baths can also bring on orthostatic hypotension. Some patients may need help in walking if they get dizzy spells from the antihypertensive.

Antihypertensives are used for long-term control of high blood pressure. Because there are no dramatic symptoms of high blood pressure, yet many possible side effects from the drugs, people may not want to take their medicine. Patients need education and encouragement to comply with their medication regimen so as to avoid potentially serious consequences of hypertension.

CALCIUM CHANNEL BLOCKERS

Calcium channel blockers are the newest group of cardiac drugs that inhibit the transport of calcium into the myocardial and vascular smooth muscle cells, which decreases myocardial contractibility and the demand for oxygen. They also dilate the coronary arteries. They are generally used to treat hypertension and angina. The calcium channel blockers include amlodipine (*Norvasc*), bepridil (*Vascor*), diltiazem (*Cardizem*), felodipine (*Plendil*), isradipine (*DynaCirc*), nicardipine (*Cardene*), nifedipine (*Procardia*), and verapamil (*Calan*).

The most frequent side effects of calcium channel blockers are headaches, dizziness, fatigue, edema of the extremities, and shortness of breath. *Procardia* has the greatest effect on lowering blood pressure. Before administering calcium channel blocker drugs, it is important to take the patient's blood pressure and pulse. Caution patients to move slowly from a lying to a sitting position because of the hypotensive effect.

ANTILIPEMICS

Although the link between high cholesterol levels and heart disease is not completely understood, lowering cholesterol levels is usually considered as part of the course of prevention and treatment. Diet and exercise are frequently all that is necessary. However, several drugs can help lower cholesterol levels. Several lipid-lowering (**antilipemic**) agents exist: fenofibrate, gemfibrozil (*Lopid*), probucol (*Lorelco*), pravastatin (*Pravachol*), simvastatin (*Zocor*), clofibrate (*Atromid-S*), cholestyramine (*Questran*), colestipol (*Colestid*), niacin (*Nicobid*), and lovastatin (*Mevacor*).

CARDIAC GLYCOSIDES

Cardiac glycosides strengthen the myocardium, increase the force of contraction, slow the heart, and improve the muscle tone of the myocardium. They also stimulate the pacemaker cells that control the rate (not the force) of the heartbeat. They are products of the digitalis plant. Digitalis is given to relieve some arrhythmias. Digoxin (*Lanoxin*) is by far the most commonly used digitalis product.

Digitalis therapy is begun with large doses to bring the blood level up to a certain point. This is called the period of digitalization. Thereafter, smaller doses are given—just enough to maintain the proper level of digoxin (*Lanoxin*) in the blood. Doses are adjusted carefully according to the needs of the individual patient.

Before giving digoxin (*Lanoxin*), the patient's apical pulse must be checked for one minute, as digoxin doses are cumulative. If the pulse is below about 60 (see the doctor's order), or if it has noticeably changed in any way, do not give the drug; instead, notify the nurse.

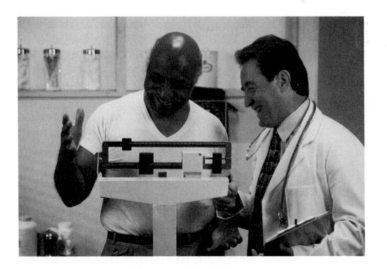

Figure 9.5
Patients on digitalis must be weighed daily.

Patients on digitalis are weighed every day (Figure 9.5). A careful record is also kept of their fluid intake and output (see Chapter 12). These measures tell the medical team whether digoxin (*Lanoxin*) is taking effect and whether the kidneys are working properly. People who have low potassium levels are more prone to the toxicities of digoxin. This fact, along with the fact that CHF patients are commonly also taking the potassium-losing diuretic furosemide (*Lasix*), makes potassium supplements important for these patients.

Digoxin (*Lanoxin*)–specific antibody fragments, also known by its product-name, *Digibind*, is an antidote for life-threatening digoxin intoxication.

ANTIDYSRHYTHMICS

Antidysrhythmia medications also act on the heart's pacemaker cells. They are used mainly to treat dysrhythmias. They stabilize the heart muscle so that it does not flutter or beat too rapidly. Examples are quinidine (*Quinora*), propranolol (*Inderal*), and procainamide (*Pronestyl*). (Propranolol is also used in the control of both hypertension and angina pectoris.)

Used improperly, antidysrhythmics can have serious side effects. The dosages must be adjusted individually to each patient. When an order for an antidysrhythmic says "give three times a day," check with the physician or pharmacist for the correct timing. These drugs should be given every 8 hours to ensure a constant blood level. Before administering antidysrhythmics, pulse and blood pressure usually must be taken. The response to the drug may be checked on the ECG.

ANTICOAGULANTS

Anticoagulants prevent blood from clotting. This helps prevent or reduce the formation of a thrombus. There are two main groups of anticoagulants: those that are administered orally and those that are administered parenterally. Warfarin (*Coumadin*) is an example of an oral anticoagulant. Another anticoagulant, heparin, is given only parenterally. Enoxaparin (*Lovenox*) is a low-molecular-weight heparin used to prevent deep vein thrombosis after surgery. It is given subcutaneously for 7 to 20 days following surgery.

If the physician wants continuous IV infusion of heparin to control the rate and volume of administration, the prescribed amount of heparin is added to 1000 ml of normal saline and an infusion pump is used.

For subcutaneous administration, use a 25- to 26-gauge, 1/2- or 5/8-inch needle to withdraw heparin from the container. Preferably, inject into the fatty layer of the abdomen just above the iliac crest. Pinch up a skinfold and insert the needle at a 90-degree angle; do not aspirate the syringe but inject the drug slowly. If you do not use a 90-degree angle, there will be a greater possibility of **hematoma** (collection of blood caused by a break in a blood vessel) formation. After injection, apply pressure (do not rub) for 1 minute. Be sure to rotate administration sites.

Anticoagulants are strong drugs. Dosages must be adjusted carefully because they can lead to internal hemorrhage. Patients taking such drugs must regularly be given blood clotting tests (prothrombin time) to determine the proper dosage. They must also be observed for signs of blood in the urine and feces (red or dark brown urine and tarry stools) and bleeding from the skin or mucous membranes, which indicate overdosage. Many other drugs (including OTC drugs such as aspirin, oral contraceptives, and antacids) affect the action of warfarin. Careful records must be kept of the various drugs a patient is taking.

THROMBOLYTICS

Whereas anticoagulants prevent blood from clotting, **thrombolytics** are drugs that are used to dissolve clots. They are used only in a hospital setting by health care providers experienced in caring for patients with thrombosis. Thrombolytics are effective for the treatment of myocardial infarction if given within 6 hours of the onset of chest pain. Available thrombolytic agents include streptokinase (*Streptase*), urokinase (*Abbokinase*), alteplase (*Activase*), and anistreplase (*Eminase*).

HEMOSTATICS

Hemostatics help the formation of blood clots. This is useful when much blood is being lost due to injury or disease, or when a patient has had an overdose of an anticoagulant. Vitamin K, a necessary ingredient in blood clotting, helps stop internal bleeding. It is sometimes given before surgery or childbirth. Vitamin K is also given to reverse the effects of warfarin toxicity. One form of vitamin K is phytonadione (*Mephyton*). Protamine sulfate may be administered in cases of heparin overdosing to negate heparin's effects. Aminocaproic acid is useful in some cases of acute, life-threatening bleeding.

HEMATINICS (ANTIANEMICS)

Hematinics are used where there is a lowered red blood cell count or a lack of hemoglobin in conditions such as anemia. Hematinics provide the necessary ingredients for the production of red blood cells, such as iron and cyanocobalamin (vitamin B_{12}). Meanwhile, the physician must look for the underlying cause of the iron deficiency, such as poor diet and effects of other drugs. Cyanocobalamin is used to treat pernicious anemia. Popular iron preparations are ferrous sulfate (*Feosol, Fer-In-Sol*), given orally, and iron (*Imferon*), given parenterally.

Iron taken orally can irritate the mucous membranes. Tablets must be given with plenty of liquid. Patients who have trouble swallowing may need a liquid preparation. Iron supplements can stain skin and clothing, so they must be handled carefully. Liquid preparations should be well-diluted with the liquid called for in the package insert. They should be taken with a straw and the mouth rinsed afterward to avoid staining the teeth. Patients should be warned to expect their stools to look dark and tarry. This is a harmless side effect of taking iron. However, patients should report any trouble with diarrhea or constipation.

GIVING CARDIOVASCULAR MEDICATIONS

Many of the patients to whom you will give medications suffer from some form of cardiovascular disorder. Therefore, you need to learn as much as you can about how the medications work and about how the cardiovascular system works. Read package inserts and drug references to become familiar with all the common drugs for this system.

Note that more than one dose is sometimes shown in the dosage column of the product information table. The dosage depends on whether a person is just beginning to take the drug or has been taking it for several days. When a disorder has just been discovered, the doctor may order a fairly large dose to start the drug therapy. This quickly builds up the level of medication in the patient's bloodstream. It is called the initial or loading dose. After one or more initial doses, the dosage is lowered to a maintenance dose. This is the amount that maintains the level of drug in the blood without overdosing the patient. The maintenance dose will continue to be given for as long as the doctor orders. Anticoagulants and digitalis products are both given in this way, but a loading dose of an anticoagulant is used less frequently now.

Occasionally an initial dose is lower than a maintenance dose. This is true, for example, of some antihypertensives. They must be given in small doses at first to let the body adjust to them gradually. Once the body has adjusted, the normal larger dose can be given.

Side effects and adverse reactions are of special concern when giving cardiovascular drugs. The medications are strong and can be dangerous. The dosages must be absolutely correct. Most side effects of these drugs come from a sensitivity to the medication or too strong a dose.

Observe your patients, and question any who are taking a cardiovascular drug for any unusual sensations such as headache, lightheadedness, and **palpitations** (rapid, throbbing heartbeats). Chart any unusual signs in the nurses' notes and report them to your supervisor. Remember also to take and chart the pulse and/or blood pressure as ordered.

Patients who have trouble with the cardiovascular system may be very anxious. They need all the emotional support you can give. Explain procedures carefully and answer their questions as best you can. Do not rush them. Try to gain their confidence so they will cooperate with any special procedures you need to do.

Many patients with cardiovascular diseases must change their lifestyles if they wish to survive. The doctor has probably ordered them to give up lifelong habits like smoking or eating rich and salty foods. They may have to start exercise programs to lose weight and strengthen the heart. These new ways of doing things are sometimes hard to accept. Patients may be depressed or fearful. You can help by teaching them, by reassuring them, and by focusing on the benefits of their lifestyle changes.

REPRESENTATIVE DRUGS FOR THE CARDIOVASCULAR SYSTEM

CATEGORY, NAME[a], AND ROUTE	USES AND DISEASES	ACTIONS	USUAL DOSE[b] AND SPECIAL INSTRUCTIONS	SIDE EFFECTS AND ADVERSE REACTIONS
Vasodilators				
Nitroglycerin, *Nitro-Bid, Nitrostat* Sublingual, buccal, oral, topical, ointment, patches	Angina pectoris	Reduces myocardial oxygen demand by causing peripheral vasodilation	*Sublingual:* 0.15–0.6 mg repeated at 5-minute intervals; if no relief after 15 minutes or 3 tablets, notify physician *Ointment:* 1–2 inches every 8 hours and at bedtime *Patch:* apply 1 patch every 24 hours	Headache, dizziness, flushing, orthostatic hypotension, nausea, rapid pulse
Clonidine hydrochloride (*Catapres*) PO, topical, patch	Hypertension	Suppresses sympathetic outflow from the brain and decreases cardiac output	0.2–0.8 mg in divided doses daily, PO; one patch effective for 7 days	Rebound hypertension if discontinued abruptly, dry mouth, drowsiness, dizziness, constipation, pruritis
Prazosin (*Minipress*) Oral	Hypertension	Decreases peripheral vascular resistance	1 mg BID or TID PO	Weakness, nausea, headache, palpitations, dizziness, orthostatic hypotention
Hydralazine (*Apresoline*) Oral, IV, IM	Hypertension	Vasodilates vascular smooth muscle	10–50 mg PO q6h; take with meals	Lupuslike syndrome, headache, diarrhea, increased pulse, coma, angina, hypersensitivity, impotence; avoid abrupt discontinuance; blood dyscrasis (disease)
Antidysrhythmics				
Quinidine Oral, IV, IM	Dysrhythmias (atrial fibrillation, flutter)	Lessens excitability of the myocardium; slows heart rate; lowers blood pressure	200–300 mg PO TID or QID; take pulse and blood pressure before administering; give with meals to avoid gastrointestinal irritation	Gastrointestinal distress, hypersensitivity (esp. fever or rash), hypotension, severe headache, blurred vision, dizziness, tinnitus

REPRESENTATIVE DRUGS FOR THE CARDIOVASCULAR SYSTEM

CATEGORY, NAME[a], AND ROUTE	USES AND DISEASES	ACTIONS	USUAL DOSE[b] AND SPECIAL INSTRUCTIONS	SIDE EFFECTS AND ADVERSE REACTIONS
Cardiac Glycosides				
Digoxin (*Lanoxin*) Oral, IV, IM (avoid intramuscular injections because they are painful; also bioavailability of IM injection is low and has unpredictable absorption)	CHF, arrhythmias	Slows and strengthens heartbeat; increases cardiac output	Daily maintenance dose: 0.125–0.5 mg PO; usually 0.25 mg; take apical pulse for 1 minute prior to administering	Nausea, vomiting, slow or irregular pulse, loss of appetite, extreme fatigue; increased risk of side effects when blood levels are greater than 2 mg/dl, hypokalemia, and worsening renal functioning; yellow-green halos around images, blurred vision
Antihypertensives/Diuretics				
Atenolol (*Tenormin*) Oral, IV	Hypertension, angina pectoris	Decreases cardiac output, peripheral resistance, and cardiac oxygen consumption	50 mg/day in single or divided doses; maintenance dose: 50–100 mg/day	Respiratory distress, bradycardia, dizziness, fatigue, diarrhea, nausea, hypotension
Metoprolol tartrate (*Lopressor*) Oral	Management of hypertension; most effective when used with a thiazide diuretic or another antihypertensive	Beta blocker, lowers blood pressure	100 mg/day in single or divided doses; maintenance dose: 100–450 mg/day	Respiratory distress, bradycardia, dizziness, fatigue, diarrhea, nausea
Nifedipine (*Procardia, Adalat, Procardia XL*) Oral, sublingual	Vasospastic angina; coronary artery spasm; hypertension	Inhibits calcium ion influx across the cell membrane of cardiac and vascular smooth muscle, causing modest hypotension	30–90 mg/day; obtain blood pressure and pulse immediately before administration (use same arm and place patient in same position each time)	Dizziness, lightheadedness, flushing, peripheral edema, nausea, weakness, myocardial infarction
Diltiazem hydrochloride (*Cardizem, Cardizem SR*) Oral	Angina and hypertension	Inhibits calcium ion influx across the cell membrane during depolarization of cardiac and vascular smooth muscle	30–120 mg (up to 240 mg/day) SR	Edema, arrhythmias, drowsiness, nausea, lightheadedness
Verapamil hydrochloride (*Calan*) Oral, IM, IV	Angina and hypertension: paroxysmal atrial tachycardia, atrial fibrillation or flutter	Inhibits calcium ion influx and slows atrioventricular conduction; reduces supraventricular tachycardia due to atrial flutter or fibrillation	120–480 mg/day PO, 5–10 mg slow IV push. Titrate doses: 80 mg 3 or 4 times a day; up to 240–480 mg. Obtain blood pressure, pulse, and respirations immediately before giving drug	Peripheral edema, bradycardia, dizziness, headache, constipation
Hydrochlorothiazide (*Diuril*) Oral	Management of hypertension	Diuretic; increases water and sodium excretion	Initially, 25 mg/day PO to patient's response; potassium supplement may be needed	Hypokalemia, weakness, dizziness, fatigue, dry mouth, confusion
Triamterene (*Dyrenium*) Oral	Used to counteract potassium-losing effect of thiazides	Potassium-sparing diuretic	50–100 mg/day; do not give potassium supplement	Hyperkalemia, renal stones, nausea and vomiting

(continued)

REPRESENTATIVE DRUGS FOR THE CARDIOVASCULAR SYSTEM (continued)

CATEGORY, NAME[a], AND ROUTE	USES AND DISEASES	ACTIONS	USUAL DOSE[b] AND SPECIAL INSTRUCTIONS	SIDE EFFECTS AND ADVERSE REACTIONS
Dysrhythmics (Arrhythmia Medications)				
Propranolol (*Inderal*) Oral, IV	Arrhythmias (especially tachycardia), hypertension, migraine prophylaxis, angina	Both procainamide and its active metabolite (NAPA) lessen excitability of the myocardium; slows heart rate, lowers blood pressure	Arrhythmias, 10–30 mg PO TID or QID; give before meals and at bedtime; take pulse and blood pressure before administering	Diarrhea, nausea, dry mouth, dyspnea, hypotension, confusion, slow pulse
Procainamide (*Pronestyl, Procan-SR*) Oral, IM, IV	Premature ventricular contractions, ventricular tachycardia; atrial fibrillation and paroxysmal atrial tachycardia	Lessens excitability of the myocardium; slows heart rate; lowers blood pressure	PO, SR 0.5–1 g/6 hr; IV, 25–50 mg/min; method depends on patient's condition; blood tests needed when on maintenance dose; adjust dosage to appropriate level	Hypotension, anorexia, nausea, urticaria, chills, fever, agranulocytosis, lupus syndrome after prolonged use
Anticoagulants				
Warfarin sodium (*Coumadin*) Oral	Thrombus, pulmonary embolism, phlebitis, coronary occlusion	Prevents or slows formation of blood clots; prevents enlargement of existing thrombus	Dosage must be adjusted individually; 2–10 mg PO daily for maintenance (initial dose may be given IM, IV, or PO); adjust doses weekly until blood coagulation (prothrombin time) tests are 1.5–2 times normal; not to be used when there is a risk of hemorrhage (e.g., with surgery, ulcers, pregnancy); watch for signs of bleeding	Hemorrhage (blood in urine, feces, and tissues, bruising, nosebleed, bleeding gums)
Heparin (*Calciparine*) IV, SC, IV bolus	Thrombosis, embolism, prophylaxis for deep venous thrombosis	Inhibits reactions that lead to clotting	5000–40,000 units; do not give IM due to pain or risk of hematoma formation; doses adjusted to individual patient	Hemorrhage, chills, fever, hypersensitivity reactions, alopecia

[a] Trade names given in parentheses are examples only. Check current drug references for a complete listing of available products.
[b] Average adult doses are given. However, dosages are determined by a physician and vary with the purpose of the therapy and the particular patient. The doses presented in this text are for general information only.

Administering Oral, Sublingual, and Buccal Medications

■ **EQUIPMENT**

Medication orders for three patients

- Patient 1: digoxin, 0.25 mg PO qd.
- Patient 2: ferrous sulfate, 220 mg PO QID with juice
- Patient 3: nitroglycerin, 0.4 mg subl PRN

Medications

- *Lanoxin* (0.125-mg or 0.25-mg tablets)
- *Feosol* elixir (220 mg ferrous sulfate per teaspoonful)
- *Nitrostat* (0.4-mg sublingual tablets)

Apple juice, water, cups

Medication tray or cart with appropriate charts and records

■ **PROCEDURE**

1. Set up medications one at a time. Read drug labels as you reach for bottles, then again as you pour, and again as you put drugs away. Check and double-check the medication orders for the "five rights."

2. Wash your hands and wear gloves.

3. Go to Patient 1. Identify the patient. Explain what you are going to do. Assist the patient into a position for oral administration.

4. Administer digoxin (*Lanoxin*).

   - Check the apical pulse first to make sure that it is over 60.
   - Administer one 0.25-mg tablet or two 0.125-mg tablets.
   - Give water to drink. Assist the patient if necessary.
   - Chart drug, dose, time, and apical pulse.
   - Make the patient comfortable before leaving.
   - Wash your hands.

5. Go to Patient 2. Identify, explain, and assist (as in Step 3).

6. Administer ferrous sulfate (*Feosol*).

   - Mix one teaspoonful of *Feosol* elixir with apple juice, if the patient is unable to take elixir without juice.
   - Administer it to the patient (helping the patient to use a straw).
   - Chart drug, dose, and time.
   - Make the patient comfortable before leaving.
   - Wash your hands.

7. Go to Patient 3. Identify the patient. Explain that you are leaving a packet of nitroglycerin tablets by the bedside. As you leave, the patient complains of angina pain.

8. Administer nitroglycerin (*Nitrostat*).

   - Place one tablet (0.4 mg) of *Nitrostat* under the patient's tongue or in the buccal pouch (Figure 9.6 on page 178). Instruct the patient not to swallow until the tablet is completely dissolved.
   - Do not give liquids.
   - Chart drug, dose, time, and reason for administration.
   - Make the patient comfortable before leaving.
   - Wash your hands.

9. Return equipment and charts to the proper location.

Demonstrate this procedure for your instructor.

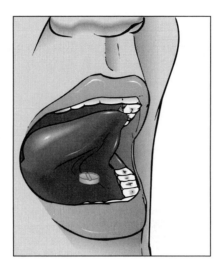 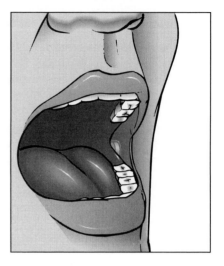

Figure 9.6
Sublingual (left)
and buccal (right)
administration.

Define each of the terms listed below.

1. Edema _____

2. Tachycardia _____

3. Bradycardia _____

4. Hypertension _____

5. Hypotension _____

From Column 2, select the term that best matches each description in Column 1.

_____ 6. Blood pressure instrument

_____ 7. Graphic record that shows the spread of electrical excitation to different parts of the heart

_____ 8. Important in clotting process

_____ 9. Surround and destroy microorganisms and foreign matter

_____ 10. Liquid portion of blood and lymph

a. electrocardiograph

b. sphygmomanometer

c. plasma

d. white blood cells

e. platelets

Complete the following statements by filling in the blanks.

11. An important landmark when taking the apical pulse before administering cardiac drugs is the _____.

12. The tiny vessels that connect arterioles to venules are called _____.

13. Veins carry _____ blood.

14. Arteries carry _____ blood.

Select the cardiovascular disorder that best matches each description. Write the name of the disorder in the blank.

Angina pectoris   Arteriosclerosis   Myocardial infarction   Atherosclerosis

Thrombophlebitis   Shock   Embolism

15. Collapse of the circulatory system, signaled by severe hypotension; high pulse rate; pale, clammy skin; and mental confusion.

_____

16. Fat deposited along vessel walls reduces circulation.

_____

17. Most common arterial disorder, characterized by thickening, loss of elasticity, and calcification of arterial walls.

_____

18. Formation of a blood clot in a blood vessel, associated with inflammation.

_____

19. A blood clot or air bubble travels through the bloodstream and cuts off circulation to a vital organ.

_____

20. Chest pain that may be relieved by giving nitroglycerin.

_____

21. Death of a part of the heart muscle resulting from lack of blood circulation to that area.

_____

Tell what these types of drugs do; for example, diuretics help the body eliminate excess fluids through the urine.

22. Vasopressors _____

23. Vasodilators _____

24. Cardiac glycosides _____

25. Antidysrhythmics _____

26. Anticoagulants _____

27. Hemostatics _____

28. Hematinics _____

Match drug names to drug categories.

_____ 29. Verapamil, *Procardia*   a. calcium channel blockers

_____ 30. *Lopressor,* hydralazine, *Aldomet*   b. antihypertensives

■ CASE STUDIES FOR CRITICAL THINKING

Complete the following statements by filling in the blanks.

31. Patients taking heparin or warfarin (*Coumadin*) must be watched for signs of _____ in the urine, feces, and mucous membranes.

32. _____ may be left at a patient's bedside for angina pain.

33. Because digitalis slows as well as strengthens the heartbeat, an adult patient's pulse rate must be at least _____ in order to give the drug.

34. Patients on antihypertensives may feel _____ when they get up from bed because of orthostatic hypotension.

35. Some hematinics can _____ clothing and skin, so they must be handled with care.

■ APPLICATIONS

Obtain a current copy of a drug reference book or the PDR®. Use it to answer the questions that follow in a notebook or on file cards.

36. Use Section 4 of the *PDR®*, Generic and Chemical Name Index, to find another product name for each of the drugs on the Representative Drug List on pages 174–176 of this text.

37. Use Section 3 of the *PDR®*, Product Category Index, to locate Cardiovascular Preparations; then find the subheading Anginal Preparations. List all of the drugs named.

If you have a problem finding some drugs in the *PDR®*, look in the back under Discontinued Products.

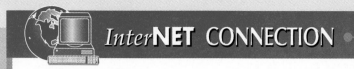

InterNET CONNECTION

To learn more about the cardiovascular system and cardiovascular disease, go to www.intelihealth.com. This site, operated by Johns Hopkins Hospital, offers detailed information on health and medicine. Click on The Cardiovascular System to learn about the risk factors, tests and procedures, and medications.

Drugs for the Respiratory System

In this chapter you will review the parts and functions of the respiratory system. You will learn how breathing takes place and how common respiratory disorders affect this process. You will study the types of drugs used to treat respiratory disorders and their actions. You will learn to administer drugs in the form of nose drops and sprays to the mucous membranes of the nose and throat.

OBJECTIVES

After studying this chapter, you should be able to

- name and describe the parts of the respiratory system.
- give the normal respiration rate for an adult.
- explain why coughing is important for maintaining a patient's airway.
- list and describe common symptoms of respiratory disorders, using correct medical terms.
- recognize descriptions of the major respiratory disorders.
- describe the actions and give examples of the following drug groups: antitussives, expectorants, decongestants, antihistamines, and bronchodilators.
- define the three chest physiotherapy procedures.
- administer nose drops using correct procedure.
- correctly administer oxygen therapy as ordered.

KEY TERMS

acute: short term, usually less than six months

alveoli: tiny air sacs in the lungs that permit the exchange of oxygen and carbon dioxide through capillary walls (singular: alveolus)

antihistamine: drug that counteracts the effects of histamine, relieving allergy symptoms

antitussive: drug that decreases coughing

apnea: stoppage of breathing; may be temporary or fatal

bronchi: air passages leading from the trachea to the bronchioles in the lungs (singular: bronchus)

bronchiole: branch of the bronchi leading to alveolar ducts

bronchodilator: drug that increases the vital capacity of the lungs by dilating the bronchi and relaxing the smooth muscles

bronchopulmonary: pertaining to the lungs and the air passages

chronic: long term, usually more than six months

decongestant: drug that reduces congestion or swelling, especially in nasal passages, by constricting blood vessels and restricting blood flow to the area

dyspnea: labored or difficult breathing

emphysema: condition in which the air sacs dilate and are unable to contract to their original size; the alveoli lose their elasticity, causing residual air to be trapped in them

epiglottis: leaf-shaped structure on top of the larynx that seals off the air passages to the lungs during swallowing

expectorant: drug that breaks down mucus to enable the patient to cough it up more easily (also called mucolytic)

Fowler's position: position in which the patient's upper body is raised 45° to 60° by means of pillows or by adjusting the head of the bed

hemoptysis: spitting of blood

hyperpnea: breathing too rapidly or deeply; also called hyperventilation

hypoxia: absence or decrease in oxygen

larynx: voice box; joins the pharynx with the trachea

mucolytic: drug that liquifies or breaks down tenacious mucus so it can be coughed up more easily; also called expectorant

nebulizer: device that produces a drug mist for inhalation

orthopnea: abnormal condition in which the patient must sit or stand to breathe deeply and comfortably

percussion: physical therapy for respiratory patients; tapping of various body organs and structures

pharynx: tubelike structure that extends from the base of the skull to the esophagus; serves both respiratory and digestive tracts

pleura: membranes lining the lungs and lung cavities

postural drainage: physical therapy for respiratory patients; use of positioning along with vibration and percussion to drain secretions from specific areas of the lungs, bronchi, and trachea

productive cough: cough that brings up large amounts of mucus

pulmonary: pertaining to the lungs

rebound effect: reappearance of symptoms in even stronger form after a drug dose has worn off

respiration: breathing

semi-Fowler's position: position in which the patient's upper body is elevated to 30°

sputum: abnormally thick fluid formed in the lower respiratory tract that may contain blood, pus, or bacteria

stethoscope: instrument for listening to the heartbeat and breathing sounds

tachypnea: rapid breathing

trachea: windpipe; connects larynx to bronchi

unproductive cough: cough that brings up nothing from the lungs; a dry cough

ventilator: machine that assists breathing

vibration: physical therapy for respiratory patients; a fine, shaking pressure applied to the chest wall during exhalation

viscosity: thickness

RESPIRATORY SYSTEM

The respiratory system consists of the organs that make it possible for blood to exchange gases with air. They are the nose, pharynx, larynx, trachea, bronchi, and lungs (Figure 10.1). These structures constitute the lifeline of the body, supplying a continuous, uninterrupted source of oxygen. The exchange of gases between blood and air is called **respiration.** If anything jeopardizes the functioning of this vital system, death is certain within a short time.

Air enters the body through the mouth or the nose. Like all of the respiratory system, the nose is lined with mucous membranes. As air enters the nose, very small hairs, cilia, warm and moisten the air and trap dust particles and bacteria. The **pharynx** is a tubelike structure that extends from the base of the skull to the esophagus and serves both the respiratory tract and the digestive tract. The **larynx,** or voice box, lies at the upper end of the trachea just below the pharynx.

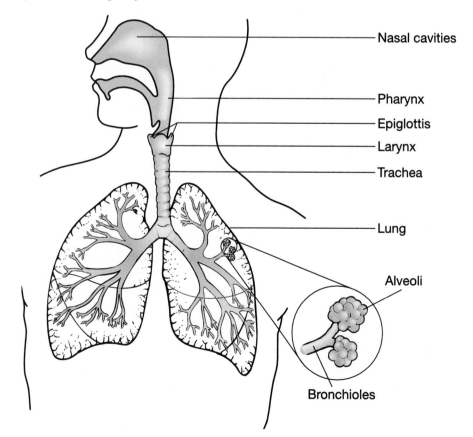

Figure 10.1
The respiratory system.

The larynx is responsible for making sounds. The larynx serves a protective function because the **epiglottis,** a leaf-shaped structure on top of the larynx, closes the airway when a person swallows. The epiglottis thus keeps food and saliva from entering the lungs.

The larynx joins a tube that leads into the lungs called the **trachea,** or windpipe. C-shaped pieces of cartilage line the trachea to keep it firm and prevent it from collapsing and shutting off the airway. The trachea branches off into two tubes: the right and left **bronchi,** which lead to the right and left lungs. The right bronchus is slightly larger and more vertical than the left. This is why, when an individual aspirates, the aspirated object generally lodges in the right bronchus. The bronchi branch into increasingly smaller tubes, the **bronchioles,** that subdivide into smaller tubes. The smaller branches further divide into alveolar ducts. These terminate in several alveolar sacs whose walls consist of **alveoli,** small sacs that are the functional units of the lungs.

The alveolar sacs are tiny air sacs with thin walls. They are in close contact with many capillaries. This is where inhaled oxygen is picked up from the air by the red blood cells. At the same time, carbon dioxide is released from the blood into the air sacs and travels back up the air passages. During exhalation, the carbon dioxide and other waste gases pass out of the body.

The lungs are cone-shaped organs that fill the pleural portion of the thoracic cavity. They provide a place where the exchange of gases can take place between blood and air.

The average person breathes in and out about 18 times per minute. The normal respiration rate varies between 12 and 25 times per minute. Children tend to breathe more quickly, and elderly patients more slowly, than the average adult.

Breathing is accomplished by the muscles around the ribs and by the diaphragm, a layer of muscle tissue that separates the chest cavity from the other internal organs. When a person inhales, the respiratory muscles contract to lift the rib cage, and the diaphragm flattens out. These actions create a downward and outward pull on the lungs that forces them to draw in air (inhalation). When the muscles relax, the lung cavity collapses and forces the air back out (exhalation). Inside the lungs, the elastic walls of the bronchioles and the alveoli expand and contract with each breath. When this elasticity is decreased by disease, proper breathing is no longer possible.

RESPIRATORY SYSTEM DISORDERS

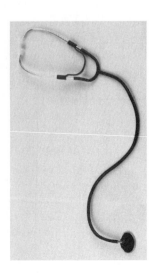

Figure 10.2

Respiration is crucial to sustaining life. A person cannot live more than a few minutes without oxygen. Brain damage begins after only 6 minutes without oxygen. This is why respiration rate is one of the four vital signs. The other vital signs are body temperature, blood pressure, and pulse.

As a routine part of a physical examination, the doctor examines the patient with a **stethoscope,** an instrument that amplifies breathing sounds (Figure 10.2). Auscultation is the process of listening to the lung sounds to evaluate lung function. Listening to the lung sounds with a stethoscope helps to assess the movement of air throughout the trachebronchial tree. Normally, air flows through the airways without obstruction. To the examiner, it sounds like a swish of air. Variations in lung sounds are often characteristic of certain lung diseases.

Several other tests help in diagnosing respiratory diseases. A chest X ray may be taken. A patient may cough up sputum to be sent to the laboratory for microscopic examination. Blood tests called blood gases are done to check oxygen and carbon dioxide content. A pulse oximetry is a technique whereby a probe is attached to the ear, finger, toe, or bridge of the nose to measure the oxygen concentration of the blood.

SYMPTOMS

Coughing. Coughing is a protective reflex to clear the trachea, bronchi, and lungs of secretions and irritants. Respiratory diseases often cause secretion of mucus, pus, or other fluids in the lungs. Coughing can be persistent or it can come in uncontrolled fits. A patient may deny or underestimate the extent of the cough, making a cough difficult to evaluate.

Sputum. Coughing brings up secretions known as **sputum.** The sputum itself contains clues to possible disease. It varies in color and consistency. Blood in the sputum **(hemoptysis)** is usually a signal that bleeding is occurring in the respiratory or gastrointestinal tract.

Hoarseness. This symptom may be caused by an abnormal growth on the larynx, or it may be the result of an infection in the throat.

Wheezing. Wheezing is a high-pitched, musical sound that occurs through a narrowed airway. It is frequently seen with asthma and bronchitis or in patients with allergies.

Chest Pain. Pains in the chest area occur in various forms during respiratory disorders: for example, chest tightness, pain when taking a deep breath, or stabbing pain that comes unexpectedly.

Certain types of breathing can be symptoms of disorders. **Dyspnea** is shortness of breath or labored breathing. **Tachypnea** is rapid breathing. **Apnea** is the cessation of breathing, which often occurs during sleep. **Hyperpnea,** or hyperventilation, is breathing that is too rapid or deep. A patient who has great difficulty breathing when lying down but who can breathe more easily when in a sitting or standing position demonstrates **orthopnea.** More general symptoms of respiratory disorders are loss of appetite, weight loss, fever, fatigue, cyanosis, clubbing of the fingers, and sweats and chills.

MAJOR DISEASES

Some respiratory problems are caused by disturbances in the control centers of the brain or in the nerves that send messages to the respiratory muscles in the ribs and the diaphragm. These problems, and the drugs used to treat them, are discussed in Chapter 16. Here we will focus on disorders that affect the air passages and the lungs, or **bronchopulmonary** disorders (**pulmonary**, pertaining to the lungs).

Pneumonia. There are many types of pneumonia, each named for the agent (bacterium, virus, fungus, etc.) that causes it. All pneumonias are infections of the lower respiratory tract (bronchi, bronchioles, and alveoli). Factors that predispose an individual to pneumonia include smoking, air pollution, malnutrition, bed rest, immobility, and other diseases.

Some pneumonias are caused by bacteria that normally live in the human air passages. At times of low resistance, these bacteria may multiply and infect the lungs. Such bacterial growth may occur after surgery, anesthesia, diseases that interfere with lung drainage, and use of drugs that suppress the body's immune system. As soon as the type of bacteria is identified, antibiotics can be given to fight the infection.

Bronchitis. Bronchitis is an inflammation of the air passageways caused by irritants (e.g., smoke or chemicals), allergic reactions, flu, or viruses. It can be **acute** (short-term) or **chronic** (long-term). The main objective of bronchitis treatment is to keep the air passages open. They are easily plugged by sputum and pus produced by the infected bronchi. The main symptoms of bronchitis are fever, cough, tachypnea, purulent sputum (containing pus), and pleuritic chest pain. Treatment is with a broad-spectrum antibiotic, such as ampicillin, tetracycline, or erythromycin, for 7 to 10 days. The patient must drink large amounts of fluids and take drugs that keep the sputum moist and thin **(expectorants).**

Emphysema. **Emphysema** is the result of the enlargement of and damage to alveolar sacs. These two problems reduce the surface of the alveoli and limit the exchange of oxygen and carbon dioxide. "Stale" air becomes backed up in the alveoli, which, in turn, makes it impossible to take in much air on the next breath. The alveoli are hyperinflated and overdistended. The trapped air gives the patient a "barrel chest" appearance. Although the cause of emphysema is not always understood, smoking, chronic bronchitis, and advanced age are commonly found in an emphysema patient's history. Dyspnea that continually worsens is an early symptom of emphysema.

There is no cure for emphysema, although breathing exercises are sometimes helpful. Antibiotics can be given for specific infections. Drugs that thin the sputum (expectorants) and drugs that expand the bronchioles (**bronchodilators**) are given to promote coughing up sputum that may be clogging the air passages.

Pleurisy. Pleurisy is an inflammation of the linings (the **pleura**) of the lungs and lung cavities. The most common causes are pneumonia, tuberculosis, chest trauma, pulmonary infarctions, and tumors. The patient feels a knife-sharp pain in the chest that is worse on inspiration (inhalation). Pleurisy usually clears up with rest, mild sedatives, pain medication, and treatment of the primary disease. The patient is frequently taught to splint the affected side when coughing or to lie on the affected side.

Asthma. Asthma is characterized by airway obstruction, inflammation, and increased response to stimuli. Asthma attacks can be caused by substances in the environment, food additives, exercise, drug allergies, illness, or emotional upset. The attacks may occur from time to time or may last for several days (the most dangerous form). During an attack, the muscles around the bronchioles contract, narrowing the air passages. Inhaled air cannot be exhaled properly. The alveoli become plugged with unusually thick sputum that is hard to cough up. There is wheezing, shortness of breath, and coughing. The individual often has a feeling of suffocating and sits straight up or bends forward in an attempt to get more air.

The goal of asthma treatment is to relieve the constriction of the bronchioles. Bronchodilators are the drugs of choice. Theophylline was the preferred drug, but it has been replaced by other bronchodilators and anti-inflammatory drugs. Currently, B_2-adrenergic agonists such as metaproterenol (*Alupent*) and albuterol (*Proventil*) are used. Prevention is important in the treatment of asthma. Patients are taught to avoid the triggers of an attack. An inhaled corticosteroid such as Prednisone may be given for its anti-inflammatory effect.

Cancers of the Respiratory Tract. Cancers of the upper respiratory tract include cancers of the head and neck. Although cancers of the oral cavity and larynx account for only 5 percent of all cancers, their effects are devastating. Disability is great because of the loss of voice and disfigurement. The cause of head and neck cancers is unknown, but smoking and alcohol are high on the list of contributing factors. Symptoms range from pain that is aggravated by food to hoarseness. Persistent hoarseness is one of the first signs of upper respiratory cancer. It is treated by removing the growth surgically.

Cancer of the lung is the most common cancer of the lower respiratory tract. It is the leading cause of all cancer deaths. A well-known risk for lung cancer is the inhalation of cigarette smoke. Lung cancer may also spread from another cancer elsewhere in the body. It is difficult to detect because the symptoms are vague. Generally, the first symptom is a persistent, productive cough. Hemoptysis, spitting of blood, may occur late in the disease process because of bleeding caused by the malignancy. Dyspnea and wheezing occur if the bronchials become obstructed. Surgery to remove the cancerous tissue is the major form of treatment. Radiation and chemotherapy may also be used.

Pulmonary Embolism. Pulmonary embolism is the most common complication found in hospitalized patients. It generally begins as a thrombus deep in the vein of a leg. This is why maintaining mobility in patients is essential to prevent pulmonary embolisms, which can be fatal. Symptoms include sudden, unexplained dyspnea, tachypnea, or tachycardia. Oxygen and anticoagulant therapy are often effective in treatment.

Tuberculosis. Tuberculosis (TB) is an infectious disease caused by *Mycobacterium tuberculosis.* The body becomes sensitive to this bacterium when it is first exposed. Coughing spreads airborne droplets that contain rod-shaped bacteria known as tubercle bacilli; when droplets are inhaled, the bacteria multiply in the lungs. After initial infection, tuberculosis germs can remain dormant for long periods and then reactivate when the immune system weakens. The patient weakens, coughs up blood, and eventually dies without early treatment. Treatment consists of drugs that attack the tubercle bacillus (e.g., rifapentine, isoniazid, rifampin, ethambutol, pyrazinamide), rest, and proper disposal of sputum in a designated waste receptacle. Rifapentine (*Priftin*) is the first new drug developed against the disease in over 25 years. It is a longer-acting form of rifampin, which has been a standard part of the treatment of TB.

Although the occurrence of tuberculosis in the United States fell steadily from 1953 until 1985, the number of new cases is rising. The main reasons are the prevalence of the human immunodeficiency virus (HIV) infection, which impairs immunity, and new strains of tuberculosis that are resistant to drug therapy. Risk factors for tuberculosis are immigration from countries where tuberculosis is prevalent, poverty, overcrowding, poor nutrition, and homelessness. Because many cases of tuberculosis are left untreated, the disease can spread at an alarming rate. In the early stages, the patient may be free of symptoms. TB may be found accidentally on a routine chest X ray. Later, fatigue, weight loss, anorexia, low-grade fever, and night sweats may develop. If it is thought that a patient might have tuberculosis, the patient should have a tuberculin skin test and chest X ray.

Treatment of tuberculosis consists of a combination of at least three drugs. In high-risk areas or areas known to have a high incidence of drug resistance, three or more drugs are used. The four most commonly used drugs are isoniazid, rifampin, streptomycin, and ethambutol. The current protocol for treatment is to use isoniazid, rifampin, and ethambutol for two months, followed by four months of isoniazid and rifampin. Therapy is continued for three months even after a negative culture. Hospitalization is generally not necessary. If it is required, it is very brief. The patient is placed in respiratory isolation and on drug therapy for 2 weeks. Patients must show a positive response to treatment before discharge.

Inflammations of the Nose, Sinuses, and Throat. Rhinitis, sinusitis, and strep throat are some of the most common inflammations of the upper respiratory tract. They are caused by bacterial infections, allergies, or irritating substances. "Seasonal rhinitis," for example, is an allergic reaction to the pollen in the air during the late summer and fall. Signs of rhinitis and sinusitis include runny nose, sneezing, headache, sore throat, watery eyes, fever, and redness and swelling of mucous membranes. The symptoms can be controlled with decongestants and antihistamines. To treat strep throat, the disease-causing bacterium may need to be identified by means of a throat culture. Then a systemic antibiotic is prescribed to kill that specific bacterium.

DRUGS FOR RESPIRATORY DISORDERS

ANTITUSSIVES

Antitussive drugs are cough suppressants. They act on the control center in the brain that stimulates coughing. Remember that not all coughing is harmful or undesirable. Coughing clears the respiratory tract of foreign objects and sputum that interfere with breathing. A cough that brings up sputum is called a **productive cough.** A cough that brings up nothing is called "dry," or

unproductive cough. Unproductive coughing occurs when mucus is clogged in the lower respiratory tract or when irritation in the throat stimulates repeated coughing. Despite the fact that no mucus is being brought up, a person may have a repeated urge to cough. Frequent and prolonged coughing can be exhausting, painful, and stressful to the circulatory system. Antitussives are given to suppress the cough reflex somewhat (never completely). There are narcotic antitussives, such as codeine, and nonnarcotic antitussives, such as dextromethorphan (*Dimetapp-DM*). Increasing fluids and inhalation of steam are also utilized to thin and increase the production of secretions. Patients should be monitored for drowsiness.

MUCOLYTICS/EXPECTORANTS

Mucolytic drugs, also called expectorants, have a disintegrating effect on mucus. They increase the amount of fluid in the respiratory tract to help liquefy and reduce the **viscosity** (thickness) of secretions. One of the most commonly used mucolytics is acetylcysteine (*Mucomyst*).

DECONGESTANTS

Decongestants are vasoconstrictors used for nasal congestion because they shrink engorged mucous membranes that are frequently present in respiratory infections.

Decongestants only relieve symptoms; they do not cure the underlying cause of congestion. They are available as nasal solutions. Examples are phenylephrine hydrochloride (*Neo-Synephrine*) and oxymetazoline (*Afrin*). Most decongestants are available OTC, but patients should not overuse them.

A **rebound effect** can occur with decongestants after continued use; when the drug effect wears off, the mucous membranes swell even more than before. Decongestants can also irritate the nasal passages.

ANTIHISTAMINES

Antihistamines are drugs that work against the effects of histamine, which is why they are used in allergic conditions such as hay fever. Recall that histamine is released by certain cells whenever there is a foreign "invader," such as an irritating substance, a microorganism, or an injury. Histamine causes the blood vessels to dilate and the smooth muscle in the bronchi to contract. Antihistamines, in contrast, shrink the blood vessels and relax the bronchial muscles.

Antihistamines are administered orally because they are easily absorbed through the intestinal lining. The major antihistamines used for respiratory problems are diphenhydramine (*Benadryl*), astemizole (*Hismaral*), chlorpheniramine maleate (*Chlor-Trimeton*, *Teldrin*) and related drugs (*Dimetane*, *Actidil*), and cyproheptadine (*Periactin*).

Antihistamines have the side effects of drowsiness, sedation, dizziness, dry mouth, and insomnia (Figure 10.3). Caution patients about driving or operating hazardous equipment because of the sedative effect. Antihistamines should also be used with caution in patients with asthma, glaucoma, or urinary retention, because the side effects are potentiated (intensified). Side effects are also enhanced in the elderly.

BRONCHODILATORS

Bronchodilators cause the bronchioles to relax and expand (dilate). This is a useful effect in conditions like asthma, bronchitis, and emphysema. B_2-adrenergic agonists are the most effective bronchodilators. They act by relaxing the smooth muscle of the airways and increasing the cleansing of

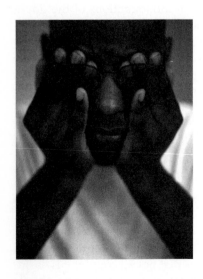

Figure 10.3
One of the common side effects of antihistamines is drowsiness.

the airways by the cilia and mucus. The most common side effects are tachycardia, nervousness, palpitations, tremors, and nausea. The B_2-adrenergic agonists are most effective in the inhaled form. The main B_2-adrenergic agonist bronchodilators are metaproterenol (*Alupent*), albuterol (*Proventil, Ventolin*), pirbuterol (*Maxair*), epinephrine (*Primatine Mist*), isoproterenol (*Isuprel*), ephedrine (*Quibron Plus*), and terbutaline (*Brethine*). A different type of bronchodilator is the anticholinergic agent ipratroprium (*Atrovent*). Many patients are prescribed a combination of an inhaled regimen of ipratroprium and one of the B_2-adrenergic agonists.

The methylxanthine derivatives, such as theophylline, aminophylline, and oxtriphylline (*Choledyl*), are another type of bronchodilator. They are considered less effective than the B_2-adrenergic agonists. These drugs are taken orally or intravenously but not by inhalation. Examples of standard theophyllines for oral administration are *Elixophyllin, Theolair,* and *Slo-Phyllin,* which must be taken about four times a day. Sustained-release theophylline products that allow once- or twice-daily administration are available, including *Elixophyllin SR, Slo-Bid, Slo-Phyllin SR, Theo-Dur, Theo-24, Uniphyl,* and *Theolair.* Remember, the sustained-release products should never be crushed to give the drug. Crushing would cause toxic effects because too much of the drug would be absorbed at one time.

Bronchodilators are given by inhalation or orally, depending on the drug (and by injection in some emergencies). Besides dilating the bronchioles, these drugs have other effects, such as stimulating the heart and respiration and stopping the release of histamine. For this reason, some of these drugs are used in emergency treatment of cardiac arrest and allergic reactions. They must be used with great care, in the proper dosages, and with close attention to side effects. Epinephrine, for example, can cause anxiety, restlessness, dizziness, weakness, pallor (pale skin), palpitations, and breathing difficulty. Patients can develop tolerance to bronchodilators, and rebound effects are also possible.

Drugs for the respiratory system are often given in combination. For example, a medicine might contain a bronchodilator to open the air passages and an expectorant to loosen the sputum so that it can be coughed up. Many cold remedies are combinations of antitussives, expectorants, and decongestants. Elixir of terpin hydrate and codeine, for example, has a combined antitussive and expectorant action. Tedral combines two bronchodilators, theophylline and ephedrine, with a sedative, phenobarbital. Popular product name remedies for allergies and colds combine antihistamines with decongestants, expectorants, and antitussives—for example, *Actifed, Benylin, Dimetapp, Ornade, Drixoral,* and *Phenergan Expectorant with Codeine.*

Other drugs often used for the treatment of respiratory diseases include cromolyn and corticosteroids. Cromolyn sodium (*Aarane* and *Intal*) is classified as a mast cell stabilizer. They inhibit mass cells from releasing histamine.

Corticosteroids are potent anti-inflammatory drugs that can help control severe asthma. When administered via inhalation, steroid activity can be provided at the needed site while minimizing systemic effects. Some examples of inhaled corticosteroids are belcomethasone (*Beclovent, Vanceril*), triamcinolone (*Azmacort*), and flunisolide (*Aerobid*).

The Representative Drugs table at the end of this chapter lists uses, side effects, dosages, and special instructions for representative drugs used in treating respiratory disorders.

GIVING RESPIRATORY DRUGS

The goals of therapy in respiratory diseases are to control the rate and depth of breathing, to remove anything that may be blocking the air passages, and to clear out sputum so that it does not lead to infection. Drugs are only one part of the treatment; other important parts are to remove the source of irritation (e.g., have the patient stop smoking and avoid allergens) and to use physical techniques that promote normal mucus drainage and breathing.

You may be called on to assist in one of the three chest physiotherapy procedures when you administer medications to respiratory patients. Oxygen inhalation therapy may be ordered to prevent or relieve hypoxia. A **ventilator** may be needed to help the patient breathe regularly by mechanical means. **Postural drainage** may be ordered. The postural drainage technique consists of placing the patient in one of several positions so that gravity helps draw secretions from certain areas of the lungs and bronchi into the trachea.

Percussion is another technique for loosening clogged mucus. It involves striking the chest wall over the area being drained. Percussion is usually combined with postural drainage. Percussion is performed over a single layer of clothing and not over buttons or zippers. The single layer of clothing protects the patient's skin, but the buttons or zippers would interfere with the sensations of the percussion. Sometimes patients have to be encouraged to cough, even if it hurts, so that excess mucus does not build up in the lungs.

The third type of chest physiotherapy is **vibration,** a fine shaking pressure applied to the chest wall during exhalation. It increases the amount of air exhaled and may loosen mucus and promote a cough.

Psychological factors are important when administering respiratory medications. It is threatening and frightening to a patient to be unable to breathe properly. But this is exactly what happens with diseases of the respiratory tract, even the common cold. Patients need a calm and supportive environment.

With respiratory medications, it is especially important to watch the patient's symptoms closely. Each time you are with the patient, make a note of the rate and depth of breathing. This helps you decide which PRN drugs are needed, if any, or whether new drugs need to be ordered. Observe the patient:

- Has the patient's breathing changed since you last saw him or her?
- Has the respiration rate increased?
- Is it hard for the patient to take in a breath?

You can tell by looking at the patient's chest whether the soft tissues of the chest are retracting with each breath. Holding the mouth open while breathing, spreading the nostrils, and wheezing are other signs of respiratory problems. Some signs are so subtle that the patient may not be aware of them. Does the patient move more slowly, get excited easily, or have muscle twitches? Even stomach movements or changed speech patterns can be clues to the need for respiratory medications. Naturally, you should chart your observations.

CLINICAL CONSIDERATIONS

There are ways you can make respiratory medications work better and help patients breathe. Here are a few suggestions:

- Explain the effects of the drugs and the breathing exercises that are part of patients' treatment. The instructions that come with the drugs will help you do this.
- Assist patients into sitting or leaning positions. These positions allow the lungs to expand fully.
- Give drugs on time. Many respiratory drugs are ordered just before busy times of the day to prevent the fatigue that comes with extra activity. When getting a breath of air is an effort, any added activity can be tiring.
- Remove mucus from the nose and throat (Figure 10.4). Encourage the patient to cough. Regardless of the number of respiratory drugs a patient is taking, mucus in the respiratory tract can still prevent proper air exchange.

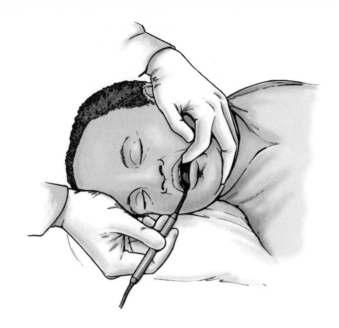

Figure 10.4
When a patient has a respiratory disorder, it is sometimes necessary to suction mucus from the throat and nose.

- Ask the patient to let you know whenever breathing begins to get difficult. Catching a problem early makes drug treatment more effective.
- Do not rush the patient while giving drugs. Rushing increases anxiety when the patient is already anxious because of the effort of catching a breath.
- Give the proper amounts of fluids (e.g., juice, water) with respiratory medications. Expectorants and antitussives should be given with extra fluids. Fluids help thin out respiratory secretions so they can be coughed up and eliminated. Do not give fluids with soothing syrups (demulcents), because they are designed to coat the respiratory tract.
- If a patient has an unproductive cough, remove irritating fumes, dust, and smoke. Provide hard candy or a demulcent to get rid of tickling in the throat.
- Add moisture to the air with a humidifier. Dry mucous membranes can become irritated and are more prone to infection.
- Remember that some respiratory drugs, especially antihistamines, may cause drowsiness. Warn patients not to drive a car or operate heavy equipment while taking them. This is true of many OTC products as well as prescription drugs. Some doctors avoid antihistamines because they tend to dry secretions, causing dry mouth and urinary retention.
- Instruct the family in taking measures to assist the patient's breathing. Well-informed family members can encourage a patient to cooperate in treatment.

RESPIRATORY THERAPY

Many patients with lung disorders are treated with some form of respiratory therapy. They inhale drugs such as bronchodilators, **mucolytics** (drugs that liquify or break down tenacious mucus so it can be coughed up more easily), corticosteroids, and antibiotics from machines that produce mists containing tiny droplets of medications.

Drugs inhaled as a mist are able to travel deep into the lungs. They are absorbed directly through the linings of the respiratory tract or through the alveoli, depending on the size of the droplets. Drugs that are absorbed by the alveoli have a rapid systemic effect because of the richness of the blood supply. Drug absorption through the linings of the respiratory tract is like that of topical applications to mucous membranes.

Most inhalation therapy is delivered to patients via pocket-sized, hand-held **nebulizers.** Because this therapy is self-administered, it is important to teach patients how to use the nebulizer properly. (See Practice Procedure 10.4 on page 198.)

Order of Administration. Many patients are prescribed more than one drug for inhalation. When this is the case, there is a preferred order in which the drugs should be taken. Inhaled drugs should be given in this order: (1) beta-agonist (metaproterenol, albuterol, or pirbuterol), (2) anticholinergic (ipratroprium), (3) corticosteroid (beclomethasone, triamcinolone, or flunisolide).

USE OF OXYGEN

Oxygen is a gas that is essential for life. It is colorless, odorless, and tasteless. Although it is not flammable, it is combustible. Without oxygen, cells die within a few minutes. Lack of oxygen is called **hypoxia.** The goal of oxygen therapy is to relieve hypoxia and maximize the blood's oxygen-carrying ability.

Too much oxygen, generally 100 percent for more than six hours, leads to oxygen toxicity. Consistently high levels of oxygen inactivate the pulmonary surfactant and lead to acute respiratory distress syndrome. Careful assessment of the patient's needs can prevent oxygen toxicity. Symptoms of oxygen toxicity are chest pain; nausea and vomiting; malaise; fatigue; nasal stuffiness; sore throat; dry, hacking cough; and numbness and tingling of the extremities.

Oxygen should be considered a drug and prescribed and administered as such. There must be specific written orders for the flow rate and the method of administration. The initial dose, as well as any changes in administration and dose, including discontinuation, should be based on blood gas analysis or pulse oximetry. Pulse oximetry allows indirect measurement of the blood's oxygen content. A probe with a light and a sensor is attached to the bridge of the nose, an ear, or a fingernail. A reading occurs within 10 to 30 seconds.

Methods of administering oxygen include the nasal cannula, nasal catheter, oxygen mask, and possibly an oxygen tent or a face tent (Figure 10.5). In some situations, incubators or respirators may be used. An oxygen tent is used mainly with children or with patients who will not tolerate other modes of administration. To prevent dryness of the nose and throat, sterile distilled water is added to the humidifying device. Because oxygen is a dry gas, adequate humidity is crucial. You must take care to keep combustible materials away from where oxygen is being used. These include woolen blankets, clothing, and electrical equipment. And, of course, no one may smoke near oxygen equipment.

Oxygen therapy is never ended abruptly. You must gradually wean the patient by alternating periods of oxygen-supplemented inspiration with periods of breathing without the oxygen.

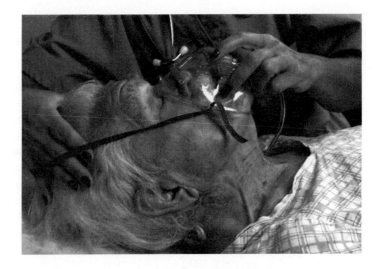

Figure 10.5
An oxygen mask is one method of administering oxygen.

DIRECT APPLICATIONS, SPRAYS, AND NOSE DROPS

Drugs may be painted, sprayed, or dropped onto the mucous membranes of the mouth, nose, and throat. They penetrate directly into the linings of the respiratory tract, but they treat only the sprayed area rather than traveling into the lungs. These topical applications are useful for localized inflammations and for symptoms such as sinus infections, stuffy nose, injuries of the mucous membranes, and sore throat. Decongestants, for example, may often be sprayed or dropped into the nasal cavities to reduce swelling so the patient can breathe more easily (Figure 10.6).

Nose drops should not be swallowed, as they are meant to give a local rather than a systemic effect. The dropper should be rinsed with hot water after use to avoid spreading germs to the medicine bottle.

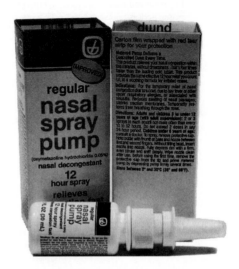

Figure 10.6
Decongestants are sprayed into the nasal cavity to reduce swelling.

REPRESENTATIVE DRUGS FOR THE RESPIRATORY SYSTEM

CATEGORY, NAME[a], AND ROUTE	USES AND DISEASES	ACTIONS	USUAL DOSE[b] AND SPECIAL INSTRUCTIONS	SIDE EFFECTS AND ADVERSE REACTIONS
Antitussives/Expectorants				
Narcotic Codeine Oral	Antitussive	Suppresses cough	10–20 mg every 4–6 hours; do not exceed 120 mg in 24 hours	Nausea, vomiting, constipation, dizziness, palpitations, drowsiness, sedation
Nonnarcotic Dextromethorphan (*Mediquell, Benylin DM*) Oral	Suppression of unproductive cough or cough at bedtime	Inhibits cough reflex	10–20 mg every 4 hours PRN	Drowsiness, dizziness, nausea, vomiting
Acetylcysteine (*Mucomyst*) Inhalant	As auxiliary therapy for patients with abnormal, viscid (thick) mucous secretions	Lowers viscosity of mucus	3–5 ml of a 20% solution or 6–10 ml of a 10% solution inhaled TID or QID	Stomatitis, nausea, vomiting, drowsiness, rhinorrhea

continued

REPRESENTATIVE DRUGS FOR THE RESPIRATORY SYSTEM (continued)

CATEGORY, NAME[a], AND ROUTE	USES AND DISEASES	ACTIONS	USUAL DOSE[b] AND SPECIAL INSTRUCTIONS	SIDE EFFECTS AND ADVERSE REACTIONS
Decongestants				
Phenylephrine (*Neo-Synephrine*) Nasal solution	Nasal congestion	Shrinks engorged mucous membranes	*Nasal spray:* 2–3 sprays into each nostril BID for 3–5 days *Drops:* 2 or 3 drops into each nostril BID for 3–5 days	Burning, stinging, sneezing, dryness of nasal mucosa
Antihistamines				
Promethazine (*Phenergan*) Oral	Allergic rhinitis, pruritus	Provides antihistaminic action	25 mg at bedtime or 12.5 mg before meals and at bedtime	Sedation, drowsiness, blurred vision, dryness of mouth, possible confusion, hypotension, urinary retention
Chlorpheniramine (*Teldrin*) Oral	Rhinitis, allergy symptoms	Provides antihistaminic action	2–4 mg every 4–6 hours	Dryness of mouth, drowsiness, dizziness, nausea, urinary retention
Bronchodilators				
Methylxanthine Derivatives Theophylline (*Elixophyllin*) Oral	Bronchial asthma, bronchitis, emphysema	Relaxes smooth muscle of bronchioles, increases mucociliary clearance	330–660 mg PO every 6–8 hours; give oral form with full glass of water; should be given with food to avoid upset stomach; do not crush sustained-release tablets	Headache, dizziness, restlessness, nausea, vomiting, insomnia, tachycardia, irritability, palpitations
B$_2$-Adrenergic Agonists Albuterol (*Proventil, Ventolin*) Oral; inhalation	Asthma, bronchitis	bronchodilation	*Oral:* 2–4 mg TID or QID, not to exceed 32 mg daily *Inhalation:* 4–6 times daily; start with one inhalation, following with second inhalation in 3–5 minutes if no relief Rinse mouth with water between doses to prevent throat irritation and cough	Tremor, anxiety, nervousness, and restlessness
Epinephrine (*Primatene Mist*) Inhalation	Bronchodilation	Relaxes smooth muscles of bronchioles, increases mucociliary clearance	1 inhalation, wait at least 1 minute; if not relieved, use once more; do not repeat for at least 4 hours; if still no relief, call physician	Nervousness, headache, restlessness, palpitations, tachycardia

CATEGORY, NAME[a], AND ROUTE	USES AND DISEASES	ACTIONS	USUAL DOSE[b] AND SPECIAL INSTRUCTIONS	SIDE EFFECTS AND ADVERSE REACTIONS
Antitubercular Drugs				
Isoniazid (*INH*) Oral, IM	Treatment and prevention of tuberculosis	Bactericidal, interferes with lipid and DNA synthesis	5 mg PO or IM daily in active TB; 300 mg once daily; used for 1 year alone for TB prevention; used in conjunction with effective agents, rifampin and ethambutol for active TB	Peripheral neuropathy most common adverse effect (treated with vitamin B$_6$), nausea, vomiting, and epigastric distress, hepatitis
Rifampin (*Rifadin, Rimactane*) Oral	Treatment of tuberculosis and for carriers of meningitis	Broad-spectrum bactericidal antibiotic that inhibits RNA	600 mg once daily	Hepatotoxicity; flulike symptoms; drowsiness, epigastric distress

[a]Trade names given in parentheses are examples only. Check current drug references for a complete listing of available products.
[b]Average adult doses are given. However, dosages are determined by a physician and vary with the purpose of the therapy and the particular patient. The doses presented in this text are for general information only.

PRACTICE PROCEDURE 10.1

Spraying Medication Onto Mucous Membranes of the Mouth or Throat

■ EQUIPMENT

Physician's medication order, Kardex, medicine card, or medication record

Medication in atomizer, plastic spray bottle, or tube applicator

Flashlight, tongue blade, and cotton-tipped applicator

Medication tray or cart with appropriate charts and records

■ PROCEDURE

1. Set up medications. Check for the "five rights."

2. Wash your hands.

3. Identify the patient, explain the procedure, and assist the patient into a position for medication administration (either sitting up or lying down).

4. Apply medication as follows:

   • Tilt the head backward and open the mouth.
   • Locate the affected area visually. Use a tongue blade and small flashlight to find the area.
   • Spray the medication directly on the affected area.

5. Assist the patient back into a comfortable position.

6. Instruct the patient not to eat or drink for a certain period of time. Allow the patient to gargle with a mouthwash after a sufficient period of time for absorption (at least 15 minutes).

7. Chart the administration of medications.

8. Wash your hands.

9. Return equipment and charts to the proper location.

Demonstrate this procedure for your instructor.

PRACTICE PROCEDURE 10.2

Instilling Nose Drops

■ EQUIPMENT

Medication orders for nose drops

Medication record, medicine cards, or Kardex

Nose drops

Cart or tray with appropriate charts and records

Tissue wipes

■ PROCEDURE

1. Set up medications. Check for the "five rights."

2. Wash your hands.

3. Identify the patient. Explain the procedure. Warm nose drops to body temperature by holding them in your hand or placing them in a bowl of warm water.

4. Instruct the patient to blow the nose to remove mucus and secretions that can block distribution of the medication.

5. Instruct the patient to assume a supine position for administration. For nose drops, the patient should lie on the back, with the head extended beyond the edge of the bed or with a pillow under the shoulders. Support the head with your hand to avoid straining the neck muscles. The head should be either tilted back at a right angle to the body or tilted back and to one side, depending on the affected area (Figure 10.7).

6. Instruct the patient on the correct administration of nose drops.

   • Measure the correct dosage on the marked dropper.
   • Hold the dropper ½-inch above the nares.
   • Instill the prescribed number of drops toward the midline of the ethmoid bone, which makes up the upper part of the nasal septum, to facilitate even distribution over the nasal mucosa. Repeat with the other nostril, if ordered.
   • Instruct the patient to stay in the supine position for at least 5 minutes to prevent loss of medication through the nares.
   • Give tissue wipes to blot any flow from the nose. Instruct the patient to avoid blowing nose for several minutes.

Continued

7. Give further instructions to the patient according to the package directions or the physician's orders.

8. Chart the medication administration, including whether you treated one or both nostrils.

9. Wash your hands.

10. Return equipment and charts to the proper location.

Demonstrate this procedure for your instructor.

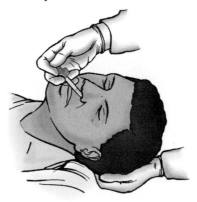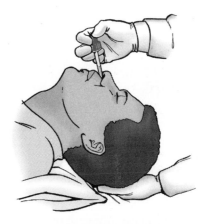

Figure 10.7
Instilling nose drops.

PRACTICE PROCEDURE 10.3
Using a Nasal Spray

■ EQUIPMENT

Medication orders for nasal spray

Medication record, medicine, or Kardex

Nasal spray

Cart or tray with appropriate charts and records

Tissue wipes

■ PROCEDURE

1. Set up medications. Check for the "five rights."

2. Wash your hands.

3. Identify the patient. Explain the procedure.

4. Instruct the patient on the proper position for administration. For nasal spray, the patient should be in a sitting position.

5. Teach the patient correct administration of the nasal spray.

- Instruct the patient to breathe through the nose with the mouth open. The patient must breathe this way as the medication is administered.
- Instruct the patient to place the tip of the bottle at the opening of the nose, taking care not to touch the mucous membrane.
- Tell the patient to take a deep breath and, at this time, spray the bottle two or three times quickly.
- Wipe any excess medication from the nose.

Continued

6. Give further instructions to the patient according to the package directions or the physician's orders.

7. Chart the medication administration.

8. Wash your hands.

9. Return equipment to the proper location.

Demonstrate this procedure for your instructor or the nurse in charge.

PRACTICE PROCEDURE 10.4

Oral Inhalation of Metered-Dose Inhalers

■ EQUIPMENT

Physician's medication order, Kardex, medicine record

Medication in atomizer, plastic spray bottle, tube applicator, or metered-dose inhaler

Medication tray, cart, or equipment with appropriate charts and records

■ PROCEDURE

1. Set up medications. Check for the "five rights."

2. Wash your hands.

3. Identify the patient, explain the procedure, and assist the patient into a position for medication administration (either sitting up or lying down).

4. Apply medication as follows:
   - Shake the inhaler.
   - Hold the inhaler upright.
   - Instruct the patient to tilt the head back and breathe out.
   - Instruct the patient to position the inhaler in one of two ways:
     (1) Tell the patient to open the mouth, with the inhaler 1 to 2 inches away. The patient may attach a spacer to the mouthpiece of the inhaler. (A spacer is a device that traps the medication released from the inhaler. The patient then inhales the drug from the spacer. Spacers deposit 80 percent of the medication in the lungs instead of in the oropharynx. Spacers are especially effective for patients who have trouble learning the correct way to use an inhaler, and for weak or elderly patients.)
     (2) Instruct the patient to place the mouthpiece of inhaler or spacer in the mouth.
   - Tell the patient to press down on the inhaler while inhaling.
   - Tell the patient to breathe in slowly for 2 to 3 seconds and hold breath for 10 seconds.
   - Wait 1 minute before administering additional puffs.

5. If two inhaled medications are ordered, wait 5 to 10 minutes between inhalations.

6. Assist the patient back into a comfortable position.

7. Instruct the patient to rinse the mouth and throat with a drink of water.

8. Chart administration of medications.

9. Wash your hands.

10. Return equipment and charts to the proper location.

Demonstrate this procedure for your instructor.

Administering Oxygen by Mask

■ **EQUIPMENT**

Physician's order and appropriate charting record

Oxygen (tank or wall oxygen outlet system)

Humidifier equipment as ordered

Mask as ordered (Figure 10.8)

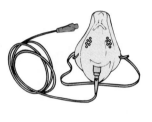 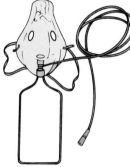 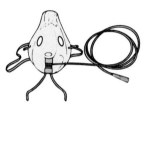 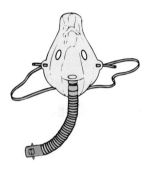

Simple face mask
(Low-flow system)

Partial rebreather mask
(Low-flow system)

Nonrebreather mask
(Low-flow system)

Venturi mask
(High-flow system)

Figure 10.8
Masks for oxygen administration.

EQUIPMENT	PERCENTAGE OXYGEN	FLOW RATE
Simple face mask	35%	Low flow: 6–10 liters/min
Partial rebreather mask	60–90%	Low flow: 10 liters/min
Nonbreather	80–95%	Low flow: 10 liters/min
Venturi mask	24, 28, 35, 40%	High flow: 4, 6, 8, 10 liters/min
Face tent with Venturi mask	30–55%	High flow: 4–8 liters/min

■ **PROCEDURE**

1. Set up oxygen equipment.

2. Wash your hands.

3. Identify the patient and explain the procedure.

4. Assist the patient into an appropriate position (**semi-Fowler's position**—the patient's upper body is elevated to 30°—or **Fowler's position**—45° to 60°).

5. Inflate one-half of a rebreather bag with oxygen. (The rebreather bag conserves oxygen.)

6. Place the top of the mask over the nose and then over the mouth.

7. Mold the mask to the face so that oxygen does not escape from it.

8. Turn on oxygen as ordered (see above).

Continued

9. After 30 minutes, check the flow rate and rebreather bag.

10. Chart the procedure.

Demonstrate this procedure for your instructor.

PRACTICE PROCEDURE 10.6

Administering Oxygen by Cannula

■ EQUIPMENT

Physician's order

Oxygen (tank or wall oxygen outlet system)

Humidifier equipment as ordered

Paper tape

Gauze pads (2 × 2)

Rubber gloves (nonsterile)

Cannula (Figure 10.9)

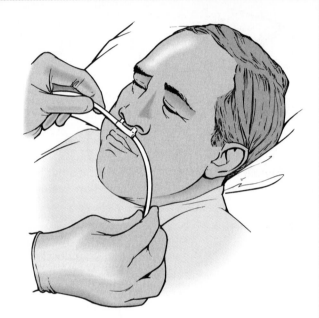

Figure 10.9
Cannula for
oxygen
administration.

■ PROCEDURE

1. Set up oxygen supply equipment.

2. Wash your hands.

3. Put on rubber gloves.

4. Identify the patient and explain the procedure.

5. Assist the patient into a semi-Fowler's or Fowler's position.

6. Turn on the oxygen at the ordered rate flow system (usually 1 to 6 liters/min of a 23 percent to 40 percent concentration of oxygen for the cannula).

7. Check the tubing to be sure it is not twisted.

8. Place your fingertips near the opening of the cannula to check for oxygen flow.

9. Turn the nasal prongs upward and curved toward the tip of the nose.

10. Place one prong in each nostril.

11. Place tubing from the prongs over the ears.

12. Pull remainder of tubing under the patient's chin and tighten at "Y".

13. Ask the patient if tubing is comfortable.

Continued

14. Tape tubing in place on the cheeks if necessary.

15. Place gauze pads under tubing going over the ears if necessary.

16. After 30 minutes, check flow rate and humidifier water level.

17. Chart the procedure.

Demonstrate this procedure for your instructor.

PRACTICE PROCEDURE 10.7

Administering Oxygen by Nasal Catheter

■ EQUIPMENT

Physician's order and appropriate charting record

Oxygen (tank or wall oxygen outlet system)

Humidifier equipment as ordered

Paper tape

Gauze pads (2 × 2)

Lubricating jelly (water-soluble)

Flashlight

Tongue blade

Container of sterile water

Nasal catheter as ordered for an adult or child (Figure 10.10)

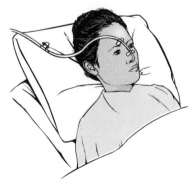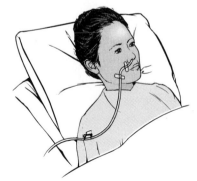

Figure 10.10
Nasal catheter
for oxygen
administration.

■ PROCEDURE

1. Set up oxygen equipment.

2. Wash your hands.

3. Put on rubber gloves.

4. Identify the patient and explain the procedure.

Continued

5. Assist the patient into a semi-Fowler's or Fowler's position.

6. Lubricate catheter with water-soluble lubricating jelly.

7. Pass catheter through the nose until tip is just above the epiglottis.

8. Do not insert the catheter too far, or the patient will swallow air.

9. Tape the catheter to the forehead or nose.

10. Turn on oxygen at the ordered slow rate flow (commonly 4 to 8 liters/min of a 25 percent to 40 percent concentration of oxygen).

11. After 30 minutes, check flow rate and humidifier water level.

12. Chart the procedure.

Demonstrate this procedure for your instructor.

Define each of the terms listed below.

1. Pulmonary _____

2. Dyspnea _____

3. Tachypnea _____

4. Apnea _____

5. Hyperpnea _____

6. Hyperventilation _____

7. Pleura _____

8. Rebound effect _____

Complete the following statements by filling in the blanks.

9. Inhaling and exhaling air so that gases can be exchanged in the lungs is called _____ _____.

10. The part of the respiratory tract that is shared with the digestive system is the _____ _____.

11. The part of the respiratory system that produces speech sounds is called the _____ _____.

12. The flap of tissue that keeps food from going down into the lungs when it is swallowed is the _____.

13. The tube that leads to the lungs and is known as the windpipe is the _____ _____.

14. The two tubes that branch from the windpipe and lead into the right and left lungs are the _____.

15. The tiny sacs where gases are exchanged between the blood and inspired air are the _____ _____.

16. The instrument used to listen to breathing sounds is the _____ _____.

17. A hand-held device that produces a drug mist for inhalation is called a(n) _____ _____.

Tell what these types of drugs do; for example, Demulcents coat mucous membranes and soothe irritation that causes coughing.

18. Antitussives _____

19. Mucolytics _____

20. Decongestants _____

Match the drug names to the drug categories.

_____ 21. *Neo-Synephrine, Afrin*   a. decongestants

_____ 22. *Benadryl,* chlorpheniramine, *Teldrin, Periactin*   b. tuberculosis drugs

Continued

_____ 23. Isoniazid, ethambutol, rifampin, rifapentine   c. bronchodilators

_____ 24. *Slo-bid*, *Theolair*, theophylline   d. antihistamines

Match the treatment to the description.

_____ 25. Positioning the patient so that clogged mucus is drawn   a. antihistamines
out by gravity

          b. nebulizer

_____ 26. Clapping the patient's chest or back to loosen mucus   c. percussion

_____ 27. Machine that helps a patient breathe by artificial means   d. postural drainage

_____ 28. Device that produces a mist for inhalation   e. ventilator

_____ 29. May cause drowsiness as a side effect

■ CASE STUDIES FOR CRITICAL THINKING

Answer the following questions in the spaces provided.

30. Give at least three reasons why tuberculosis is becoming more common. _____

_____

_____

_____

31. Describe the difference between bronchodilators and expectorants. _____

_____

_____

_____

Select the disorder that best matches each description. Write the name of the disorder in the blank.

Bronchitis   Asthma   Pneumonia

Tuberculosis   Emphysema

32. In a small town in Asia, Grandfather Kim has had a lung disease for a long time. He is very weak and is coughing up blood. The public health worker is worried that Kim's grandchildren will catch the disease from him.

_____

33. Nancy Epstein suffers from frequent attacks of wheezing, coughing, and shortness of breath. She can control these attacks by inhaling epinephrine and avoiding dust and mold.

_____

34. Mr. Smith can never take a deep breath because he cannot exhale completely. He does breathing exercises every day and takes expectorants and bronchodilators to help his condition.

_____

35. Sue Bosworth has a viral infection of the upper respiratory tract. Her doctor instructs her to drink plenty of fluids so that she can cough up the sputum that is clogging her air passage.

_____

Continued

36. Frank Fernandez was recovering from the flu when he developed a bacterial infection. The infection has now blocked his alveoli with pus, making it difficult for him to breathe.

_____

■ APPLICATIONS

Obtain a current copy of a drug reference book or the PDR®.

37. Use Section 4 of the *PDR®*, Generic and Chemical Name Index, to find another product name for each of the drugs listed on pages 193–195 of this text.

38. In Section 3 of the *PDR®*, Product Category Index, find the Allergy Relief Products. List all the drugs named.

 *Inter*NET CONNECTION

To learn more about asthma and medications used to treat asthma, go to http://www.aaaai.org, the Web site of the American Academy of Allergy, Asthma, and Immunology. Click on Patient/Public Resource Center to get facts about asthma and allergic diseases.

11

Drugs for the Gastrointestinal System

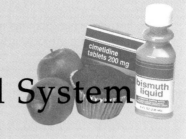

In this chapter you will learn about the organs of digestion and elimination. You will learn what they do, what happens to them when they are diseased, and how drugs are used to treat their disorders. You will also learn procedures to follow in giving gastrointestinal medications.

OBJECTIVES

After studying this chapter, you should be able to

- state the five main functions of the gastrointestinal system.
- name the major parts of the gastrointestinal system and tell what they do.
- use correct medical terms to describe symptoms of gastrointestinal disorders.
- describe the major gastrointestinal disorders for which drugs are given.
- discuss the actions and give examples of the following drug groups: antacids, histamine H$_2$-receptor antagonists, digestants, antiflatulents, emetics, antiemetics, anticholinergics and antispasmodics, antidiarrheals, laxatives, antihelmintics, and anorexiants.
- state three important conditions to be aware of when giving medications for the gastrointestinal system.
- describe and follow proper procedure for inserting rectal suppositories.
- describe and follow proper procedure for giving medications through a nasogastric or gastrostomy tube.

KEY TERMS

antacid: drug that neutralizes hydrochloric acid in the stomach

anticholinergic: drug that acts on the autonomic nervous system to reduce intestinal motility and slow production of stomach acid

antidiarrheal: drug that slows intestinal motility and helps produce formed stools instead of loose, watery stools

antiemetic: drug that prevents or relieves nausea and vomiting

antiflatulent: drug that relieves gassiness and bloating; also called carminative

antihelmintic: drug that eliminates intestinal parasites

antispasmodic: drug that acts on the smooth muscle of the intestines to relieve cramping

anus: distal (far-end) opening of the gastrointestinal tract through which feces are eliminated

astringent: drug (applied to skin) designed to shrink and dry swollen tissues

bile: digestive juice produced by the liver and stored in the gallbladder; helps digest fats

chyme: food mixed with gastric secretions

cirrhosis: chronic, progressive disease of the liver characterized by degeneration and destruction of the liver cells

colon: the main part of the large intestine

defecation: passage of feces out of the body; bowel movement

digestant: drug that aids digestion by replacing digestive enzymes that are missing due to diseases such as stomach cancer, pernicious anemia, or pancreatitis

duodenum: first portion of the small intestine, just past the stomach

dyspepsia: indigestion

emesis: vomiting; reversal of peristalsis

emetic: drug that causes vomiting

endoscope: a flexible, tubelike instrument used to view the inside of the body

enzyme: substance that assists chemical changes (e.g., digestion)

eructation: belching, burping

esophagus: portion of the gastrointestinal tract leading from the mouth and pharynx to the stomach

feces: solid waste products remaining after food is digested and nutrients are absorbed; also called stools

flatulence: gas in the stomach and intestines

gallbladder: storage pouch for bile

gastric: pertaining to the stomach

gastrointestinal (GI) tract: body tube leading from the mouth through the anus, through which food passes, nutrients are absorbed, and solid wastes are eliminated; also known as the alimentary canal or digestive tract

gastrostomy tube: tube inserted through a stoma into the stomach, used for tube feeding and administration of medications

hepatitis: inflammation of the liver

histamine H$_2$-receptor antagonist: drug that inhibits gastric acid secretion

hyperacidity: too much acid (e.g., in the stomach, esophagus)

intestinal motility: movement or excitability of the smooth muscles lining the gastrointestinal tract; speed of peristalsis

laxative: drug that promotes defecation either to relieve constipation or to clear the bowel before surgery; also called cathartic or purgative

liver: organ that filters blood, stores and releases nutrients into the blood, and is involved in biotransformation or excretion of some drugs and other substances

nasogastric tube: tube inserted through the nose and down the esophagus into the stomach, used for tube feeding and administration of medications

pancreas: organ that secretes strong digestive enzymes that empty into the duodenum; also secretes insulin that passes directly into the bloodstream

peptic: pertaining to digestion in the stomach

peristalsis: rhythmic contractions of the smooth muscles lining the gastrointestinal tract, for moving food and waste materials through the system

rectum: distal (far-end) portion of the large intestine

saliva: digestive juice secreted by salivary glands in the mouth; breaks down certain sugars, moistens and coats food for easy swallowing

small intestine: composed of the duodenum, jejunum, and ileum, where most absorption takes place after food intake

stoma: surgically produced opening in the stomach or the abdomen

ulcer: open sore or break in the lining of the stomach (peptic ulcer) or duodenum (duodenal ulcer); can break through the gastrointestinal lining into the abdominal cavity (perforated ulcer)

villi: small, fingerlike projections of the intestinal lining that provide a large surface area for absorption of nutrients into the bloodstream

GASTROINTESTINAL SYSTEM

Food is vital to survival. Every cell requires nourishment to carry on its life functions. But cells cannot use the food we eat just as it enters the body. The food must first undergo mechanical and chemical changes that break it down into particles small enough to pass through cell walls. This function is carried out by the gastrointestinal (GI) system, also known as the digestive system. There are five steps in the digestive process.

Step 1. Breaking up food into smaller pieces. This is a mechanical action. It is performed by the mouth and its accessory parts, the tongue and the teeth, with the aid of the salivary glands.

Step 2. Transporting food through the GI tract. The **gastrointestinal (GI) tract** (also known as the digestive tract or alimentary canal) is one long tube passing from the mouth to the rectum. Rhythmic contractions of the lining of the GI tract push food along this passageway. These muscle movements are called **peristalsis.** By moving food along, peristalsis puts the food in contact with physical and chemical processes that take place in different parts of the system.

Step 3. Secreting digestive enzymes. Glands in the mouth, in the lining of the stomach, and in the accessory organs (liver, small bowel, and pancreas) all secrete **enzymes,** which are chemical substances that aid digestion. Digestion is a series of chemical changes that break down food particles into basic nutrients that can be used by cells: namely, amino acids (proteins), fats, minerals, vitamins, sugars, and water.

Step 4. Absorbing nutrients into the blood. After being broken down into its smallest parts, food is absorbed from the small intestine into the bloodstream. From there it circulates to all the cells of the body to supply fuel for energy production and growth.

Step 5. Excreting solid waste products. This function takes place in the large intestine and the rectum. Undigested substances, like plant fibers, are not absorbed into the blood but pass into the large intestine. The large intestine prepares these substances for elimination from the body.

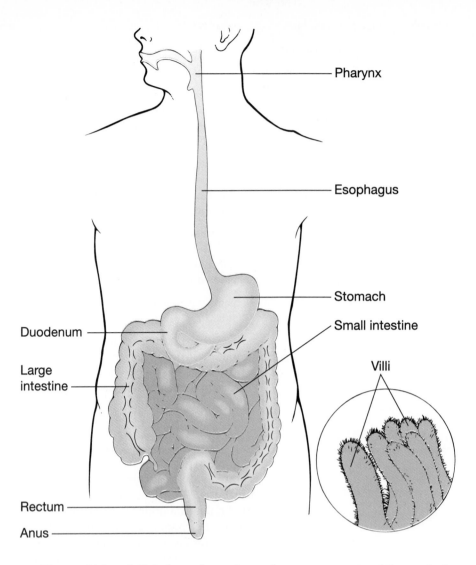

Figure 11.1
The gastro-
intestinal tract.

Pharynx

Esophagus

Stomach

Small intestine

Villi

Duodenum

Large
intestine

Rectum

Anus

Figures 11.1 and 11.2 show the major and accessory parts of the gastrointestinal tract.

ORGANS OF DIGESTION

Mouth. The teeth and the tongue work together to break food into small pieces. The tongue moves food into position so it can be chewed by the teeth. Teeth have different shapes that make them suitable for cutting, tearing, and grinding food. Even before chewing begins, the salivary glands start to produce a fluid called **saliva.** Saliva helps dissolve food and coats it so that it can be easily swallowed. Saliva also begins to act on carbohydrates (starchy foods) to turn them into sugars.

Esophagus. Recall from Chapter 10 that when a person swallows, the epiglottis closes to prevent food from entering the lungs. The food then passes into the **esophagus,** the part of the GI tract that extends from the pharynx to the stomach. Chunks of food are pushed down the esophagus by peristaltic movements of the tube lining. When the stomach is irritated, peristalsis may take place in the opposite direction, and vomiting will probably result.

Stomach. The stomach is a gourd-shaped pouch that can expand to hold up to 2 quarts of food and liquid. Valves at the entrance and exit of the stomach control the intake and outlet of food. The stomach lining is dotted with over 35 million tiny glands that secrete **gastric** (pertaining to the stomach) juice. Gastric juice consists of stomach acid and digestive enzymes. Stomach acid is an important factor in digestion. It dissolves food, destroys bacteria, and breaks down connective tissue in meats. After entering the stomach, food

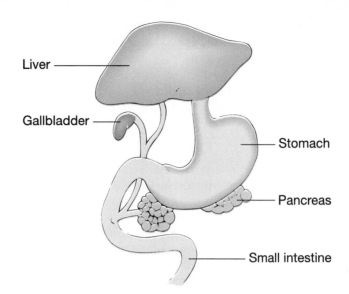

Figure 11.2
Accessory organs of the gastrointestinal system.

is churned around by muscles in the stomach wall and mixed with gastric juice. Food remains in the stomach for about 3 hours, with a range of 1 to 7 hours. By this time it has become an acidic, liquified mass (**chyme**).

Small Intestine. The section of the small intestine closest to the stomach is called the **duodenum.** As soon as food enters the duodenum, it is doused with strong digestive enzymes from the liver and pancreas. These juices complete the process of breaking down food into molecules of protein, sugar, fat, minerals, and so on. The **small intestine** is a long, coiled tube about 20 feet long. It also secretes a fluid rich in digestive enzymes that helps to break down fats, proteins, and carbohydrates. Its walls are lined with tiny fingerlike projections called **villi.** The villi are responsible for absorbing nutrients into the bloodstream. They have thin walls, and, because of their shape, provide a huge surface area for absorption to take place. Tiny capillaries and lymph ducts in the villi take in the nutrients and transport them to the liver. From there they are released into the bloodstream as needed. By the time food has passed through all 20 feet of the small intestine, most of the nutrients have been absorbed. All that is left is indigestible materials mixed with water. The other sections of the small intestine include the jejunum and ileum. The jejunum is the middle part of the small intestine and makes up two-fifths of the whole small intestine. The lowest part of the intestine is the ileum. It connects two folds of intestinal membrane, which make up an exit and entryway or valve. This is the ileocecal valve, which prevents the backflow of contents of the colon, feces, into the ileum.

Large Intestine. The large intestine, also known as the **colon,** is much shorter and wider than the small intestine. It is about 5 to 6 feet long. In the large intestine, excess water is absorbed into the bloodstream, leaving undigested wastes. These are collected and compacted into semisolid masses, called **feces** or stools. The feces leave the body by way of the **rectum** and its opening, the **anus.**

Liver and Gallbladder. The **liver** is the largest gland in the body and serves many functions. Its role in the GI system is to secrete **bile,** a substance that aids in digesting fats. Bile is collected in a storage pouch called the **gallbladder** until it is needed for digestion. The liver stores nutrients absorbed from the small intestine. The liver also removes certain waste products from the blood, and it produces important substances for blood clotting and the immune system.

The liver is important in drug action because it breaks down or inactivates many drugs. Patients with poor liver function can become overdosed with some routinely administered drugs because their livers are unable to break down the drugs quickly.

Pancreas. The **pancreas** is another large glandular organ that has several functions. It produces digestive juices that complete the chemical changes that turn fats, proteins, and carbohydrates into particles that can be absorbed. The pancreas also secretes insulin, a hormone that regulates the amount of sugar used by the cells (see Chapter 14). Insulin is released directly into the bloodstream. It does not enter into digestion.

AUTONOMIC CONTROL

Peristalsis and the secretion of digestive enzymes are both under the control of the autonomic nervous system. This means that people cannot consciously control what goes on in their stomachs and intestines. It also means that digestion is affected by stress.

When the autonomic nervous system prepares the body to meet danger or stress, the muscular movements of the stomach and intestine slow down. Digestive enzyme production slows down, too. In other cases, peristalsis and enzyme secretion are stimulated needlessly by nervous tension. Therefore, chronically nervous or anxious people tend to have overactive digestion. Mild sedatives or tranquilizers are sometimes used to calm these reactions and restore normal digestion.

DISORDERS OF THE GASTROINTESTINAL SYSTEM

SYMPTOMS

The symptoms of GI disorders are quite familiar. Hardly anyone has escaped occasional nausea, vomiting, constipation, diarrhea, indigestion (**dyspepsia**), heartburn (**hyperacidity**), gassiness, stomachache, and abdominal cramps. The symptoms have many causes. They can be the result of passing irritations, flu, mild food poisoning, psychological stress, or side effects of drugs. Or they can signal more serious underlying diseases. Drugs can relieve some GI symptoms, but the underlying disease must be treated to achieve permanent relief.

Nausea is a queasy feeling in the stomach arising from many causes, such as infection, radiation treatment, psychological stimulation, reaction to a drug, pregnancy, poisoning, or stomach irritation. Sometimes this feeling leads to vomiting, or **emesis.** Vomiting is a protective mechanism to rid the body of spoiled or irritating foods and liquids. The contents of the stomach are emptied as peristalsis switches direction and carries food back up the esophagus. Too much vomiting is dangerous because it can remove essential fluids and electrolytes, such as potassium, from the body. It is also dangerous because it keeps the body from digesting and absorbing needed nutrients.

Heartburn is a burning sensation in the pit of the stomach that may be felt in the esophagus and the throat as well. It is often felt along with sour belching. Indigestion is a gassy or bloated feeling in the stomach. Both heartburn and indigestion may be the result of poor eating habits or psychological tension. A bland diet, mild sedatives, and simple antacids help to relieve passing symptoms. Of course, if symptoms persist, an underlying cause must be looked for.

Burping, belching (**eructation),** and passing gas are common symptoms of GI irritation. The gas (flatus) comes from chemical reactions that release gases into the GI system. It also comes from swallowing air along with food and drink. Excess gas can cause pressure, pain, and a bloated feeling. Cramping or griping of the digestive tract is also common with many disorders. Cramps are the result of muscle spasms in the walls of the stomach and intestines.

Constipation is the failure to have regular bowel movements. It can be due to hardened feces, slow movement of the intestine, lack of fiber and fluids in the diet, psychological factors, or lack of physical activity. Constipation is of concern when it causes straining at stool or when it threatens to block the intestines. Normal bowel elimination may vary from 3 times a day to once every 3 days. Different people have different schedules, and no one should be concerned if he or she does not have a bowel movement every single day. **Laxatives** (drugs that promote bowel movement) are much overused. Elderly people who do not have a daily bowel movement may take laxatives every day and become dependent on the drug, which can cause serious problems. Laxatives can further potentiate constipation and irregularity but may cause lazy bowel syndrome, which means the colon needs a laxative to artificially cause stimulation to produce a bowel movement.

Diarrhea means passing loose, watery stools or passing stools too often. It is often accompanied by abdominal cramps, which signal irritation in the large intestine. Diarrhea is the result of increased peristalsis. It has many underlying causes, including these:

- Intestinal infection
- Psychological factors (stress, anxiety)
- Food allergies
- Food intolerance (greasy and spicy foods; alcohol; coffee)
- Certain medications (antacids containing magnesium; antibiotics; antineoplastics)
- Certain diseases (irritable bowel syndrome; diverticulitis; cancer)

As in the case of diarrhea, many disorders either result from or cause changes in the speed at which nutrients are carried through the GI tract. The term used to refer to the speed of peristalsis is **intestinal motility.** Changes in motility lead to either diarrhea or constipation. Nervous tension, infections, drugs, and many other factors affect intestinal motility.

Abdominal or stomach pain sometimes accompanies GI disorders. The pain can be the result of gas pressure, irritation, or more serious problems. Especially in the case of abdominal pain, it is important not to give medications until a search has been made for an underlying cause. Treating abdominal pain with an analgesic may delay discovery of something serious like appendicitis.

Other symptoms to look for are difficulty in swallowing (dysphagia), loss of appetite (anorexia), sudden or severe weight loss, and change in the appearance of the stools (bloody, tarry, clay-colored, or containing excess mucus).

MAJOR DISORDERS

GI symptoms can be about the same for minor problems and serious problems. A physician may order tests (X rays, blood tests, etc.) to find an underlying cause for the symptoms. Special flexible fiberoptic instruments (**endoscopes**) may be used to visually examine the walls of the stomach, intestine, or rectum.

Tooth and Gum Disorders. Problems with the teeth, gums, or dentures can lead to GI problems. Unless the teeth and gums are in good condition, eating and drinking may be painful or inefficient. Patients may avoid hard-to-chew foods, including foods that would help keep their bowel movements regular (e.g., fruits, vegetables, and grain products high in bulk and fiber content). Some of the main tooth and gum disorders are dental abscess (which can result from neglect or severe tooth decay), gingivitis, pyorrhea, trench mouth (Vincent's infection), and stomatitis. They are treated with antibiotics, surgical removal of diseased tissue, or special cleaning procedures. Many toothpastes have fluoride added to them and are recommended by the American Dental Association. Fluoride rinses and tablets are also available. Fluoride helps prevent tooth decay (caries). Elderly persons, patients in long-term care, and people who are being fed with a tube may require your help in maintaining their oral hygiene.

Gastritis. Gastritis is an inflammation of the stomach, signaled by epigastric tenderness, nausea, vomiting, and a sense of fullness. It may be caused by accidentally swallowing caustic substances. It also results from normal use of irritants such as coffee, alcohol, and tobacco. The condition may be temporary, or it may persist for months, causing damage to the stomach lining. Treatment involves removing the cause as well as treating the symptoms.

Peptic Ulcer Disease. Peptic ulcer disease is a broad term encompassing both gastric (stomach) and duodenal (duodenum) ulcers. (**Peptic** pertains to digestion in the stomach.) An **ulcer** is an open sore in the stomach or duodenal lining. The mucous membranes have been broken down by digestive acids so that the underlying tissue is exposed and can be destroyed by the acids.

The causes of ulcers are excessive secretion of hydrochloric acid (HCl), insufficient stomach protection—a breakdown in the gastric mucosal barrier (normally this protects the stomach from autodigestion)—or the presence of Helicobacter pylori (H. pylori). Hypersecretion of hydrochloric acid can be caused by prolonged use of alcohol, cigarettes, coffee, drugs such as aspirin, ibuprofen, and corticosteroids, and by psychological factors. Part of the treatment is to remove the source of irritation (food sources or psychological causes). Drug therapy is aimed at reducing the stomach acid or improving stomach protection. **Antacids** (drugs that neutralize HCl in the stomach) are the initial drugs of choice in the treatment of peptic ulcer disease. **Histamine H_2-receptor antagonists** (drugs that inhibit gastric acid secretion) are also used. Anticholinergics and tricyclic antidepressants are occasionally used. There is divided opinion as to their efficacy in preventing recurrences and in alleviating symptoms. They also have a high incidence of undesirable side effects and must be used with caution.

Liver Disorders. A symptom of many liver disorders is jaundice, a yellowing of the skin. This is due to bilirubin (a yellow pigment) entering the bloodstream, usually because the bile duct is blocked. **Cirrhosis** is a chronic, progressive disease of the liver characterized by degeneration and destruction of the liver cells. This condition is accompanied in the early stages by nausea, weight loss, vomiting, and difficulty in digesting fats. Jaundice, anemia, spiderlike markings on the skin, and a loss of sensation occur in the later stages. Cirrhosis is caused by drinking too much alcohol, toxins to the liver such as large doses of drugs, obstruction of the biliary ducts, and advanced heart failure. Complications include enlarged veins, fluid in the abdomen, and renal and liver failure. It is treated with rest and a high-calorie, high-carbohydrate, low-fat diet. There is no specific drug therapy for cirrhosis. Colbenemid has been used to reduce the scarring of the liver that occurs.

Hepatitis is inflammation of the liver. The most common cause is viral. The types of viral hepatitis are A, B, C, D, and E. Noninfectious hepatitis may be caused by drugs and chemicals. Occasionally, hepatitis is caused by bacteria. Hepatitis B is of major concern to the health care worker because it is bloodborne and may be spread by accidental needle sticks. Both treatment and recovery can take a long time. The Centers for Disease Control and Prevention recommend immunization with the hepatitis B vaccine for all health care workers.

Gallbladder Disorders. Gallstones are small granules, primarily of cholesterol, in the gallbladder. They are thought to be the result of extra concentrated bile. They are common in people over the age of 40, but they do not necessarily cause symptoms. Gallstones can cause trouble if they block the opening of the gallbladder or the tube that carries bile to the intestine. Inflammation of the gallbladder (cholecystitis) most commonly occurs with stones. Cholangitis (inflammation of the biliary ducts) is a complication of stones. Symptoms of gallbladder disease include fever, vomiting, jaundice, and pain in the upper right quadrant of the abdomen. Surgery is frequently indicated for cholelithiasis (gallstones) only. Treatment for cholecystitis is aimed at treating the symptoms. Analgesics and anticholinergics are the most common drugs used to control gallbladder disease. Drugs used to dissolve certain types of gallstones include chenodeoxycholic acid (*Chenix*) and ursodiol (*Actigall*).

Pancreatitis. Pancreatitis is an inflammation of the pancreas that causes severe pain in the left upper quadrant of the abdomen, vomiting, fever, hypotension (low blood pressure), tachycardia (rapid pulse), and jaundice. Shock may occur as a result of hemorrhage. Pancreatitis is treated with analgesics to relieve the pain, IV fluids, bed rest, withdrawing foods, and antibiotics to prevent infections. (Two other disorders of the pancreas, diabetes and hypoglycemia, are described in Chapter 14.)

Enteritis and Ulcerative Colitis. These are inflammations of the small and large intestine, respectively, resulting in diarrhea, fever, pain, anemia, and weight loss. They are treated with antidiarrheals, antibiotics, sulfasalazine (*Azulfidine*), corticosteroids, rest, and a bland diet.

Peritonitis. This is an acute inflammation of the membranes that line the abdomen. Peritonitis is caused by trauma or rupture of an organ releasing bacteria into the abdominal cavity. Abdominal pain and tenderness are the main symptoms. The treatment is surgery to repair the damage and antibiotics to stop the infection.

Irritable Bowel Syndrome. Irritable bowel syndrome (IBS) is not a disease but a group of symptoms characterized by intermittent abdominal pain associated with changes in bowel patterns (diarrhea or constipation). It seems to be related to an intolerance to certain foods or to psychological factors. The condition is generally harmless. Anticholinergics such as dicyclomine (*Bentyl*) may be given before meals to relieve the pain associated with food. A mild sedative may be given, but only for a short time.

Diverticulosis. This is a condition in which multiple pouches (diverticula) develop in the walls of the large intestine. There are generally no symptoms until the pouches become inflamed (diverticulitis). The main symptoms are crampy, left-sided abdominal pain and alternating diarrhea and constipation. Treatment of diverticulitis consists of rest, a high-fiber diet, antibiotics, and bulk laxatives such as psyllium (*Metamucil*). Anticholinergics such as *Bentyl* and *Donnatol* are used to decrease cramping.

Hemorrhoids. Hemorrhoids are enlarged hemorrhoidal veins. They can become swollen and painful, and blood clots may form in them. Problems with hemorrhoids can be averted by not straining during bowel movements and avoiding heavy lifting and prolonged sitting and standing. Suppositories, ointments, and warm sitz baths (immersion of thighs, buttocks, and abdomen) are used to relieve pain in severe cases. Some hemorrhoid preparations, such as *Anusol-HC*, include anti-inflammatory ingredients as well as soothing and lubricating ingredients. Stool softeners such as ducosate (*Colace*) may be given to promote regular bowel movements.

Tumors. Tumors, either benign or malignant, may grow in any part of the GI tract, causing obstruction, bleeding, pressure or rupture, and producing a variety of symptoms. Small outgrowths on the inside of the large intestines, most often found in the rectum or sigmoid colon, are called polyps. All polyps are abnormal and should be biopsied or removed because of their link to colon cancer.

Intestinal Parasites. Intestinal parasites are worms that live in the intestines, such as tapeworms, hookworms, trichina worms, pinworms, and roundworms. Some of these parasites are quite common, and others are found only in certain parts of the world. Most may be prevented by eating properly cooked meats (especially pork), by keeping the hands and nails clean, and by wearing shoes. Children may pick up parasites from playing in dirt or sandboxes.

ANTACIDS

Antacids relieve gastritis and ulcer pain by neutralizing hydrochloric acid in the stomach. Many people take OTC antacids to relieve indigestion as well. Remember, however, that stomach acid is necessary to digestion. Overuse of antacids may actually interfere with proper digestion.

The substances used to neutralize stomach acid are alkaline. When these substances are combined with acids, they cancel each other out chemically. Certain antacids are absorbable. If too much of these are taken, there will be excess alkali that can pass into the intestine and be absorbed. This may cause an imbalance in the body's natural chemistry called alkalosis (see Chapter 12).

The major ingredients in antacids include aluminum salts, calcium carbonate, magnesium salts, and sodium bicarbonate, alone or in combination. Sodium bicarbonate is seldom prescribed because of its high sodium content and because it causes an increase in gastric acid. Common antacids are calcium salts (e.g., calcium carbonate), aluminum salts (e.g., aluminum hydroxide), and magnesium salts (e.g., magnesium hydroxide, oxide, carbonate, and trisilicate). Aluminum hydroxide is sold both generically and under the trade name *Amphojel*. Magnesium hydroxide is the familiar preparation milk of magnesia.

Aluminum salts and calcium salts tend to cause constipation as a side effect. Magnesium salts, on the other hand, tend to cause diarrhea. It is generally believed that combining these substances cancels out the side effects, so there are many preparations that contain both. *Maalox, Gelusil,* and *Mylanta,* for example, are combinations of magnesium salts and aluminum hydroxide. Because antacids are over-the-counter drugs and require no medical supervision, patient education is important.

PATIENT EDUCATION

Antacids

- Aluminum- and calcium-based antacids cause constipation
- Magnesium-based antacids cause diarrhea
- When using chewable antacids, chew them thoroughly
- Avoid milk and milk products when using calcium carbonate antacids

- Avoid antacids containing sodium if one has high blood pressure or cardiac or renal disease
- Antacids may interact with certain antibiotics, such as tetracycline, and reduce the absorption of the antibiotic.
- Do not take extra doses of antacids without a physician's direction

HISTAMINE H₂-RECEPTOR ANTAGONISTS

These drugs block the action of histamine, which produces hydrochloric acid secretion, and promote ulcer healing. Examples of histamine H$_2$-receptor antagonist drugs include cimetidine (*Tagamet*), ranitidine (*Zantac*), famotidine (*Pepcid*), and nizatidine (*Axid*). Another drug, omeprazole (*Prilosec*), is an inhibitor of the gastric acid pump and is used for short-term therapy in gastritis and peptic ulcer disease.

DIGESTANTS

The category of **digestants** includes a variety of drugs that promote the process of digestion in the gastrointestinal tract and serve as replacement therapy in deficiency conditions. Pancreatic enzyme replacement may be necessary for people with certain pancreatic diseases, such as pancreatic insufficiency and cystic fibrosis. Pancreatin (*Entozyme, Donnazyme*) and pancrelipase (*Viokase, Cotazym, Pancrease*) aid in the digestion and absorption of fats, carbohydrates, and triglycerides.

ANTIFLATULENTS (CARMINATIVES)

The main function of **antiflatulents** is to reduce the gas in the stomach and intestines (**flatulence**) that accompanies indigestion. They facilitate the passing of gas by mildly stimulating intestinal motility. Simethicone (*Mylicon*), a common antiflatulent, relieves flatulence by dispersing and preventing the formation of gas pockets in the gastrointestinal tract. Other examples of simethicone are *Phazyme, Gas-X,* and *Mylanta*. Patients can reduce the need for antiflatulants by avoiding gas-forming foods, such as cabbage, onions, and beans, and by avoiding the use of straws to drink liquids, because straws cause air to be swallowed.

EMETICS

Emetics are drugs that produce vomiting in cases of poisoning. Syrup of ipecac is often kept in home medicine chests for accidental swallowing of pills, plant leaves, and noncaustic cleaning substances. Syrup of ipecac usually works after about 15 to 30 minutes. Give 8 ounces of water to promote vomiting. If vomiting does not occur after the first dose, ipecac may be administered once more. Because syrup of ipecac is an over-the-counter product, individuals must be educated as to its correct usage. Another emetic is apomorphine hydrochloride, which is given by injection and stimulates the brain center that controls vomiting.

PATIENT EDUCATION

Syrup of Ipecac

- Do not induce vomiting if someone is unconscious, has swallowed a corrosive substance, or has depressed gag or cough reflexes
- Do not give with milk, because it delays the emetic effect

- The dose for adults and children over 12 is 15 to 30 ml (1 oz) orally
- The dose for children 1 to 12 years is 15 ml orally
- Never administer to infants

ANTIEMETICS

Antiemetics suppress nausea and vomiting by acting on the brain's control center to stop the nerve impulses. They have various uses, including motion sickness, "morning sickness" of pregnancy, and nausea and vomiting that occur with various diseases, after surgery, and with chemotherapy and radiation treatments.

The main antiemetics are antihistamines and phenothiazines. For example, dimenhydrinate (*Dramamine*), frequently used for motion sickness, is an antihistamine. Other antiemetics are cyclizine (*Marezine*), buclizine (*Bucladin-S*), and meclizine (*Antivert, Bonine*). The phenothiazines include *Compazine, Thorazine,* and *Phenergan*. Drowsiness is their main side effect. An anticholinergic, scopolamine, is especially effective against motion sickness. Ondansetron (*Zofran*) is a powerful drug for the prevention of nausea and vomiting associated with cancer chemotherapy. Other antiemetics include trimethobenzamide (*Tigan*), the marijuana-derived agent dronabinol (*Marinol*), propantheline bromide (*Pro-Banthine*), thiethylperazine (*Torecan*), benzquinamide (*Emete-Con*), and metoclopramide (*Reglan*).

ANTICHOLINERGICS AND ANTISPASMODICS

These drugs act on the autonomic nervous system to slow peristalsis in the GI tract. They make the smooth muscle contract less often and less forcefully. This is useful in the treatment of ulcers and irritable bowel syndrome because it allows the bowel to rest.

In addition to slowing intestinal motility, **anticholinergics** block the action of acetylcholine, a chemical substance that helps transmit nerve impulses, including those that stimulate the acid-secreting glands of the stomach. By blocking these nerve impulses, anticholinergics cause less stomach acid to be produced. This action is important in ulcer treatment.

The anticholinergics are a group of natural and synthetic alkaloids. The major natural alkaloids are atropine sulfate, belladonna, and scopolamine hydrobromide. Examples of synthetic anticholinergics are methantheline bromide (*Banthine*) and propantheline bromide (*Pro-Banthine*). Because these drugs affect the entire autonomic nervous system, they have many side effects. Blurred vision, dilated pupils, dry mouth, heart palpitations, constipation, and inability to urinate are some of the effects.

Antispasmodics have an effect on the smooth muscle and very little effect on the secretion of acid. An example is dicyclomine hydrochloride (*Bentyl*). Because of the seriousness of the side effects, special care must be taken with the elderly.

Many combinations of anticholinergics or antispasmodics with sedatives are available, including *Donnatal, Librax, Milpath,* and *Bellergal.* Changes in diet and eating habits to decrease the stimulation of colon or peristalsis are usually ordered along with these drugs.

CAUTION: Anticholinergics and the Elderly

Use extreme caution when administering anticholinergic drugs to geriatric patients who have hypertension, or coronary artery, renal, or liver disease.

Anticholinergics are also contraindicated for patients with glaucoma, urinary retention, and obstruction in the gastrointestinal tract.

Anticholinergics can aggravate the above conditions by drying out both the urinary (UA) and GI tract, which in turn causes further UA retention and constipation, fecal impaction, and possible obstruction.

ANTIDIARRHEALS

Antidiarrheals work by

- absorbing the bacteria and toxins causing the diarrhea and passing them out with the stools (absorbent action).
- inhibiting intestinal motility, which slows the movement of fecal material through the intestine so that there is more time to absorb water and make formed stools.
- coating the walls of the gastrointestinal tract.

Before treating diarrhea, it is important to identify the cause. Some antidiarrheals also contain ingredients that shrink swollen tissues (**astringent** action) or coat and soothe the tissues (demulcent action).

Examples of absorbents are kaolin, bismuth (*Pepto-Bismol*), and pectin (ground apples). These are found in many combinations, for example, *Kaopectate* (kaolin and pectin).

Drugs that slow intestinal motility also have a depressant effect on the central nervous system. One such drug is loperamide (*Imodium*). The main group is the opiates, including opium tincture (paregoric) and codeine. Use caution when administering codeine and paragoric to patients who are receiving other CNS depressants causing sedation because of the cumulative effects.

Anticholinergics such as atropine are often used as adjuncts in the treatment of diarrhea because they relieve painful intestinal spasms. They are found in combination with absorbents and opiates; for example, *Lomotil*, *Donnagel*, *Arco-Lase Plus*, and *Cantil*. Other preparations suppress the growth of diarrhea-causing pathogens and reestablish the normal lining of the intestinal tract. Two examples of this type of drug are *Lactinex* and *Bacid*.

ANTI-INFLAMMATORY AGENTS

Diarrhea can also be caused by inflammation of the GI tract, such as enteritis or colitis. Steroids such as methylprednisolone (*Solu-Medrol*) and prednisone are one way to decrease inflammation. Sulfasalazine (*Azulfidine*) taken orally is changed into mesalamine, an aspirinlike drug, when it reaches the colon. Olsalazine sodium (*Dipentum*) is used with patients who have an intolerance for *Azulfidine*. The anti-inflammatory activity provided by these drugs makes them commonly used drugs for the treatment of colitis. Colitis closer to the anus can be treated with either mesalamine (*Rowasa*) suppositories or enemas, or with a hydrocortisone retention enema (*Cortenema*) or intrarectal foam (*Cortifoam*).

LAXATIVES

Laxatives (also called cathartics or purgatives) are drugs that promote **defecation** (bowel movement). There are different types: stimulants, saline, bulk-forming, lubricants, stool softeners, and combination stool softener/stimulant.

Stimulants. One group of laxatives stimulates peristalsis in the intestines to push fecal material through faster. When intestinal motility is increased, there is less time for water to be absorbed by the large intestine, so the stools are watery. Drugs that stimulate peristalsis include castor oil (*Neoloid*), senna (*Fletcher's Castoria, Senokot*), cascara sagrada (*Cas-Evac*), and several synthetics including bisacodyl (*Dulcolax*). Foods and beverages such as prunes, prune juice, and coffee also act as stimulants.

Saline. Another group of laxatives holds liquid in the large intestine to soften feces and stimulate bowel movements. These are the saline cathartics, or salts of sodium, magnesium, and potassium. Milk of magnesia (taken in higher doses than when used as an antacid) and Epsom salts are members of this group.

Bulk Forming (High Fiber). A third family of laxatives includes drugs that increase bulk. They absorb water to increase the bulk and moisture content of the stools. Bulk-forming laxatives are indigestible substances. They take from 12 hours to 3 days to be effective. Whole-grain cereals and breads that contain bran and other fibers relieve constipation in this way. So do extracts of the plantain weed (psyllium) found in such preparations as *Metamucil* and *Citrucel*. There are also several synthetic compounds. These should be taken with plenty of water to prevent constipation and possible fecal impaction.

Lubricants. A fourth group of laxatives coats the surface of the stools and softens the stool to ease defecation. Lubricants such as mineral oil allow the feces to pass more easily through the intestine, but they are thought to interfere with the absorption of some vitamins.

Stool Softeners. Drugs in this category incorporate the liquid in the bowel to soften stool. Examples of stool softeners are docusate sodium (*Surfak*) and docusate calcium (*Colace*). These drugs may cause throat irritation when administered in liquid form and should be diluted with fruit juice.

Combination of Stool Softener and Stimulant. These drugs combine the action of both a stool softener and a stimulant. An example is docusate sodium (*Peri-Colace*).

CAUTION: Laxative Abuse

Regular laxative use leads to laxative abuse. Excessive laxative use develops over some years, and dependency goes unnoticed. This situation is especially common in elderly patients.

Laxative abuse is also seen in patients with eating disorders, such as anorexia nervosa and bulimia. Patients generally deny the overuse of laxatives. If laxative abuse is not discovered, permanent bowel and bone damage and electrolyte imbalances (particularly potassium) result. Arrythymia (irregular heartbeat) and cardiac arrest can result from severe and prolonged potassium depletion.

ANTIHELMINTICS

Antihelmintics are drugs given for helminthiasis, an intestinal infestation of worms. These parasites belong to the animal group helminths (worms). The drugs are effective against worms, but they can be toxic to the body, so they must be used with care and according to the doctor's orders. Usually a doctor instructs an infected person on hygienic practices to prevent future episodes. Drugs used for pinworms and roundworms are diethylcarbamazine (*Hetrazan*), thiabendazole (*Mintezol*), and pyrantel pamoate (*Antiminth*).

PATIENT EDUCATION

Hygienic Practices to Prevent Helminthiasis

- Wash hands before and after eating and using the toilet
- Avoid walking barefoot (hookworm)
- Take showers instead of baths

- Change underclothes, bedclothes, and towels daily
- Wash perianal area daily
- Take medicine for the full course of therapy to prevent reinfestation
- Avoid tasks that require mental alertness, such as driving

ANOREXIANTS

Anorexiants, also called appetite suppressants, help the patient eat less and lose weight. (Recall that the term "anorexia" means loss of appetite.) They are used only to treat extreme obesity. The main anorexiants are amphetamines or related drugs. These act by stimulating the central nervous system, which has an appetite-suppressing effect. Examples of these drugs are diethylpropion (*Tenuate*) and phentermine (*Fastin*). These drugs are not prescribed frequently because they are potentially harmful and often abused. Appetite suppressants should be prescribed only in combination with an increase in physical activity, behavior modification, and caloric restriction. Many over-the-counter diet products contain caffeine or phenylpropanolamine, both mild central nervous system stimulants.

Table 11.1 lists common over-the-counter products that affect the GI system.

TABLE 11.1: Selected Over-the-Counter Medications for Gastrointestinal Disorders

CONDITION	PRODUCTS	ACTIONS
Toothache, cold sores, canker sores	*Benzodent, Blistex, Numzident, Orabase, Betadine*	Anesthetic/astringent
Diarrhea	*Kaopectate, Pepto-Bismol, Donnagel*	Antidiarrheal
Acid indigestion, heartburn	*Amphojel, Di-Gel, Maalox, Gelusil, Mylanta, Phillips' Milk of Magnesia, Rolaids, Tums*	Antacid/antiflatulent
Constipation	*Haley's M-O, Metamucil, Senokot, Dulcolax, Correctol*	Laxative
Motion sickness	*Bonine, Dramamine, Marezine*	Antiemetic
Poisoning	Ipecac syrup	Emetic
Hemorrhoids	*Anusol, Nupercainal, Preparation H*	Antiseptic/astringent/anesthetic/protectant

GIVING GASTROINTESTINAL MEDICATIONS

With most GI disorders, drug therapy is only an adjunct to physical measures. Someone with constipation needs to get on a regular bowel-movement schedule; eat a high-fiber diet consisting of fresh fruits and vegetables, whole-grain cereals and breads; take in 1500 to 2000 ml of fluids daily; and increase physical activity. Likewise, someone with diarrhea may get relief by eating small portions of bland foods that are low in fiber and high in calories and protein; avoiding very hot or very cold drinks; resting; and replacing lost fluids. People with ulcers or gastritis should follow a bland diet consisting of six small meals daily and eliminate irritating substances like tobacco, coffee, and alcohol. As a health care worker, your role is to make sure that patients understand how these practices will help them feel better and make the drugs work better.

Avoiding stress is also important for good digestion. Psychological factors such as stress and anxiety can worsen constipation, nausea, ulcers, and many other disorders. You should strive to create a pleasant, unstressful atmosphere around the patient. Arrange the environment for comfort and privacy, with empathy for the patient's worries and fears, and be supportive and encouraging.

There are some general principles to remember when giving medications for the GI system:

- *Time.* Time of administration is particularly important. Medications that help digestion must be given before, during, or after mealtime, as ordered. Otherwise, they may not be of any use. Other medications must be given between meals when no food is present. Read and follow instructions carefully. These are common abbreviations for GI medications:

a.c. = before meals
p.c. = after meals
h.s. = bedtime

- *Liquids.* Give the recommended amount of liquids with each medication, according to the physician's instructions or your drug reference book.
- *Abdominal pain.* If a patient requests medication for abdominal pain, check with your supervisor before administering a PRN analgesic. Abdominal pain may signal some other undiagnosed GI disturbance that should be evaluated by a doctor.

SUPPOSITORIES

Suppositories may be ordered when a patient is unconscious or cannot take oral medication and is nauseated, has a fever, or is in pain. They may also be ordered when a laxative effect on the large intestine is desired, to promote defecation within 15 to 60 minutes.

The insertion of a suppository can be unpleasant and embarrassing for a patient. Close the room curtain or door to maintain privacy and minimize embarrassment. Explain what you are doing and why it is necessary. Remove the wrapper, and lubricate the rounded end of the suppository to make it enter the rectum as smoothly and gently as possible. The suppository must be inserted gently through the anus, past the internal sphincter and against the rectal wall. Insert the suppository, with your gloved index finger, 4 inches in an adult and 2 inches in infants and children. To be effective, the suppository must be placed along the wall of the rectum, rather than into fecal matter, to increase absorption.

If the patient has pain or irritation in the rectal area after you have inserted the suppository, chart it and inform the nurse in charge or the physician. Either reaction may be a sign of local inflammation caused by the drug. When the patient has a bowel movement, note and chart the appearance of the stools.

FEEDING TUBES

When a patient is unable to ingest, chew, or swallow food but still has a functioning GI tract, a feeding tube is ordered. Many conditions can call for a feeding tube, such as facial fractures; head and neck cancers; neurological conditions, such as stroke; psychological conditions, such as anorexia nervosa; extensive burns; and chemotherapy. There are two types of tubes: (1) a **nasogastric tube** is inserted through the nose or mouth and passes through the esophagus to the stomach (Figure 11.3); (2) a **gastrostomy tube** is inserted directly into the stomach through a surgical opening (**stoma**) in the left upper quadrant of the abdomen.

When feeding tubes are in place, oral medications are also given through them. These medications must be in liquid form. For this reason, tablets and capsules must be crushed and mixed with water before administering. Crush them with a pill crusher, a mortar and pestle, or between two nested spoons (Figure 11.4). They should be mixed with about 1 ounce of water. (Remember, in no case should you crush or dissolve a buccal, sublingual, timed-release, or enteric-coated pill. If this is the prescribed medication, consult the doctor or the nurse in charge as to what to do.)

Before beginning medication administration, put on disposable gloves and elevate the head of the bed 30 degrees. This is to prevent aspiration into the lungs. It is also important to check the placement of the tube. Attach the 30 cc cone-tipped syringe to the end of the tube and gently pull back on the

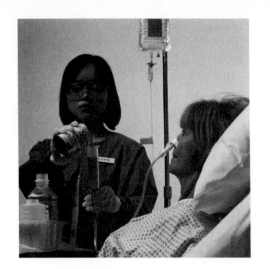

Figure 11.3
When a patient must use a feeding tube, medications are also administered through the tube.

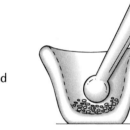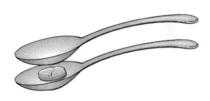

Figure 11.4
Use a mortar and pestle or two spoons to crush pills.

syringe to obtain gastric contents. If you obtain 100 cc or more of gastric contents, notify your supervisor and do not proceed with the medication administration. This amount indicates the stomach has too much fluid in it and you may cause the patient to aspirate.

After determining that the tube is in the stomach, flush the tube with 30 to 60 cc of warm tap water to establish patency or that the tube is open and not blocked. Administer one medication at a time. Never mix medications. Mixing medications may cause incompatability among the medications and render them useless. Administering medications together can also cause the tube to become clogged. After administering one medication, flush the tube with 5 to 10 cc of warm tap water to wash any residual medication down the tube and to maintain patency of the tube. Following the last medication, flush the tube again with 30 to 60 cc of warm tap water. It is important to keep track of how much water you use during the medication administration procedure because it is part of the patient's intake for the day. Record the intake on the patient's intake and output sheet and report it, as well as how the patient tolerated the procedure. This is particularly important in patients with certain cardiac or renal diseases, to prevent fluid overload. The same procedure is followed for the gastrostomy tube. Observe for redness, pus, or drainage around the insertion site of the tube and report to your supervisor.

Keep in mind that tube-fed patients are dependent on others for eating and taking medications. This is not a pleasant experience for them. Try to make them as comfortable as possible and maintain a calm environment. Explain the procedure to patients to alleviate their fears.

Tube-fed or unconscious patients need special care with oral hygiene because they are mouth breathers and the tube is in one side of the nose. Their mouths are usually open, allowing the mucous membranes to dry out. Be alert to the need for rinsing their mouths and caring for their teeth. Cleanse the patient's mouth with a swab containing a solution of sorbitol, sodium, carboxymethycellulose, and electrolytes. These swabs are effective in treating dry mouth. Do not use glycerin or lemon swabs. Glycerin swabs further dry the mouth and cause the gums and mucous membranes to shrink. They also promote bacterial growth. Lemon swabs change the chemical composition of the mouth and wear away tooth enamel.

REPRESENTATIVE DRUGS FOR THE GASTROINTESTINAL SYSTEM

CATEGORY, NAME[a], AND ROUTE	USES AND DISEASES	ACTIONS	USUAL DOSE[b] AND SPECIAL INSTRUCTIONS	SIDE EFFECTS AND ADVERSE REACTIONS
Antacids				
Riopan Oral	Hyperacidity with peptic ulcer disease	Reduces gastric acid	5–10 ml suspension or 1–2 tablets QID	Infrequently, constipation or diarrhea; with prolonged use, hyper-magnesium
Antiflatulents				
Simethicone (*Mylicon*) Oral	Flatulence in the digestive tract, diverticulitis, peptic ulcer	Defoaming action; prevents formation of gas pockets	40–160 mg PO; 1 or 2 tablets QID after meals and at bedtime, as needed	Excessive expulsion of gas, belching
Antiemetics				
Ondansetron hydrochloride (*Zofran*) Oral	Nausea and vomiting associated with chemotherapy; postoperative nausea and vomiting	Serotinin antagonist	8 mg PO, 30 minutes before chemotherapy, then 8 mg q 8 hours PO	Diarrhea, headache
Dimenhydrinate (*Dramamine*) Oral, IM, dermal patch	Nausea, vomiting, motion sickness	Exact mechanism of action unknown	Give 30 minutes to 1 hour before activity; 50–100 mg every 4 to 6 hours; 50 mg IM PRN; advise against driving and other activities that require mental alertness	Dizziness, drowsiness, confusion, dry mouth
Prochlorperazine (*Compazine*) Oral, rectal, IM	Severe nausea, vomiting; also used for severe anxiety and psychosis	Controls vomiting reflex by depressing CNS	5–10 mg 3 PO or 4 times a day; 10–20 mg IM once, repeat in 1–4 hours if needed	Orthostatic hypotension, drowsiness, blurred vision, urine retention, constipation, dry mouth
Meclizine (*Antivert*) Oral	Motion sickness, dizziness, nausea, and vomiting; management of vertigo associated with diseases affecting vestibular system	Antihistamine properties	5–10 mg PO TID or QID; 25 mg rectally bid; 5–10 mg IM every 3–4 hours	Drowsiness, dry mouth, blurred vision
Antispasmodics/Anticholinergics				
Propantheline bromide (*Pro-Banthine*) Oral	Adjunctive therapy in treatment of peptic ulcer disease, irritable bowel syndrome	Inhibits gastrointestinal motility, diminishes acid secretion	15 mg PO 30 minutes before meals and 30 mg at bedtime	Dry mouth, decreased sweating, blurred vision, mydriasis (excessive pupil dilation), urinary retention, tachycardia, headache, nervousness
Dicyclomine (*Bentyl*) Oral, IM	Adjunctive therapy in treatment of peptic ulcer disease, irritable bowel syndrome	Unknown; appears to relieve smooth muscle spasm, reduce intestinal motility	20–40 mg QID	Constipation, drowsiness, dizziness

REPRESENTATIVE DRUGS FOR THE GASTROINTESTINAL SYSTEM

CATEGORY, NAME[a], AND ROUTE	USES AND DISEASES	ACTIONS	USUAL DOSE[b] AND SPECIAL INSTRUCTIONS	SIDE EFFECTS AND ADVERSE REACTIONS
Antidiarrheals				
Diphenoxylate HCl and atropine sulfate (*Lomotil*) Oral	Diarrhea	Reduces intestinal motility	5 mg PO QID; do not exceed 20 mg/day; maintenance dose lower; adjusted individually	Abdominal distention, dry mouth, sedation, urine retention, dizziness
Laxatives				
Bisacodyl (*Dulcolax*) Oral, rectal	Chronic constipation, preparation of bowel for surgery or examination	Increases intestinal motility through direct effect on smooth muscle of intestine	*Tablets* (enteric-coated): 10–15 mg PO at bedtime or early morning; to be swallowed whole; do not give within 1 hour of giving an antacid or milk (these can dissolve the enteric coating) *Suppository:* 10 mg	Abdominal cramps, nausea, vomiting, burning sensation in rectum
Psyllium (*Metamucil*) Oral	Chronic constipation; bowel management	Bulk-forming; absorbs water and expands to increase bulk and moisture content of stool	Give 1–2 rounded tsp PO stirred into 8-oz glass of liquid; give 1–3 times a day followed by another full glass of liquid	Nausea, vomiting, diarrhea after excessive use; obstruction of colon if not taken with plenty of water
Docusate sodium (*Colace*) Oral	Constipation and hard stools, in patients with painful anorectal conditions, and after a heart attack, and in cardiac and other conditions where patients should not strain during defecation (Note: stool softener, not a laxative)	Stool softener; decreases surface tension by increasing liquid content of stool	50–300 mg/day PO; full effect may take 1–3 days	Bitter taste, throat irritation; mild abdominal cramping; diarrhea

[a]Trade names given in parentheses are examples only. Check current drug references for a complete listing of available products.
[b]Average adult doses are given. However, dosages are determined by a physician and vary with the purpose of the therapy and the particular patient. The doses presented in this text are for general information only.

PRACTICE PROCEDURE 11.1

Inserting a Rectal Suppository

■ EQUIPMENT

Physician's order for a rectal medication

Kardex, medicine card, medication record, patient chart

Medicine tray or cart

Continued

Rectal suppository

Disposable gloves

Lubricating jelly (water-soluble)

Protective pad or paper towel

■ PROCEDURE

1. Assemble the equipment and set up the medication. Check for the "five rights."

2. Identify the patient according to agency policy. Explain the procedure. Make sure that the patient understands that the suppository must be held in for at least 20 minutes. You will need the patient's cooperation.

3. Wash your hands. Unwrap the suppository and place it on the wrapper.

4. Assist the patient into a side-lying (lateral) position with the upper leg bent. Drape the patient so as to expose only the anal area. Place a paper towel or pad under the hip to protect the sheet. Help the patient relax in preparation for the procedure.

5. Put on gloves. Lubricate the smooth or rounded tip of the suppository. Also lubricate your gloved index finger on your dominant hand.

6. Insert the suppository as shown in Figure 11.5.

   • With the nondominant hand, spread the buttocks apart and locate the anus.
   • Instruct the patient to breathe through the mouth. This will help relax the anal sphincter.
   • With the dominant hand, insert the suppository through the anus, past the internal sphincter and against the rectal wall. The suppository must be placed against the wall of the rectum for proper absorption and therapeutic action. Insert the suppository 4 inches in adults and 2 inches in children and infants. Withdraw finger and wipe the anal area.

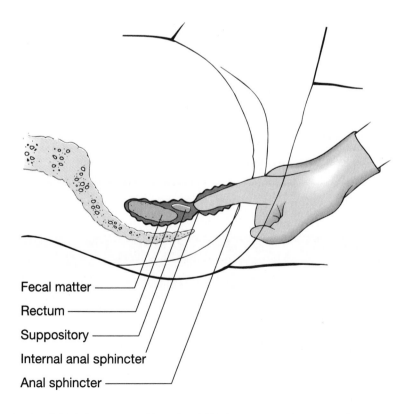

Fecal matter

Rectum

Suppository

Internal anal sphincter

Anal sphincter

Figure 11.5
Administering a
rectal suppository.

Continued

7. Instruct the patient to remain flat on the side for 5 minutes to prevent expulsion of the suppository.

8. Remove gloves by turning them inside out. Wash your hands.

9. Return in 5 minutes to determine if the suppository remained in place.

10. Chart the medication.

11. After this procedure has been completed, watch for signs of pain or irritation in the rectal area; chart and report them. Observe for the effects of the suppository, such as a bowel movement or relief of nausea or pain 30 minutes after administration.

Demonstrate this procedure for your instructor.

PRACTICE PROCEDURE 11.2

Administering Medication Through an Installed Nasogastric or Gastrostomy Tube

■ EQUIPMENT

Physician's order

Medication (tablet, capsule, powder, or liquid; no timed-release or enteric-coated forms)

Medication record, medicine card, Kardex, patient chart

Medicine tray or cart

Pitcher containing 2–4 oz of water at room temperature

30 cc cone-tipped syringe

Protective cover such as a small towel or disposable protective pad

Tube clamp on patient tubing

Disposable gloves

■ PROCEDURE

1. Assemble the equipment and set up the medication. Check for the "five rights."

2. Wash your hands.

3. Prepare the medication. Crush one tablet or pill with a pill crusher, mortar and pestle, or between two spoons, using the top spoon to press down on the tablet. Never crush buccal, sublingual, or time-release capsules or enteric-coated tablets. Then mix with 10 to 20 cc of lukewarm tap water in a medicine cup. If the medication is in capsule form, empty capsule contents into water and mix.

4. Identify the patient according to agency policy. Explain the procedure.

5. Place the patient in the proper position for administration.

   • In bed: semi-Fowler's or Fowler's position; elevate head of bed at least 30 degrees
   • In a chair or wheelchair: sitting position

6. Put on disposable gloves.

7. *Nasogastric:* Place a towel over the patient's chest and remove the clamp from the tube.

   Gastrostomy: Remove the dressing from the abdomen and unclamp the tube.

8. Check placement of the tube by attaching a 30 cc cone-tipped syringe to the end of the tube. Aspirate gently back on the syringe to obtain gastric contents.

9. Before administering medications, flush the tube with 30-60 cc of water.

10. Administer each medication separately. (Never mix medications together.) Between each medication, administer 5–10 cc of tap water.

11. After administering the last medication, flush the tube with 30–60 cc of warm tap water.

12. Clamp the tube. With a corner of a towel, wipe the end clean of any liquid.

13. *Nasogastric:* Tape the tube to the forehead or cheek.

    Gastrostomy: Replace the dressing over the stoma. Check for leakage and report it to the supervisor. Lay the tube down over the abdomen.

14. Keep the patient in the semi-Fowler's position for 30–45 minutes following the procedure.

15. Wash your hands and clean the equipment.

16. Chart the medication. Chart any signs of redness, pus, or drainage around the insertion site of the tube and report to the supervisor.

17. Chart the amount of water used during the procedure on the patient's intake sheet.

Demonstrate this procedure for your instructor.

Match the medical terms to their definitions.

_____ 1. Yellow color of the skin due to liver bile in the bloodstream

_____ 2. Instrument for looking into the stomach

_____ 3. Belching

_____ 4. Tube inserted into the stomach through a hole

_____ 5. Tube inserted into the stomach through the nose and esophagus

_____ 6. Moving the bowels

_____ 7. Vomiting

a. emesis

b. eructation

c. jaundice

d. nasogastric tube

e. gastrostomy tube

f. gastroscope

g. defecation

Complete the following statements by filling in the blanks.

8. Another name for the gastrointestinal system is the _____ system.

9. The opening that passes through the body from the mouth to the rectum is the _____.

10. The muscular movement that carries food through the gastrointestinal system is called _____ _____.

11. Glands in the mouth, stomach, liver, and pancreas secrete _____ that help break down food.

12. Nutrients are absorbed into the blood mainly from the _____.

13. The fluid that coats and dissolves food in the mouth is called _____.

14. The body tube that connects the mouth to the stomach is the _____.

15. When peristalsis moves in the opposite direction, the result is _____.

16. Powerful juices from the pancreas and liver are mixed with food in the _____ _____ , which is the entryway to the small intestine.

17. Because of their fingerlike shape, the _____ of the small intestine provide a huge area for absorption.

18. Undigested waste products that collect in the large intestine are called _____.

19. The opening that allows material from the rectum to pass out of the body is the _____ _____.

20. Bile, an enzyme that breaks down fat, is produced in the _____.

21. Bile is stored in the _____.

22. Powerful digestive juices that complete the digestion of carbohydrates, fat, and protein are produced in the _____.

Answer the following questions in the spaces provided.

23. What are the five functions of the gastrointestinal system?

_____

_____

_____

24. How is digestion related to psychological stress?

_____

_____

25. List all the symptoms you can think of that signal some disorder of the digestive tract.

_____

_____

26. What is intestinal motility, and what happens if it is too fast or too slow?

_____

_____

27. How can tooth and gum disorders lead to other gastrointestinal problems?

_____

_____

Describe what each of the following drug groups does; for example, Emetics cause vomiting.

28. Antacids   _____

29. Digestants   _____

30. Antiflatulents   _____

31. Antiemetics   _____

32. Anticholinergics _____

33. Antidiarrheals   _____

34. Laxatives   _____

35. Antihelmintics   _____

36. Anorexiants   _____

Match these drugs to their categories.

_____ 37. *Hetrazan,* quinacrin, *Mintezol*

_____ 38. *Senokot, Metamucil,* bisacodyl, *Neolid*

_____ 39. Kaolin, pectin, bismuth, paregoric, *Lomotil*

_____ 40. *Pro-Banthine,* atropine, *Bentyl*

_____ 41. *Zofran, Dramamine, Compazine*

_____ 42. Simethicone, *Mylicon*

_____ 43. *Viokase,* pancreatin

_____ 44. *Maalox,* aluminum hydroxide, *Gelusil,* sodium bicarbonate

_____ 45. *Tagamet, Zantac,* famotidine

_____ 46. Apomorphine, syrup of ipecac

_____ 47. Metoclopramide, *Reglan*

_____ 48. *Solu-medrol,* sulfasazine

a. anticholinergics and antispasmodics

b. laxatives

c. antacids

d. antiflatulents (carminatives)

e. antidiarrheals

f. antihelmintics

g. digestants

h. antiemetics

i. histamine H_2-receptor antagonists

j. emetics

k. GI stimulants

l. anti-inflammatory

■ CASE STUDIES FOR CRITICAL THINKING

49. State the four ways that laxatives (cathartics) work.

_____

_____

_____

50. What are some of the physical measures that help gastrointestinal drugs work better?

_____

_____

51. List three things to remember when giving gastrointestinal medications.

_____

_____

_____

_____

_____

52. How can you ease the discomfort and embarrassment of the patient when you are inserting a rectal suppository?

_____

_____

_____

53. What signs should you look for, chart, and report after inserting a suppository?

_____

_____

54. How should you prepare a tablet or capsule for administration through a nasogastric or gastrostomy tube?

_____

_____

55. What signs should you look for, chart, and report when administering medications through a nasogastric or gastrostomy tube?

_____

_____

56. Explain what a laxative does.

_____

_____

57. List two different antacid combinations.

_____

_____

Continued

Choose the gastrointestinal disorder that best matches each description below and write it in the space provided.

Gastritis	Gallstones	Hepatitis	Peritonitis
Duodenal ulcer	Cirrhosis	Hemorrhoids	Irritable bowel

58. Mrs. Phillips has been straining at stool. The large veins around her anal opening are swollen, itching, and beginning to bleed.

_____

59. Following a transfusion of blood, Mr. Mann develops a liver infection. The doctor suspects that the blood donor also had the infection and passed it on to Mr. Mann through the transfusion.

_____

60. Mrs. Merriweather has small grains of cholesterol building up in her gallbladder. They cause mild spasms from time to time. The doctor will not remove them unless they begin to block the tube that leads to the intestine. The doctor prescribes a drug to reduce the intestinal spasms.

_____

61. Mr. Hale is an alcoholic. His doctor has been warning him about the damage to his liver for years. Now Mr. Hale has developed a severe inflammation of the liver. The doctor orders rest, a high-calorie, high-carbohydrate, low-fat diet, and Colbenemid.

_____

62. Ms. Yang has an inflammation of the stomach. The epigastric tenderness and nausea have been coming and going for several weeks. Her doctor suggests that she cut out smoking and coffee to give her stomach relief.

_____

63. Mr. Hruban has developed an open sore at the entrance of the small intestine. The doctor prescribes antacids to calm his nervous tension. She also orders Mr. Hruban to quit smoking.

_____

64. Because of an injury to the Nelson child's intestine, bacteria is released into the abdominal cavity. This has caused a serious inflammation of the abdominal linings. Surgery and antibiotics are ordered at once.

_____

65. Miss Perez is troubled by abdominal cramping and flatulence. She is under a great deal of stress in her job as a junior high school teacher. After a careful examination, the physician reassures her that the condition is not serious and prescribes an antispasmodic to reduce the cramping.

_____

■ APPLICATIONS

Obtain a current copy of a drug reference book or the *PDR*®. Use it to answer the following questions in a notebook or on file cards.

66. Where would you look in the *PDR*® to find other product names for the antacids listed in the Representative Drug table in this chapter? Find another product name for each antacid listed.

67. In Section 3 of the *PDR*®, Product Category Index, find Antacids. Make a list of any antacid and combination drugs that are not on the Representative Drug list on pages 222–223 of this text.

Continued

68. In Section 2 of the *PDR®*, Product Name Index, look up the page number and locate the detailed information about one of the antacids you listed in item 67. What is the adult dosage? Child dosage? How is the drug supplied? Who is the manufacturer of this drug?

69. Find the picture of your antacid and combinations in Section 5 of the *PDR®*, Product Identification Section.

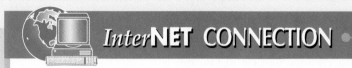

*Inter*NET CONNECTION

To learn more about medications and digestive disorders, go to http://www.intelihealth.com. Click on Digestive Disorders. This will give information on the gastrointestinal system including the role of medications and GI procedures and treatments.

12 Drugs for the Urinary System and Fluid Balance

In this chapter you will learn how the urinary system excretes liquid wastes from the body. You will study how the kidneys maintain the proper balance of fluids and salts to meet the needs of the cells. You will learn about the disorders that arise in the urinary system and how drugs are used to control them. You will learn how to administer drugs into an indwelling catheter and how to give diuretics.

OBJECTIVES

After studying this chapter, you should be able to

• state three functions of the urinary system.

• name the parts of the urinary system and tell what they do.

• describe how abnormal alteration in the urine gives an indication to disorders in the urinary system.

• give the correct medical terms for symptoms of urinary system disorders and fluid imbalances.

• identify descriptions of the main disorders that affect the urinary system.

• describe the actions and give examples of the following drug groups: urinary antiseptics, diuretics, and replacement electrolytes and fluids.

• describe the patient care and education that goes with giving diuretics.

• state the purposes of a urinary catheter.

• describe the causes of dehydration and treatment in the pediatric patient.

• follow proper procedure for administering medications through an indwelling catheter.

KEY TERMS

acid: substance with a low pH (below pH 7); opposite of base or alkali

acidifier: drug that makes the body's pH more acid

acidosis: condition in which there is an excessive proportion of acid in the blood

alkalizer: drug that makes the body's pH more basic or alkaline

alkalosis: condition in which there is an excessive proportion of alkali in the blood; opposite of acidosis

anuria: no measurable production of urine; less than 100 ml in 24 hours

base: substance with a high pH (above pH 7); opposite of acid; also called alkali

bladder: muscular organ for storage of urine, and primary organ of secretion

catheter: tube inserted through the urethra into the bladder to allow urine drainage, bladder irrigation, or instillation of medication

cystitis: inflammation of the bladder caused by bacterial infection

cystoscopy: direct visualization of the interior of the bladder through a flexible scope

dehydration: excessive loss of water from the tissues

dialysis: technique that moves substances from the blood through a semipermeable membrane and into a dialysis solution; used to correct fluid and electrolyte imbalances and remove waste products in case of kidney failure

diuretic: drug that reduces the body's fluid volume by stimulating urine flow

dysuria: difficult or painful urination

edema: abnormal accumulation of fluids in the interstitial spaces of the tissues

electrolyte: substance that has the ability to carry an electrical charge

frequency (urinary frequency): the need to urinate more often than normal

glomeruli: tiny structures in the kidney that filter acids, urea, uric acids, water, glucose, amino, creatine, and major electrolytes

hematuria: blood in the urine

homeostasis: maintaining a state of equilibrium of the body's internal environment, as with body fluids

hypercalcemia: high blood calcium level, greater than 11 mg/dl

hyperkalemia: high blood potassium level, greater than 5.5 mEg/l

hypernatremia: high blood sodium level, greater than 145 mEg/l

hypocalcemia: low blood calcium level, less than 9 mg/dl

hypokalemia: low blood potassium level, less than 3.5 mEg/l

hyponatremia: low blood sodium level, less than 135 mEg/l

incontinence: inability to control urination

indwelling catheter: catheter designed to be held in place over a period of time until the patient can urinate voluntarily; also called Foley catheter or retention catheter

irrigation: flushing out with a solution

nephritis: kidney inflammation

nephrons: functional units of the kidney responsible for homeostasis

oliguria: decreased urinary output in a given time period (100–400 ml in 24 hours)

ozotemia: accumulation of nitrogenous waste products in the blood

pH: measure of the acidity or alkalinity of a solution

pyelonephritis: kidney infection

pyuria: pus in the urine

residual urine: urine remaining in the bladder after voiding (volumes of 100 ml or more)

retention: inability to urinate even though urine is present in the bladder

symphysis pubis: junction of the pubic bones in front on midline

urea: a waste product contained in urine

ureteritis: inflammation of the ureter

ureters: two tubes that carry urine from the kidneys to the bladder

urethra: tube leading from the bladder to the outside of the body

urethritis: inflammation of the urethra

urgency: feeling the need to urinate immediately

urination: release of urine through voluntary control of the bladder; also called voiding or micturition

urine: fluid formed in the kidney, that flows through the ureters to the bladder, where it is stored and then expelled voluntarily from the body; consists of 95 percent water and 5 percent solutes

voiding: act of urination

URINARY SYSTEM

The urinary system includes two kidneys, two ureters, a urinary bladder, and a urethra (Figure 12.1). The system has three major functions: excretion, maintaining homeostasis, and regulating pH balance.

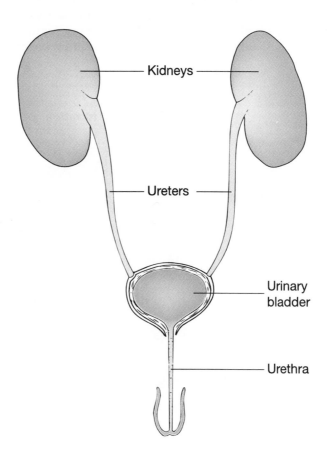

Kidneys

Ureters

Urinary bladder

Urethra

Figure 12.1
The urinary system.

- *Excretion of waste products.* The kidneys excrete waste products by filtering them out of the blood. The main waste products are **urea,** a by-product of the use of proteins by body cells; certain mineral salts; and water.
- *Regulating the amount of water.* By eliminating excess water, the urinary system helps maintain a proper balance of fluids in the body tissues **(homeostasis).**
- *Regulating the pH balance.* Body cells work best in a neutral or slightly basic environment. The kidneys help maintain the proper balance of acids and bases no matter what types of foods one eats.

All three functions of the urinary system are carried out through the same process of filtering the blood. This process takes place in the kidneys. Urine is produced and leaves the body by way of the ureter, the bladder, and the urethra, which are the organs of elimination. The two kidneys are bean-shaped organs located on either side of the vertebral column, posterior to the peritoneum and against the deep muscles of the back. They are supported by a layer of fatty connective tissue and are partially protected by the ribs. An adrenal gland lies on top of each kidney. Each kidney has two layers, the cortex (the outer layer) and the medulla (the inner layer). The functional unit of the kidney is the **nephron.** Each kidney contains one million nephrons. Each nephron has a bulb at one end, the **glomerulus,** which contains many capillaries (Figure 12.2). The glomerulus is the initial site of urine formation.

As blood circulates through the glomerulus, water and dissolved substances pass out of the blood through the capillary walls and into the nephron. This liquid then travels through the coils of the nephron tube, and some of the water, nutrients, and minerals are reabsorbed into the bloodstream through the nephron walls. This process leaves behind only waste products, certain salts, and varying amounts of water. The resulting liquid is called **urine.** The nephrons dip into the second layer of the kidney, the medulla. There urine collects in a tube called the **ureter** that leads out of the kidney. The ureter is about 10 to 13 inches long.

The two ureters, one from each kidney, carry the collected urine to the **bladder,** a collapsible storage bag for urine. Located directly behind the **symphysis pubis** (junction of the pubic bones in front), the muscular walls of the

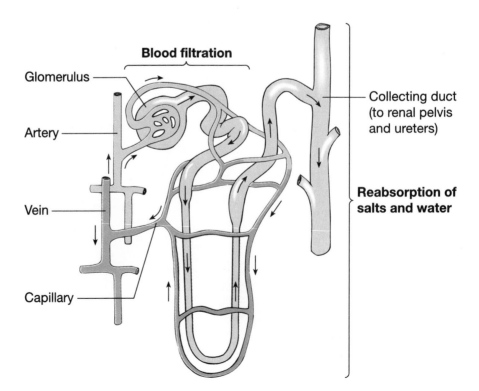

Figure 12.2
Nephrons are the functional units of the kidney where filtration and reabsorption take place.

bladder are able to stretch out and hold as much as 600 ml of urine. Nerve endings in the bladder signal to the nervous system when the bladder contains about 250 ml of urine. This signal creates the urge to **urinate,** or **void.**

During urination, urine passes out of the body by way of the **urethra.** The urethra is about 1½ inches long in the female. It opens to the outside of the body between the labia in the female genital area, just above the vaginal opening. The urethra is about 8 inches long in the male and opens to the outside at the tip of the penis. The male urethra is shared by the urinary and reproductive systems.

Urine is a medically important substance. Examining and testing urine give clues to many types of diseases and disorders, shows how well the kidneys are functioning, and indicates imbalances in the body's water and pH levels. It is about 90 to 95 percent water and 5 to 10 percent salts, urea, and other waste products. Normally, urine is amber or straw-colored and clear. When allowed to stand for any period of time, urine becomes cloudy. It normally has an ammonia odor. The kidneys produce about 1500 to 2000 ml (or cc) of urine in a 24-hour period. The bladder voids approximately 250 ml at a time. When there is an excess of water, the kidneys allow more water to be eliminated. This shows up in urine tests because there is a smaller percentage of waste products per unit of liquid.

DISORDERS OF THE KIDNEYS AND THE URINARY TRACT

TESTS AND SYMPTOMS

There are several ways to tell if the kidneys and other parts of the urinary tract are working properly. The urine is inspected for color, clarity, and odor. Normal urine is pale yellow to amber, clear, and has an ammonia odor. Abnormalities in the appearance or smell of urine may indicate possible illness. Red urine may indicate bleeding from the kidney or bladder. Cloudy or foamy urine may alert the physician to possible renal disease or infection. A patient whose urine sample has a sweet, fruity odor may be showing a sign of diabetes mellitus or starvation. A routine urinalysis is also useful to measure other elements (Table 12.1). If any of the results of the urinalysis are abnormal, further tests may be ordered to evaluate the functioning of the urinary system.

When patients cannot empty the bladder on their own, catheterization may be necessary. Catheterization of the bladder involves passing a rubber or plastic tube, the **catheter,** through the urethra into the bladder. The catheter allows the bladder to empty. The amount of urine obtained from catheterization can

TABLE 12.1: Routine Urinalysis Values

	NORMAL VALUE	ABNORMAL RESULTS
pH	4.6–8.0	Acid/base balance
Protein	Negative	Renal disease (may occur temporarily after activity)
Glucose	Negative	Diabetes mellitus
Ketone	Negative	Diabetes mellitus; starvation; dehydration
RBCs	Up to 2	Trauma
Specific gravity	1.010–1.030	*High values:* dehydration, renal disease
		Low values: overhydration
WBCs	0–8	Infection
Bacteria	Negative	Infection
Casts	Negative	Infection

be an indication of a medical problem. Finally, much can be discovered just by examining the urine. A visual examination of a urine sample may reveal traces of blood (hematuria) or pus (pyuria) in the urine.

X rays may be ordered. A kidney, ureter, bladder X ray (KUB) is used to evaluate the structures of the urinary system. It may detect trauma to a structure, such as a lacerated kidney following an auto accident, or the presence of stones, such as kidney stones. Another test, intravenous pyelogram (IVP), uses a radiopaque dye to visualize the kidneys, renal pelvis, ureters, and bladder. X-ray films are taken over a 30-minute period to evaluate the flow of dye through the kidneys, ureters, and bladder. A defect in the passage of the dye through the various structures may indicate a tumor, or a problem with the glomerular filtration. Other X rays the physician may order are a renal scan, ultrasound, or a CT scan. These procedures are noninvasive.

Invasive tests may also be used to evaluate the blood supply to the kidney (renal arteriogram), microscopic examination of the renal tissue (renal biopsy), and direct visualization of the interior of the bladder (cystoscopy).

Outward signs of urinary tract disorders are changes in the act of urinating. Inability to completely empty the bladder is called retention. Urine remaining in the bladder after voiding (volumes of 100 ml or more) is called residual urine. Inability to control urination is incontinence. Having to urinate very often (frequency) or feeling a great urge to urinate even when the bladder is empty (urgency) are common symptoms of disorders. Urination may be difficult or painful (dysuria). There may be a burning sensation during urination. Or there may be decreased urine output of 100–400 ml in a 24-hour period (oliguria) or less than 100 ml in 24 hours (anuria).

These symptoms may be the result of urinary tract disorders or of more serious kidney disease, as is the case with anuria. Some symptoms may appear as a side effect of a drug; for example, frequency may be a side effect of taking a diuretic. When these conditions appear after giving a drug, they should be charted.

MAJOR DISORDERS

Obstructions. Obstructions of the urinary tract may occur at any point in the urinary system, from the urinary meatus to the kidney. They may be congenital or caused by tumors or injuries. Kidney stones are also responsible for some obstructions. These stones are formed from salts in the urine. Crystals form and precipitate the formation of a stone. Kidney stones may be large enough to block the ureters. Typically the patient experiences severe abdominal or flank pain. A procedure, lithotripsy, may be performed to crush the stone.

In men, the prostate is a donut-shaped gland that surrounds the urethra. An enlarged or inflamed prostate can squeeze the urethra, which also impairs normal urination.

Infections. Urinary tract infections (UTIs) may occur in the kidneys, ureters, bladder, and urethra. Women are more often affected by urinary tract infections than men because of the close proximity of the urethral meatus to the anus. Men are somewhat protected because prostatic secretions contain an antibacterial substance. The elderly are especially prone to urinary tract infections because of underlying conditions such as obstructions, catheterization, or nosocomial infection (hospital-acquired infection).

Personal cleanliness is important to prevent microorganisms from entering the urinary tract. Once microorganisms gain entry, they can cause infections that may travel up the urethra to the bladder and other parts of the system. Bladder infections are frequently accompanied by pain or burning on urination. These are other infections of the urinary tract:

- pyelonephritis—kidney infection
- nephritis—inflammation of the kidney

- **cystitis**—inflammation of the bladder
- **ureteritis**—inflammation of the ureter
- **urethritis**—inflammation of the urethra

In addition to treating urinary tract infections with antibiotics and analgesics for pain, educating the patient about prevention is essential.

PATIENT EDUCATION

Preventing Urinary Tract Infections

- Good perianal hygiene reduces the risk of infection
- Wash hands after every trip to the bathroom
- Females should always wipe from front to back to avoid contaminating the urinary tract with stool
- Void following intercourse, because urinating flushes out bacteria that may have entered the urethra
- Wear cotton underwear; avoid synthetic undergarments because they encourage bacterial growth
- Drink 6 to 8 glasses of water per day
- Take showers instead of baths
- Avoid bath salts, oils, and vaginal sprays

Renal Failure. Renal failure is the severe impairment or total lack of kidney function. There is an inability to excrete metabolic waste products and water. Renal failure may be acute or chronic. Acute renal failure has a rapid onset and may be reversible. Chronic renal failure is a progressive, irreversible destruction of both kidneys. Renal failure is characterized by an accumulation of nitrogenous waste products in the blood, **ozotemia.** This buildup of waste products leads to uremia, in which the patient starts to exhibit signs of the disease. In acute renal failure, the urinary output decreases to less than 400 ml in 24 hours. Initially, there is an increase in urine, followed by oliguria and anuria. Unless kidney function can be restored, patients with renal failure often undergo **dialysis.** Mechanical filtering of the blood using a machine is called hemodialysis. Peritoneal dialysis involves the clearing of waste products by means of fluid exchanges across the abdominal lining, the peritoneum. Continuous ambulatory peritoneal dialysis (CAPD) frees the patient from having to sit for hours while attached to a machine. CAPD is done by the patient instilling the dialysis solution from a collapsible bag into the peritoneal cavity through a disposal plastic tube. The patient does this four times a day. The bag is on an IV pole so the patient can be ambulatory. In between treatments, the patient is completely free of all equipment. This can be done easily at home.

Another danger in renal failure is that drugs are not excreted from the body as rapidly as with healthy kidneys. This is important to remember when giving medications. The renal system is one of the main ways drugs are removed from the body. A kidney that does not work properly fails to eliminate the drugs as expected, and the drugs build up (accumulate) in the body with each dose. Dosages must thus be carefully adjusted and the patient watched closely for drug toxicity whenever there is a suspected problem with the kidneys.

Some drugs, especially antibiotics, are damaging to the kidneys. Infections also cause damage. Either kind of damage can lead to kidney failure. But kidney function is also affected by diseases in other parts of the body. These diseases may slow the work of the kidneys, even though the kidneys themselves are not damaged. For example, if a patient is in congestive heart failure, not enough blood flows through the kidneys. As a result, the kidneys cannot do a proper job of excreting water and salts. Water is retained in the tissues and edema occurs.

The body of an average adult ranges from 50 percent to 60 percent water (more in children and less in the elderly). Most of this water is contained within the body cells, but about a quarter of it is in the spaces between cells or in the blood plasma. Maintaining enough water in the body tissues is important, because water is the medium for many chemical exchanges that are crucial to life.

To ensure adequate water, a balance is kept between fluids taken in (through food and drink) and excreted (through sweat, urine, and exhalation). The body usually does this naturally. But when there is disease, especially disease of the kidneys, the body may not be able to maintain a balance between intake and output. This is why it is sometimes necessary to keep track of fluid intake and fluid output.

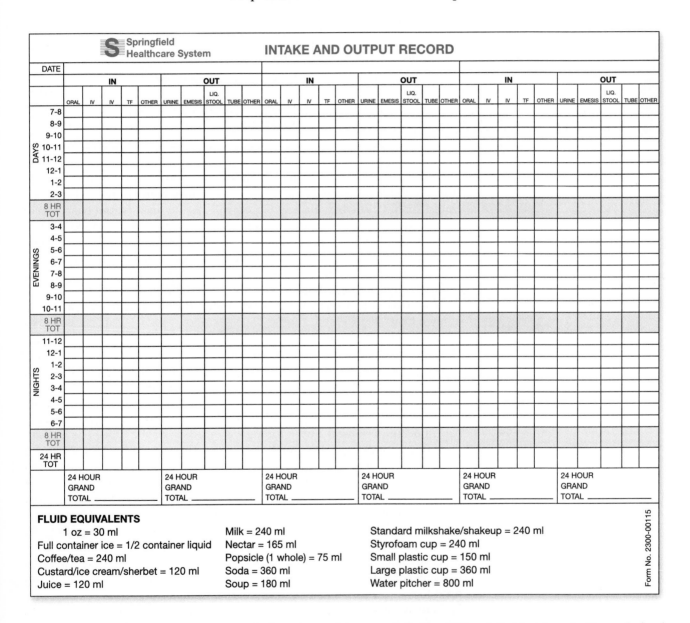

Figure 12.3
An intake/output record charts fluids taken in and excreted.

A chart is used to record the quantity of fluids taken in through food, drink, IV infusion, and so on (Figure 12.3). The chart is also used to record the quantity of fluid excreted in the urine and during vomiting. To maintain balance, each day's intake should equal the day's output. If water taken in exceeds water lost, an abnormal accumulation of fluids in the interstitial spaces of the tissues, or **edema**, results. If too much water is excreted, the body may experience **dehydration.** Either condition interferes with proper functioning. By keeping track of fluid intake and output, the medical staff can decide what treatment is necessary to maintain proper balance. A vomiting patient who loses too much water this way may need IV infusions. A patient with edema may need a **diuretic** to make the kidneys excrete more urine.

For the important chemical exchanges of living cells to take place, the water must contain the proper amount and kind of **electrolytes.** Electrolytes are electrically charged particles (ions) of dissolved salts. They are a means of carrying chemicals through the body fluids. Because salt attracts water, these salt ions are also a way to hold fluids in the body tissues. The electrolyte ions are potassium, calcium, sodium, magnesium, chloride, bicarbonate, phosphate, and sulfate. All the electrolytes must be present in proper amounts for adequate body functioning.

In addition, there must be proper balance between the amount of fluids (water) and the amounts and kinds of salts. The kidneys are sensitive to both water and salts. They compensate for an excess of salts by not allowing salts to be reabsorbed after the blood has been filtered. The unabsorbed salts, in turn, attract water. Thus, both salts and water remain in the kidney tubules, to be carried away through the urinary tract.

The kidneys, then, regulate both the amount and the makeup of body fluids. Ordinarily, the kidneys are able to keep the right proportion of salts and fluids. In disease, kidney malfunction, improper diet, or unusual physical activity, however, fluid/electrolyte imbalances occur. The types of imbalances are shown in the following table:

Hypercalcemia	High blood calcium level	Greater than 11 mg/dl
Hyperkalemia	High blood potassium level	Greater than 5.5 mEg/l
Hypernatremia	High blood sodium level	Greater than 145 mEg/l
Hypocalcemia	Low blood calcium level	Less than 9 mg/dl
Hypokalemia	Low blood potassium level	Less than 3.5 mEg/l
Hyponatremia	Low blood sodium level	Less than 135 mEg/l

Another type of necessary balance is the body's acid/base balance. This is the rate at which the body produces acids and bases equivalent to the rate at which acids and bases are excreted. This balance results in a stable concentration of hydrogen ions in body fluids. The concentration of hydrogen ions in a body fluid is called the pH value. The **pH** is a scale for measuring acidity and alkalinity of fluid. Normal pH is 7.0. A pH below 7.0 is **acid;** above 7.0 is alkaline, or **base.** The body cannot tolerate more than very small changes in pH. The body has balancing mechanisms to ensure that strong acids and bases do not upset this balance. The kidneys are very much a part of this process. They are responsible for getting rid of excess acids or bases when required. The lungs also assist in this process. When they exhale carbon dioxide, they are eliminating acids from the bloodstream.

Disorders of the acid/base balance are called acidosis and alkalosis. **Acidosis** means too acid an environment for the cells; **alkalosis** means too alkaline an environment. Drugs may be administered to restore proper pH. **Acidifiers** (e.g., ammonium chloride and sodium biphosphate) make the pH more acid, in the case of alkalosis. **Alkalizers** (e.g., sodium bicarbonate) make the pH more alkaline, in the case of acidosis. Acidifiers and alkalizers may be given to prevent pH imbalances caused by certain drugs. They are also given to help certain drugs produce their strongest effects. For example, sodium bicarbonate is given with certain sulfonamides that work best in an alkaline pH. Acidifiers such as cranberry juice or ascorbic acid (vitamin C) may be given with methenamine (*Mandelamine*) to provide an acid urine, which enhances the action of the drug.

DRUGS FOR THE URINARY TRACT AND FLUID IMBALANCES

ANTIBIOTICS

The primary drugs used to treat urinary tract infections include penicillins, cephalosporins, sulfonamides, and fluoroquinolones. Ampicillin and amoxicillin are two penicillin drugs used for UTIs. Cefaclor (*Ceclor*) and cefadroxil monohydrate (*Duricef*) are just two of the many cephalosporins used with UTIs.

Sulfonamides are among the most widely used antibiotics, particularly for UTIs. Sulfonamides are primarily bacteriostatic and effective against a wide variety of organisms. Sulfamethoxazole and trimethoprim (*Bactrim, Septra*) are frequently prescribed for UTIs. Newer sulfonamides such as sulfisoxazole (*Gantrisin*) have also proven effective. Urinary tract antiseptics such as methenamine (*Mandelamine*) and nalidixic acid (*NegGram*) are commonly used. Ciprofloxacin (*Cipro*) and ofloxacin (*Floxin*) are two broad-spectrum antibacterials that are effective against a wide range of microorganisms.

Special analgesics are sometimes given with the antibiotic to relieve the low back pain that accompanies infection. A frequently used urinary analgesic is phenazopyridine (*Pyridium*). You should warn the patient that phenazopyridine may cause the urine to become orange and may stain clothing. Urine discoloration is normal and not a reason for concern.

Urinary antimicrobials are sometimes administered directly into the bladder through a urinary catheter. (See Practice Procedure 12.1 on page 245.)

DIURETICS

Diuretics are drugs that increase the output of water from the body. They decrease reabsorption of salts and water from the kidney tubules, with the result that more urine is produced. Increased urination removes excess water from the system. Diuretics are used to control edema in congestive heart failure. They are also used in the treatment of hypertension. In kidney disorders, diuretics are given to promote normal urine production. There are many types of diuretics with different modes of action. Examples of thiazide diuretics are chlorothiazide (*Diuril*) and hydrochlorothiazide (*HydroDIURIL, Esidrix*).

The thiazides act primarily by inhibiting reabsorption of sodium in the distal tubules of the nephron. They therefore promote excretion of sodium, chloride, and water. When the increased sodium is presented to the distal tubules, there is a corresponding increase in potassium excretion. Although the thiazide diuretic achieves the goal of reducing edema, excretion of potassium can cause other problems.

The body cannot stand to lose too much potassium, because potassium is needed for chemical processes inside the cells. Too low a level of potassium (hypokalemia) results in fatigue, muscle weakness, and cardiac changes such as disturbances in the electrical impulses that stimulate the heartbeat. Hypokalemia also potentiates (increases the effect of) the action of digitalis. To avoid these problems, the patient should be instructed to eat potassium-rich foods (Table 12.2).

There are also diuretics available that prevent potassium loss. These are called potassium-sparing diuretics. Examples are spironolactone (*Aldactone*) and triamterene (*Dyrenium*). Potassium-sparing diuretics can lead to an excess of potassium (hyperkalemia), and patients are instructed to avoid potassium-rich foods. *Aldactazide* and *Dyazide* combine a potassium-sparing diuretic with a thiazide.

Two strong loop diuretics that inhibit reabsorption of both sodium and chloride are furosemide (*Lasix*) and bumetanide (*Bumex*). Like the thiazide

TABLE 12.2: Potassium-Rich Foods

FOOD	AMOUNT	POTASSIUM (MG)
Avocado	1	1097
Banana	1	451
Beets	1 cup	532
Cantaloupe	1 cup	494
Lima beans (frozen)	1 cup	694
Orange juice	1 cup	474
Potato	1	610
Prunes	1 cup	706
Raisins	1 cup	1089
Spinach (fresh)	1 cup	838
Squash (acorn)	1 cup	896
Tomato juice	1 cup	535

diuretics, they cause a corresponding excretion of potassium. Because loss of potassium in the urine can be so extensive, potassium supplements are often prescribed in combination with these potent loop diuretics. There are also carbonic anhydrase inhibitors such as acetazolamide (*Diamox*), and osmotic diuretics such as mannitol (*Osmitrol*).

Elderly patients are more susceptible to the effects of diuretics and should be monitored closely.

CAUTION: Geriatric Implications of Diuretics

- Begin treatment with the lowest possible dose
- Diuretics increase the need to urinate, especially at night
- Increase fluid intake (many people incorrectly believe that because diuretics are "water pills," fluid intake should be restricted)
- Monitor closely when a potassium-sparing diuretic and a potassium supplement are given to prevent hyperkalemia
- Diuretics often lower blood pressure, which may cause lightheadedness, dizziness, fatigue, and muscle weakness
- When discontinuing the diuretic, withdraw it gradually to avoid development of fluid retention

REPLACEMENT ELECTROLYTES AND FLUIDS

Normally, fluids are replaced simply by drinking water and eating foods that contain moisture. Electrolytes can be replaced by eating a diet rich in potassium, calcium, sodium, and magnesium. When a patient is unable to replace lost fluids and electrolytes, they are replaced through oral supplements or IV therapy. Various parenteral and oral preparations are available. Potassium (*Slow-K, K-Lyte, Kaon*), calcium (calcium gluconate), magnesium, and other electrolytes can be given orally in the form of tablets and solutions. Or they can be prepared as IV solutions for infusion. IV fluids are given routinely before and after surgery to maintain the proper amount and composition of body fluids. Dextrose 5 percent solution, Ringer's solution, and sodium chloride (saline) solution are fluids commonly administered in IV infusions.

GIVING DRUGS THAT AFFECT THE URINARY SYSTEM

ADMINISTERING DIURETICS

The administration of diuretics must be timed so as to avoid keeping the patient up all night going to the bathroom. Check the drug's onset of action so that it takes effect during the daytime. Warn the patient that he or she will be urinating more often than normal because of the diuretic. Make it easy and comfortable for the patient to urinate frequently. Keep a urinal or bedpan close by for patients who should not or are unable to get out of bed. Keep a bell or a call button handy, too, so the patient can summon help if needed. One way to make sure that a patient gets to the bathroom often enough—and in time—is to set up a schedule. Tell the patient that you will come to help every 2 hours, or according to whatever schedule you work out together.

Keep an accurate record of fluid intake and output (Figure 12.4). A record is necessary to make sure the diuretic is working. If it is taking effect, water leaving the body should be equivalent to the water taken in. The patient should also be weighed daily to confirm that the diuretic is removing excess water. Weigh at the same time every day.

Your observations of the patient's physical condition are important: swollen arms and legs and possibly a swollen abdomen are signs of edema. If you press your finger into the patient's skin, you will leave an indentation. This is called pitting edema. When a diuretic is working, you should notice a decrease in the edema and less pitting of the skin.

Be alert for side effects that signal an electrolyte imbalance. Diuretics can remove too much potassium from the body. Observe the patient for hypokalemia, low potassium level. The patient may exhibit nausea, thirst, fatigue, dry mouth, muscle weakness, muscle cramps, and irregular pulse. It is important to chart these signs. Administer oral potassium as ordered. In severe cases, potassium chloride (KCl) may have to be given intravenously.

A possible side effect of some diuretics is hypotension. Patients should move slowly when sitting up or standing from a lying-down position, to avoid the dizziness of orthostatic hypotension.

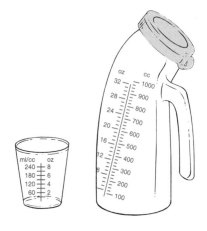

Figure 12.4
Measure fluid intake and output by means of clearly marked containers.

PEDIATRIC CONCERNS

Small children are more susceptible than adults to sudden changes in body temperature and to diarrhea, vomiting, and dehydration. An infant's body composition is approximately 75 percent water as compared to 50 percent to 60 percent in adults. Infants also have less fat content than adults. Their skin is thin and permeable, and their livers and kidneys are immature or not fully developed and therefore cannot metabolize and excrete drugs as well as those organs in older children and adults. The most accurate way to determine pediatric drug dosages is to measure body surface. As a result of the larger percentage of water in children's body weight, smaller children require larger doses of some drugs such as *Gentamicin*. Small children also have poor absorption of drugs and fluids as a result of dehydration. Drugs are most effective when administered intravenously.

Diuretics must be carefully administered to children. Obtain daily weights and vital signs to prevent fluid and electrolyte loss. Hypotension, shock, and even death can occur if children are not closely monitored. Children are more susceptible to the effects of diuretics because of their larger percentage of total body water.

Oral rehydration therapy (ORT) is a major advance in today's health care in the treatment of dehydration. Oral replacement solutions (ORS) contain glucose and carefully determined amounts of sodium. ORT is very effective, safer, less painful, and less costly than intravenous (IV) rehydration. Nutrient-based solutions such as *Pedialyte, Lytren, Ricelyte,* and *Resol* are the most frequently used solutions for oral rehydration. These solutions are rich in electrolytes and are frequently used in children with diarrhea. After rehydration, ORS is used for maintenance therapy alternating with low sodium fluids, water, breast milk, and half-strength or lactose-free formulas. ORS may be given as a supplement with older children. One cup of ORS is used as the replacement amount to be given for each diarrhea stool resulting in dehydration.

PATIENT EDUCATION

Pediatric Implications in the Management of Dehydration

- Avoid a clear liquid intake including fluids such as fruit juices, carbonated beverages, and gelatin. These fluids have a high carbohydrate content but are very low in electrolytes.

- Avoid beverages containing caffeine because the caffeine has a diuretic effect causing further loss of water and sodium.

- Avoid broths because they are high in sodium and have inadequate carbohydrate content.

- Oral rehydration solutions including *Pedialyte, Lytren, Ricelyte,* and *Resol* are the recommended therapy.

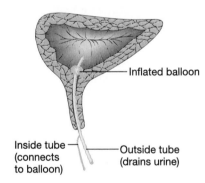

Inside tube (connects to balloon) — Outside tube (drains urine) — Inflated balloon

Figure 12.5
Bladder medication can be instilled through an indwelling catheter.

INSTILLING BLADDER MEDICATION

A bladder **irrigation,** including instillation of an antiseptic or antibiotic solution, may be ordered to wash out the bladder of a patient with a severe bladder infection.

An **indwelling catheter** (also called a retention or anchored Foley catheter) remains inside the bladder for an extended time. It allows urine to flow into a bag hung at the side of the bed. There are several types of indwelling catheters available with outlets for drainage and irrigation. The Foley catheter (Figure 12.5) is held in place by inflating a small balloon inside the bladder after inserting the catheter.

Because the catheter opens a passageway between the bladder and the outside environment, sterile technique must be used to avoid letting microorganisms enter the bladder. Special sterile kits are available containing all the equipment needed for irrigating or instilling medication into the bladder.

These are points to keep in mind when instilling bladder medications into an indwelling catheter:

- Follow aseptic procedure; do not let the catheter or medication become contaminated.
- Make sure medication is at the proper temperature. Usually room temperature is correct, but check the medication order to be sure.
- Leave the medication in the bladder for the proper amount of time, as shown on the medication order.
- Remember to hook up the drainage tube after you finish giving medication, so that urine can be carried away into the drainage bag.
- Give special consideration to the patient's privacy. Draw the curtain around the bed and drape the patient's genital area. You can ease the patient's embarrassment by being tactful and considerate.

REPRESENTATIVE DRUGS FOR THE URINARY SYSTEM AND FLUID IMBALANCES

CATEGORY, NAME[a], AND ROUTE	USES AND DISEASES	ACTION	USUAL DOSE[b] AND SPECIAL INSTRUCTIONS	SIDE EFFECTS AND ADVERSE REACTIONS
Urinary Antiseptics/Antibacterials/Analgesics				
Ciprofloxacin (*Cipro*) Oral, IV	Urinary tract infections, respiratory, bone, and skin infections	Inhibits DNA gyrase	250–500 mg PO every 12 hours; 400 mg IV every 12 hours	Nausea, headache, diarrhea, rash
Trimethoprim/sulfame-thoxazole (*Bactrim, Septra*) Oral, IV	Urinary tract infections, otitis media, bronchitis, traveler's diarrhea	Blocks two consecutive steps in the biosynthesis of nucleic acids and proteins essential for many bacteria	1 or 3 double-strength tablets taken in one dose; 2 regular-strength tablets, or 4 teaspoons (20 ml) of suspension, every 12 hours for 10–14 days. Do not give if patient is allergic to sulfa	Nausea, vomiting, diarrhea, skin rashes, anorexia, blood disorders, headache
Nitrofurantoin (*Furadantin, Macrodantin*) Oral	Urinary tract infections	Interferes with bacterial enzyme systems	50–100 mg TID or QID; give with food or milk to avoid gastric irritation; rinse mouth after giving liquid form to avoid staining teeth	Anorexia, nausea, diarrhea, may turn urine brown or darker
Cefadroxil monohydrate (*Duricef, Ultracef*) Oral	Urinary tract infections	Inhibits cell wall synthesis	500 mg PO daily	Nausea, diarrhea, dyspepsia
Ampicillin (*Omnipen, Principen*) Oral, IV	Urinary tract infections (pyelonephritis)	Bactericidal; inhibits cell wall formation	1–4 g PO daily q 4 hours	Rash, itching, shortness of breath, diarrhea, nausea, vomiting
Phenazopyridine (*Pyridium*) Oral	Pain with urinary tract irritation or infection	Anesthetizes mucous membranes of urinary tract	100–200 mg TID p.c.	Headache, vertigo, orange discoloration of urine
Diuretics				
Hydrochlorothiazide (*HydroDIURIL*) Oral	Edema, hypertension	Increases sodium and water excretion, lowers blood pressure	25–100 mg 1 or 2 times daily; give early in day because of increased urination; monitor weight and fluid intake/output	Gastric irritation, muscle weakness, hypokalemia, orthostatic hypotension, pancreatitis
Triamterene (*Dyrenium*) Oral	Edema	Conserves potassium and excretes sodium	Individualized; 100 mg BID after meals; avoid excessive intake of potassium-rich foods	Nausea, vomiting, weakness, rash, dry mouth, hypotension, dizziness
Furosemide (*Lasix*) Oral, IM, IV	Edema, hypertension, chronic renal failure	Potent loop diuretic; inhibits reabsorption of sodium and chloride	20–80 mg initially and then gradually increased to 600 mg/day in patients with severely edematous states	Dizziness, headache, dehydration, anemia, leukopenia (decreased white blood cells), rash, orthostatic hypotension, hypokalemia

CATEGORY, NAME[a], AND ROUTE	USES AND DISEASES	ACTION	USUAL DOSE[b] AND SPECIAL INSTRUCTIONS	SIDE EFFECTS AND ADVERSE REACTIONS
Replacement Electrolytes				
Potassium (*K-Lyte, Slow-K, Kaon*) Oral	Potassium deficiency	Potassium ion replacement	20 mEq/day for prevention of hypokalemia; 40–100 mEq/day or more for treatment of potassium depletion	Nausea, vomiting, diarrhea, abdominal distress, hyperkalemia, phlebitis

[a]Trade names given in parentheses are examples only. Check current drug references for a complete listing of available products.
[b]Average adult doses are given. However, dosages are determined by a physician and vary with the purpose of the therapy and the particular patient. The doses presented in this text are for general information only.

PRACTICE PROCEDURE 12.1

Instilling Medication Into the Bladder Through an Indwelling Catheter

■ EQUIPMENT

Physician's order for bladder medication

Kardex, medicine card, medication record, patient chart

Medicine tray or cart

Sterile catheter irrigation/instillation set, containing tray or basin (to catch drainage), plastic sheeting, syringe, catheter tip covers, bottle for diluting medication (in some sets), alcohol wipes, sterile gloves

Medication in sterile solution, 50 or 60 cc

■ PROCEDURE

1. Assemble equipment.

2. Read the physician's order and set up the medication. Check for the "five rights."

3. Identify the patient following agency policy. Explain what you are going to do. Curtain off the area to provide privacy.

4. Wash your hands.

5. Assist the patient to lie down on his or her back, with bent legs spread apart to expose the genital area. Drape the patient so that only the catheter is showing.

6. Open the sterile packaging of the irrigation set and establish sterile field. Protective plastic sheeting should be set down on the bed first, to prevent soiling bed. Pour desired amount of sterile solution into sterile container. Put on sterile gloves.

7. Arrange the catheter tip so that it is hanging over the edge of the tray but not touching the bottom. (This would contaminate the catheter.) Some bladder instillation sets have a notched edge on the tray to hold the catheter in place.

8. Disconnect catheter from drainage tube. (The drainage tube is the one that carries the urine to a bag at the side of the bed.) Allow urine to flow into sterile collection container. Cover the exposed end of the drainage tube with the special sterile covering in the instillation set. This keeps microorganisms from entering the tube while it is detached. Then lay the tube down on top of the bed, anchoring it with tape so that it does not slide off and drop to the floor.

9. Lift the end of the catheter and insert the sterile syringe into the opening used for irrigation. Hold the syringe and catheter tube together with the same hand. This keeps them from separating when you administer the medication.

10. Pour the measured amount of medication into the open end of the syringe. Let it drain through the catheter into the bladder. Do not force it in with the syringe bulb.

11. Follow with extra sterile water, if ordered.

12. Before putting down the catheter, clamp it if the medication is to stay in the bladder for a certain time. The physician's order should state how long the medication should be retained. If no special length of time is ordered, you may leave the tube unclamped.

13. Put down the catheter in the same position as before, with the end resting over the edge of the tray but not touching the bottom. If unclamped, the catheter will begin to drain right away. If the catheter is clamped, remember to unclamp it after the proper amount of time so that it can drain.

14. When the medication has drained out, reattach the drainage tube to the end of the catheter. Use a sterile alcohol wipe to clean both the end of the tube and the catheter as you reattach them.

15. Remove and clean or discard the equipment, supplies, and gloves.

16. Give the patient any special instructions and assist him or her into a comfortable position. Make sure that the tubing is not pinched or blocked in any way so that urine can drain freely into the collection bag.

17. Wash your hands.

18. Chart the medication. If you noticed any unusual substances draining from the bladder or irritation around the catheter, be sure to chart it and notify your supervisor.

Demonstrate this procedure for your instructor.

Define these terms that describe symptoms of urinary tract disorders.

1. Hematuria _____

2. Pyuria _____

3. Incontinence _____

4. Retention _____

5. Dysuria _____

6. Anuria _____

Match the medical terms to their definitions.

_____ 7. Mechanical filtering of blood   a. cystoscope

_____ 8. Instrument for looking into the urinary tract   b. dialysis

_____ 9. Tube for bladder irrigation and medication   c. nephritis

_____ 10. Inflammation of the kidney   d. catheter

Complete the following statements by filling in the blanks.

11. The tubes that connect the kidneys to the bladder are the _____.

12. Urine passes out of the body by way of the _____.

13. A full bladder creates the urge to _____.

14. In 24 hours, the kidneys normally produce about _____ ml of urine.

15. About _____ ml of urine is passed during normal urination.

16. When a patient is on thiazide diuretics, there is a danger of excreting too much _____, which could cause hypokalemia.

17. A lack of potassium can be corrected by giving foods such as _____.

18. A catheter that is designed to stay in place over a long period of time is called a(n) _____ _____catheter.

Answer the following questions in the spaces provided.

19. List the three functions of the urinary system.

_____

_____

_____

20. What are electrolytes? Name at least four electrolyte ions. _____

_____

_____

21. How does the kidney regulate the balance of electrolytes and fluids? _____

_____

22. List the types of fluids you would record on an input and output record.

Input: _____

Output: _____

Match the drug names to the drug categories.

_____ 23. Spironolactone, *Dyrenium*	a. alkalizers
_____ 24. *Lasix, Edecrin*	b. acidifiers
_____ 25. *Diuril, HydroDIURIL, Esidrix*	c. thiazide diuretics
_____ 26. Potassium, calcium, sodium, *Slow-K*	d. replacement electrolytes
_____ 27. *Furadantin*, methenamine, *Gantrisin, Septra*	e. potassium-sparing diuretics
_____ 28. Sodium bicarbonate	f. replacement fluids
_____ 29. Ammonium chloride, sodium biphosphate	g. very strong diuretics
_____ 30. Sodium chloride solution, dextrose solution	h. urinary antiseptics

■ CASE STUDIES FOR CRITICAL THINKING

From the list below, choose the disorder that best matches each description. Write the name of the disorder in the blank.

Renal failure	Kidney stones	Electrolyte imbalance
Pyelonephritis	Cystitis	

31. Fred Byers must be put on dialysis to eliminate toxic waste products from his bloodstream.

_____

32. Mr. Bernardi has had painful abdominal spasms for a day due to an obstruction in the ureter. Now the obstructing material has passed into the bladder. His physician will insert an instrument into the bladder to crush and flush out the material.

_____

33. Ms. Yamamoto has a severe bladder infection with painful, frequent urination. To keep the bladder empty, a urinary catheter has been inserted. The doctor has ordered regular bladder irrigation and an anti-infective to be administered into the catheter.

_____

34. Mr. Wincenz has a severe kidney infection that is damaging to the nephrons. Antibiotics are being administered with caution so as to avoid further damage that could lead to kidney failure.

_____

35. After several days on diuretics, a heart patient develops fatigue and muscle weakness. Dr. Bland then orders potassium chloride.

_____

Continued

■ APPLICATIONS

Obtain a current copy of a drug reference book or the PDR®. Use it to answer the questions that follow in a notebook or on file cards.

36. Use the *PDR®* to locate another product name for each of the urinary antibacterials listed in the Representative Drug table on pages 244–245 of this text.

37. In Section 3 of the *PDR®*, Product Category Index, find the Diuretics. Make a list of the loop diuretics listed there.

 *Inter**NET** CONNECTION*

The Agency for Health Care Policy and Research (AHCPR) at http://www.ahcpr.gov supports research designed to improve health care, reduce its cost, and broaden access to essential health services. Click on Consumer Health and go to Understanding Incontinence. This gives you information on the problem of urinary incontinence and the treatments used.

13
Drugs for the Reproductive System

In this chapter you will review the parts of the reproductive system and learn about the hormones produced by the male and female gonads. You will learn what disorders affect this system and which drugs are used to treat them.

OBJECTIVES

After studying this chapter, you should be able to

• name the main parts of the male and female internal and external genitalia.

• identify the parts and functions of the reproductive system, using correct medical terminology.

• discuss the effects of puberty on the adolescent patient and the need for contraceptive counseling.

• name the hormones produced by the male and female gonads and describe their function.

• describe the actions of gonadotropins, oxytocin, and prolactin.

• recognize descriptions of major disorders that affect the reproductive system.

• list the main uses of sex hormones in drug therapy.

• state the major side effects of sex hormone therapy.

KEY TERMS

abortifacients: anything used to terminate pregnancy

amenorrhea: failure to menstruate; missed menstrual period

cervicitis: inflammation of the cervix

cervix: entrance of the uterus

dysmenorrhea: painful menstruation

endometriosis: growth of endometrial tissue outside the uterus

endometrium: lining of the uterus

engorgement: filling up of a body part with blood or other fluid; e.g., penis engorgement prior to intercourse, breast engorgement with milk in nursing mothers

estrogen: female hormone

fetus: the developing child in utero from the third month after conception until birth

genitalia: internal and external reproductive organs

gonadotropins: pituitary hormones that stimulate the gonads (ovaries and testes) to secrete hormones

gonads: sex glands in which reproductive cells are formed; ovaries and testicles

herpes simplex (genital): sexually transmitted disease that results in painful genital lesions

labia: two sets of tissue folds, the labia majora and labia minora, surrounding the opening of the vagina

libido: sex drive

menopause: naturally occurring end of menstruation, usually between the ages of 45 and 52

menorrhea: normal menstruation; also called menses

osteoporosis: condition in which there is a decrease in total bone mass; major cause of fractures in postmenopausal women

ova: female reproductive cells (singular, ovum)

ovaries: two almond-shaped glands located in the pelvis, one on each side of the uterus, which produce ova

ovulation: release of an ovum from an ovary

oxytocic: drug that stimulates contractions of the uterus

penis: part of male external genitalia that introduces sperm into the vagina

perineum: skin-covered muscular area between the vulva and anus in the female and between the scrotum and anus in the male

postpartum: period after giving birth

progesterone: female hormone

prostate gland: gland surrounding the male urethra and ejaculatory duct; secretes a thin alkaline substance that makes up the largest part of the seminal fluid

prostatitis: inflammation of the prostate gland

puberty: age at which the reproductive organs become functional and secondary sex characteristics appear

scrotum: skin-covered pouch containing the testes; part of the male external genitalia

sexually transmitted disease (STD): infectious disease spread by intimate sexual contact; among the STDs are syphilis, gonorrhea, genital herpes, chlamydia, and AIDS

spermatozoa: male reproductive cells, also called sperm

testes: male reproductive glands (singular, testis)

testosterone: male hormone that influences development of masculine characteristics; androgen that occurs naturally in the testes

uterus: located between the bladder and rectum; contains and nourishes the embryo from time of fertilization until birth of the fetus

vagina: part of the female internal genitalia connecting the uterus to the outside of the body; passage into which sperm is introduced; canal through which a baby is born

vaginitis: inflammation of the vagina

REPRODUCTIVE SYSTEM

Creating the next generation of human life is the responsibility of the male and female reproductive systems. Of all the body systems, the reproductive system is the least alike in males and females. The two systems have different structures that must work together for reproduction to take place. One basic function of both the male and female systems is to produce sex cells. The other function is to engage in sexual intercourse, the act that makes it possible for those sex cells to join together. The female system has an added function: to nourish and protect the fetus thus created until it is fully developed for life outside the womb.

The external and internal reproductive organs in both males and females are called **genitalia.** Some of the male and female genitalia have similar functions, but their anatomy is different.

FEMALE REPRODUCTIVE SYSTEM

Internal Genitalia. The internal genitalia of the female reproductive system consist of two ovaries, two fallopian tubes, the uterus, and the vagina (Figure 13.1). The **ovaries** are two almond-shaped glands located in the pelvis, one on each side of the uterus. The ovaries produce **ova,** the female reproductive cells. Normally once a month, **ovulation** takes place. That is, a

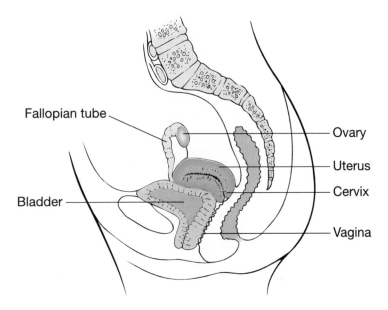

Figure 13.1
Internal genitalia
of the female
reproductive
system.

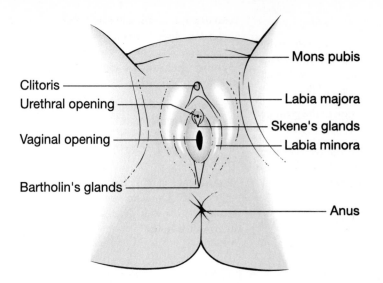

Figure 13.2
External genitalia
of the female
reproductive
system.

Clitoris
Urethral opening
Vaginal opening
Bartholin's glands
Mons pubis
Labia majora
Skene's glands
Labia minora
Anus

single ovum is expelled from the surface of one ovary and travels up the fallopian tube, where fertilization by a sperm may occur. An ovum can be fertilized for up to 72 hours after it is released from the ovary. The fertilized ovum then implants in the wall of the uterus, where it begins development into a human embryo.

The **uterus** is designed to contain and nourish the fertilized ovum as it develops. The uterus is a pear-shaped, hollow, muscular organ that lies in the pelvis between the bladder and rectum. It opens through the **cervix** into the **vagina.** The vagina is a collapsible tubular structure capable of great distention that gives access from outside the body to the internal genitalia. The vagina serves as the lower part of the birth canal and the organ that receives the seminal fluid carrying sperm from the male.

External Genitalia. The external female genitalia, commonly called the vulva, consists of the mons pubis, the labia majora, the labia minora, the clitoris, the urethral meata, the vaginal opening, Bartholin's glands, and the Skene's gland (Figure 13.2). The mons pubis is a pad of fat that lies over the pubic bone. It is covered with coarse hair. Just below it are the **labia,** the labia majora and labia minora, that surround the opening of the vagina. Farther toward the back is the opening to the rectum, called the anus. The entire female genital area between the vulva and the anus is the **perineum.**

At the forward tip of the labia is a small organ composed of erectile tissue called the clitoris. It is a sensitive nerve center that becomes engorged during sexual excitation. Two glands called Bartholin's glands are located on either side of the vaginal opening. During sexual excitement, they secrete a lubricating mucus that helps the penis enter the vagina. The Skene's gland has no known function.

Pregnancy and Childbirth. If an ovum is fertilized and attaches itself to the lining of the uterus, it begins to develop into a **fetus,** and pregnancy is the result. The fetus is nourished by the mother's blood and cushioned by a surrounding sac of fluid. After approximately 266 days, or 9 months, development is complete. Several weeks before delivery, the uterus lowers into the pelvis. This descent is called "lightening," because it gives the mother a sense of decreased abdominal pressure and distention. Labor begins with rhythmic contractions of the uterus that push the baby toward the cervix. The cervix dilates to 8 to 10 cm to allow the baby to pass through the vagina (also called the birth canal) into the outside world.

While the fetus develops inside the uterus, changes also take place in the pregnant woman's breasts. The breasts are composed of fatty tissue and mammary (milk) glands. During pregnancy, they grow larger and the mammary glands prepare to secrete the milk that will nourish the baby through the first few months of life. A few days after birth, the milk glands go into full production, and the breasts swell with milk. The baby obtains the milk by sucking on the nipples.

PUBERTY

Puberty refers to the maturational, hormonal, and growth process that occurs when the secondary sex characteristics develop and the reproductive organs begin to function. In girls, it is marked by the first menstrual flow. Breast changes, growth of pubic and axillary hair, and a rapid increase in height and weight also occur. Boys experience enlargement of the testicles, growth of pubic and axillary hair, rapid increase in height, and a change in the voice.

One in 10 adolescent girls—approximately 1 million girls under the age of 20—become pregnant every year. Of these pregnancies, 550,000 result in live births and 450,000 are terminated. Teenage pregnancy is no longer considered biologically disadvantageous to the unborn child, but it is socially, educationally, psychologically, and economically disadvantageous to the mother. Although the incidence of teenage pregnancy is high, the mortality rate has decreased. Teenage mothers and their babies are at greater risk for complications of both pregnancy and delivery, such as premature labor and low birth weight. When good care is available early in pregnancy, however, the risks to the pregnancy and its outcome are equal to those of a mature woman.

Contraceptive counseling is necessary as part of a comprehensive health education program for adolescents. The contraceptive method must be individually suited to each teenager. Motivation is essential, but sometimes difficult. The pill is effective, but the teenager must remember to take the pill. *Norplant* is a good choice for some people because it is effective and eliminates the need for compliance. It is important, however, to stress the use of condoms in the prevention of sexually transmitted diseases. All patients using contraceptive devices other than condoms should be taught that these devices do not prevent sexually transmitted diseases.

MALE REPRODUCTIVE SYSTEM

The male reproductive system consists of the external structures, the penis and scrotum, and the internal structures, the prostate gland and the seminal vesicles (Figure 13.3). The **testes** produce millions of tiny sex cells called **spermatozoa** or sperm. The sperm collect and mature in a series of coiled tubes called the epididymis. They then pass through a larger tube, the vas deferens. The vas deferens leads from the testes to several storage areas called the

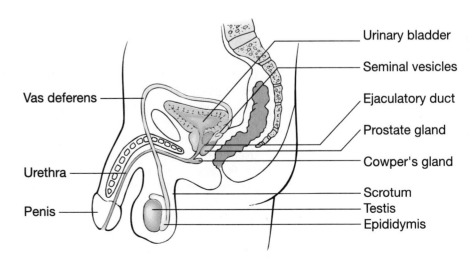

Figure 13.3
Internal and external genitalia of the male reproductive system.

Labels: Urinary bladder, Seminal vesicles, Ejaculatory duct, Prostate gland, Cowper's gland, Scrotum, Testis, Epididymis, Vas deferens, Urethra, Penis

seminal vesicles and to the two ejaculatory ducts. These two ducts pass through the **prostate gland** and terminate in the urethra, a tube that serves as the terminal portion of the reproductive tract and the passageway for eliminating the reproductive fluid, semen, from the body. The prostate gland, the seminal vesicles, and the Cowper's glands located on either side of the urethra all produce mucus and fluids that, together with the sperm, make up semen. During ejaculation, a muscular contraction that occurs with a peak of sexual excitement, the semen is propelled out of the body.

The external genitalia include the **scrotum,** a thin, loose, outer layer of skin in which the two testes are suspended, and the **penis.** During sexual excitement, the spongy tissue of the penis fills up with blood. This makes the penis lengthen and become rigid in preparation for sexual intercourse.

SEX HORMONES

A few sex hormones are secreted by the adrenal cortex (see Chapter 14), but most come from the male and female sex glands or **gonads.** These hormones, estrogen, progesterone, and testosterone, are not single hormones, but represent groups of related hormones.

The female gonads, the ovaries, secrete the hormones **estrogen** and **progesterone.** Estrogen is responsible for the higher voice, breast development, and shapeliness that are characteristic of women. It also stimulates the monthly development of an ovum. If an ovum is fertilized, the ovaries begin to produce progesterone. This prepares the uterus to carry and nourish the fetus as it grows. If the egg is not fertilized, the hormones cause the uterine lining to be shed, resulting in menstruation (**menorrhea,** or menses). Somewhere between the ages of 45 and 52, the ovaries stop producing estrogen and progesterone, and monthly menstruation ceases. This change in hormone production is known as the **menopause.**

The male gonads, the testes, produce the male hormone **testosterone.** Testosterone gives men their deeper voice and chest and facial hair. It also stimulates production of sperm cells.

A testosterone deficiency may result in erectile dysfunction (impotence), but in younger men, erectile dysfunction is most commonly attributed to an increase in substance abuse, such as alcohol and recreational drugs. In middle-aged men, erectile dysfunction is often the result of medical technologies, such as bypass surgery, chemotherapy, and organ transplants. A man over the age of 70 may experience erectile dysfunction as a result of declining testosterone levels.

Erectile dysfunction is the inability to achieve or maintain an erect penis. Treatment is based on the cause of the dysfunction. The goal of therapy is to help the male achieve a satisfactory sexual relationship after treatment. Treatment may consist of eliminating a particular drug, such as methyldopa (*Aldomet*), used for hypertension, or propanolol (*Inderal*), used for hypertension, angina, arrhythmias, and after a heart attack. Yohimbine (*Yocon*) is a vasodilator and aphrodisiac given orally. When the cause of erectile dysfunction is decreased testosterone levels, testosterone is administered intramuscularly. Research has not proven that testosterone supplementation in older men is successful. Testosterone is also contraindicated in cases of cancer of the prostate, which is common in older men.

A new drug, sildenafil citrate (*Viagra*), approved by the FDA in 1998, is used to treat impotence. *Viagra* increases the ability to achieve and maintain an erection. Men who take medications containing nitrates, such as nitroglycerin, should not take *Viagra*. The combination causes excessive hypotension. *Viagra* is commonly given orally one hour prior to sexual activity, but may be taken anywhere from 30 minutes to 4 hours before. The most common side effects are headache, flushing, diarrhea, indigestion, nasal congestion, and increased sensitivity to light.

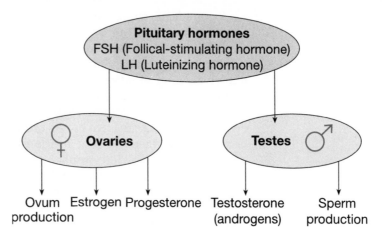

Figure 13.4
Pituitary hormones (gonadotropins) control certain functions of the gonads.

PITUITARY HORMONES THAT REGULATE REPRODUCTION

The pituitary hormones, follicle-stimulating hormone (FSH) and luteinizing hormone (LH), control several functions of the gonads. For that reason they are also called **gonadotropins.** In the female, the two gonadotropins control ovulation and the production of female hormones by the ovaries; in the male, they stimulate the testes to produce sperm and secrete testosterone (Figure 13.4).

Two other pituitary hormones are involved in childbirth. Oxytocin stimulates the uterus to start contracting at the beginning of labor. A dose of oxytocin (*Pitocin, Syntocinon*) or a similar, synthetic drug (called an **oxytocic**) may be used to bring about or strengthen labor when a delay would endanger mother or child. It may also be given to slow **postpartum** (after-childbirth) uterine bleeding. When the baby is born, prolactin signals the mammary glands in the female breast to produce milk. Then oxytocin becomes involved again. It stimulates the mammary glands to "let down" the milk each time the infant begins to nurse.

After delivery, drugs such as ergonovine (*Ergotrate*) and methylergonovine (*Methergine*) may be given to minimize bleeding or postpartum hemorrhage.

Premature labor is labor that occurs before the thirty-seventh week of pregnancy and is a major problem in obstetrics. Ritodrine (*Yutopar*) is used to prevent and treat premature labor by inhibiting uterine contractions.

Alternately, uterine contractions can be induced by prostaglandins for the purpose of pregnancy termination **(abortifacients).** Some prostaglandins include the vaginal suppository dinoprostone (*Prostin E₂*) and injectable carboprost (*Hemabate*).

DISORDERS OF THE REPRODUCTIVE SYSTEM

VAGINAL INFECTIONS

Vaginal infections are common in women because microorganisms have easy access to the internal organs through the external genitalia. Yeast infection and trichomoniasis are the two most common forms of infection. Vaginal infections cause inflammation of the vagina **(vaginitis),** and there is an unusual discharge (cheeselike, or foamy and foul-smelling). They also cause itching and burning in the vulvar area. Untreated, they may spread to other organs of the reproductive system, causing further inflammation; for example, **cervicitis,** inflammation of the cervix.

A variety of vaginal douches, creams, tablets, and suppositories are available that have antibacterial and antifungal actions. Practice Procedure 13.1 on page 262 shows how these are inserted. The specific infecting organism must be identified in the laboratory so that the proper anti-infective can be selected. Some common topical preparations are miconazole (*Monistat 7*) and clotrimazole (*Gyne-Lotrimin*).

An oral medication, metronidazole (*Flagyl*), is the drug of choice for treating trichomoniasis, a protozoan vaginal infection. Usually both sexual partners are infected with this organism, which can be identified in the vaginal secretions, prostatic fluid, and semen. To effect a cure, both partners must receive the drug simultaneously.

Endometriosis is a condition in which endometrial tissue grows outside the uterus. The most common symptom is low abdominal pain, described as dull, aching, or crampy, that occurs one to two days before menstruation and decreases after the onset of menstruation. Abnormal uterine bleeding, backache, painful sexual intercourse, and painful defecation can also occur. Treatment relies on surgery or hormonal medications, such as danazol (*Danocrine*), nafarelin (*Synarel*), and *Lupron Depot*, which is the newest and most expensive drug. The patient should be informed that hormonal therapy is not a cure. It only controls symptoms.

SEXUALLY TRANSMITTED DISEASES

Sexually transmitted diseases (STDs) are infectious diseases associated with sexual contact. Diseases associated with sexual transmission may also be contracted through blood, blood products, and accidental needle sticks.

Since 1981, when public health officials identified acquired immune deficiency syndrome (AIDS) as a new disease, it has become an increasing health concern. It is transmitted from person to person by means of infected blood, semen, vaginal secretions, and breast milk. It has been identified in both heterosexual and homosexual populations and affects all races and ethnic groups. AIDS is caused by the human immunodeficiency virus (HIV). Unlike other sexually transmitted diseases, it may be latent for as many as ten years before the onset of symptoms. Therefore, an infected person can infect another person without knowing it. Because there is currently no cure for AIDS, teaching should focus on prevention.

When symptoms do develop, they include persistent fevers, night sweats, diarrhea, headache, enlarged glands, skin rash, and fatigue. Four drugs (zidovudine, didanosine, zalcitabine, and stavudine) have been approved to treat HIV infection. They block reverse transcriptase, an enzyme required for HIV replication. As a result, they slow the disease process.

In addition to AIDS, genital **herpes simplex** and hepatitis B are sexually transmitted viral diseases. There is currently no cure for genital herpes; however, flare-ups can be prevented and treated with acyclovir (*Zovirax*). Hepatitis B can be prevented by vaccination. Venereal warts (condylomata acuminata) are also due to a virus, human papilloma virus (HPV). One common treatment is 80 percent to 90 percent trichloroacetic acid applied directly to the wart surface. Podophyllin (10 percent to 25 percent), a cytotoxic agent, is applied to each wart and left on for 1 to 4 hours before being washed off.

The older sexually transmitted infections, such as syphilis and gonorrhea, are becoming resistant to some antibiotics and are still a problem for the health care community. Ceftriaxone (*Rocephin*) is given for gonorrhea, and parenteral penicillin remains the treatment of choice for syphilis.

Chlamydial infections are caused by several strains of Chlamydiatrachomatis. Infertility and pelvic inflammatory disease (PID) are two complications of chlamydial infections. Chlamydia infections may be treated with tetracycline, doxycycline, or azithromycin.

Trichomoniasis is a vaginal infection that is usually treated with metronidazole (*Flagyl*).

Treatment of sexually transmitted diseases can be especially difficult for the health care worker. Frequently there are no symptoms, and people are reluctant to discuss existing symptoms and to involve sexual partners in the treatment plan. Prevention is preferable to trying to cure an established infection. Use of condoms (made from latex or polyurethane) by sexually active people has been

PATIENT EDUCATION

shown to help prevent the spread of these diseases. If you are concerned about transmission of STDs, especially AIDS, you can request free, up-to-date information from the Centers for Disease Control and Prevention (CDC).

PROSTATE DISEASES

The prostate is the male gland that secretes mucus and other substances that help make up semen. Inflammation of the prostate, **prostatitis,** is a disease of older men and frequently the most common urinary tract infection. Symptoms include fever, chills, painful urination, urethral discharge, and increased urination. Prostatitis is frequently associated with infection in the urethra or lower urinary tract. Treatment consists of antibiotics, anti-inflammatory drugs, and measures to promote comfort, such as sitz baths and frequent prostatic massage.

After age 40, and especially around ages 60 to 70, the prostate tends to enlarge. An enlarged prostate may indicate cancer of the prostate, which is the second leading cause of cancer deaths in men. Treatment is generally surgery and radiation.

Benign prostatic hyperplasia or hypertrophy (BPH) is a new growth of epithelial and stromal elements within the prostate gland. Hypertrophy is actually an incorrect term because it is not an enlargement of existing cells, as this term implies. Hyperplasia, an increase in the number of cells, is the correct term. As the prostate grows, it creates an obstruction of the urethra, causing a decrease in the urinary stream, dribbling, and the inability to empty the bladder. Finasteride (*Proscar*) is a new drug that inhibits a form of testosterone responsible for the hyperplasia of cells. Other drugs, such as terazosin (*Hytrin*), prazosin (*Minipress*), and doxazosin (*Cardura*), cause smooth muscle relaxation and improve urinary flow. If drug therapy fails, surgery, such as a transurethral resection, is performed to remove a portion of the prostate.

CANCER

All the organs of the male and female reproductive systems can develop malignant tumors. Cancers of the breast and uterus are common in women, as is prostate cancer in men. Eighty percent of prostate cancers occur in men over the age of 65. Tumors of the testicles are rare but often malignant. The peak age for susceptibility to testicular cancer is 20 to 40 years. The treatment of choice for these cancers is surgery to remove the cancerous growth.

INFERTILITY

Problems of infertility affect about 15 percent of couples who wish to have children. Pregnancy is ultimately achieved by about 40 percent of the couples who seek treatment.

Infertility in females can be related to cervical mucus, ovulation problems, hormonal imbalances, or endometriosis. Surgery and drugs can be used to overcome some of these problems. Infertility in the male is usually related to problems with sperm density, motility, or shape, or with seminal fluid volume or viscosity. Some of the drugs used to treat infertility are clomiphene (*Clomid*), human chorionic gonadotropin (*Pregnyl, Follutein*), and menotropins (*Pergonal*).

USE OF SEX HORMONES IN DRUG THERAPY

Although we say that there are female hormones and male hormones, both types of hormones are secreted in both the male and female bodies. The hormones secreted by the gonads—estrogen, progesterone, and testosterone—have other uses besides regulating the organs of reproduction. They are chemically related and are involved in ongoing body processes such as growth, sexual development, bone formation, the storage of minerals, and the building of proteins. They have several uses in drug therapy as well. Hormone replacement is one use, but larger doses can be therapeutic for conditions unrelated to a lack of sex hormones. Natural sex hormones for drug therapy are gathered from the bodies of domestic animals. For example, estrogen is collected from the urine of pregnant mares. Synthetic forms are also available.

Representative drugs that affect the reproductive system are shown in the table at the end of this chapter, including their uses, actions, doses, and side effects.

ESTROGEN

Estrogen is administered in drug therapy for several reasons. One is to replace female hormones after menopause or following a total abdominal hysterectomy with removal of the uterus, ovaries, and fallopian tubes. At menopause, the ovaries stop producing female hormones. The pituitary produces large amounts of gonadotropins in response to the decrease in estrogen level. As a result, the most common physical changes related to menopause are "hot flashes" and thinning and drying of the vagina. Hormone replacement therapy (HRT) reduces these symptoms.

After menopause, estrogen may also be used to prevent bone thinning, brittleness, and spontaneous fracturing **(osteoporosis).** Estrogen is also used to treat failure to menstruate **(amenorrhea),** vaginal inflammation, and breast cancer in older women and prostate cancer in men. Women who do not wish to breast-feed their newborn babies may be given estrogen to "dry up" the milk and prevent swollen breasts **(engorgement).**

The most common side effects of hormone replacement therapy are weight gain, breast and pelvic discomfort, GI disturbances, vaginal discharge, and skin pigmentation. These symptoms usually result from an excessive dose and can be reduced by decreasing the dose. Estrogens are generally administered in cycles—for example, 3 weeks on and 1 week off. The long-term use of estrogen replacement carries an increased risk of cancer of the **endometrium** (the uterine lining) and some types of breast cancer. Estrogen must not be given to pregnant women because it can cause birth defects (congenital anomalies), or it can later cause cancer in the female child. An important part of ensuring safe and effective therapy is patient education.

PATIENT EDUCATION

Hormone Replacement Therapy (HRT)

- Explore concerns about the risks of taking estrogen before beginning HRT
- Inform the physician of a family history of cancer, hypertension, cardiovascular disease, and osteoporosis
- Have regular physical exams, including a mammogram and PAP smear, every 6 months to a year during treatment
- Perform monthly breast self-examinations
- If pregnancy is suspected, immediately stop medication and contact physician
- Avoid smoking (smoking increases the side effects of HRT)
- Notify the physician if you develop severe headache, blurred vision, chest pain, shortness of breath, or leg pain

- Weigh yourself once or twice a week and report any sharp increase in weight or fluid retention to the physician
- Follow a low-sodium diet
- Maintain good oral hygiene to prevent periodontal problems
- Avoid excessive sun exposure (sun can cause blotchy, brown skin discolorations)
- Expect uterine bleeding when stopping HRT
- Apply transdermal forms of drugs to rotating sites on the abdomen, using the same site no more than once in 7 days
- Learn how to take the medication (e.g., 3 weeks on, 1 week off)
- When using the vaginal form of the drug, protect clothing with a sanitary napkin

Many chemical forms of estrogen are available generically. Common forms are estradiol, estrone, and conjugated estrogens (*Premarin*). Transdermal estradiol (*Estraderm*) is applied topically to intact skin. Topical forms of these drugs are available for application to the vagina to control inflammation (vaginitis) after menopause.

PROGESTERONE

Progesterone, the second female hormone, acts in partnership with estrogen to prepare the body for reproduction. While estrogen stimulates the production of egg cells in the ovary, progesterone helps prepare the uterus to receive and nourish a fertilized egg. During pregnancy, progesterone suppresses ovulation and relaxes the uterine smooth muscle.

Progesterone is given for conditions such as abnormal uterine bleeding, inflammation of the uterine lining (endometriosis), **dysmenorrhea** (painful menstruation), and amenorrhea. In postmenopausal women who are taking estrogen, the addition of progesterone for 1 week per month may provide protection from endometrial cancer. Side effects of progesterone—nausea, headache, and dizziness—usually go away with continued use. Occasionally a person may develop depression, edema, and apathy while on progesterone. Medroxyprogesterone acetate (*Provera, Depo-Provera*) and megestrol (*Megace*) are synthetic forms of progesterone.

CONTRACEPTIVES

Oral contraception is the most effective form of birth control presently available. "The pill" is a combination of estrogen and progestins. Advancements in contraceptive research have resulted in low-dose hormones that more closely match those in the body. Research has demonstrated that progestins are more effective when absorbed in the skin. *Depo-Provera* (DMPA) and

Norplant have high success rates, whereas the minipill or progestin-only pill (POPS) have high failure rates.

The main side effects of contraceptive pills are abdominal pain, chest pain, cough, shortness of breath, headache, weakness, dizziness, numbness, eye problems, speech problems, or severe leg pain.

The pill has been a source of controversy since it was first introduced, and many people still misunderstand and fear it. Current research proves that the new low-dose estrogen formulas have eliminated many of the earlier problems; for example, the pill is safe for women under the age of 35 who smoke. The pill also has added advantages, such as protection against pelvic inflammatory disease.

TESTOSTERONE

Like female sex hormones, male sex hormones, also called androgens, are secreted in both males and females. The main androgen, testosterone, is used in replacement therapy for men when the testes are not producing enough hormone for proper development or sexual activity. It also helps relieve the symptoms of breast cancer. Because testosterone promotes the building of body tissues, it may be used to reverse tissue wasting and loss of protein resulting from burns, surgery, and debilitating diseases that keep patients confined to a chair or bed over long periods. When used in women, testosterone can result in masculine side effects (e.g., deepening voice, increased body hair). Its use can also lead to retention of salts and thus edema, which can usually be controlled with diuretics. Examples of testosterones are methyltestosterone (*Oreton Methyl, Metandren*) and fluoxymesterone (*Halotestin*).

REPRESENTATIVE DRUGS FOR THE REPRODUCTIVE SYSTEM

CATEGORY, NAME[a], AND ROUTE	USES AND DISEASES	ACTIONS	USUAL DOSE[b] AND SPECIAL INSTRUCTIONS	SIDE EFFECTS AND ADVERSE REACTIONS
Hormones				
Conjugated estrogens (*Premarin*) Oral, Cream, IM, IV	Abnormal uterine bleeding; menopausal symptoms; breast and inoperable prostate cancer	Replaces estrogen	*Postmenopause:* 0.3–1.25 mg/day for 3 weeks, then 1 week off; repeat cycle *Cancer:* 1.25 mg TID daily as ordered by physician	Nausea, breakthrough bleeding, fluid retention
Oxytocin (*Pitocin, Syntocinon*) IV, IM	Induction or stimulation of labor, incomplete abortion, control of postpartum bleeding	Stimulation of uterine and mammary glands	10–40 units in 1000 cc D_5W or normal saline	Hypertension, arrhythmias, seizures, coma, effects on fetus, bradycardia, tachycardia, irregular heartbeat, anoxia, asphyxia
Medroxyprogesterone acetate (*Provera*) Oral, IM	Dysfunctional uterine bleeding, amenorrhea, endometrial cancer, contraception	Suppresses ovulation	5–10 mg PO for 5–10 days; administer with food if gastric upset occurs	Breast tenderness, weight changes, fluid retention, thrombophlebitis, pulmonary embolism, dizziness, migraines, breakthrough bleeding
Levonorgestrel (*Norplant*) implants	Contraception (slow release of progestin levongestrel in the bloodstream)	Prevents implantation of egg	Six capsules implanted subdermally in midportion of arm; lasts 5 years *Male:* 10–50 mg/day	Abdominal discomfort, amenorrhea, bleeding irregularities, musculoskeletal pain, breast discharge, headache

CATEGORY, NAME[a], AND ROUTE	USES AND DISEASES	ACTIONS	USUAL DOSE[b] AND SPECIAL INSTRUCTIONS	SIDE EFFECTS AND ADVERSE REACTIONS
Hormones (continued)				
Methyltestosterone (*Metandren*) Oral, Buccal	*Male:* Hypogonadism *Female:* Cancer of the breast, postpartum breast engorgement	Stimulation of spermatogenesis, development of male sex characteristics, sexual maturity	*Male:* 10–50 mg/day PO; 5–25 mg *Female:* 80 mg/day PO for 3–5 days or 40 mg/day buccal for breast engorgement; 200 mg/day PO or 100 mg/day buccal for cancer; do not swallow or chew buccal medications; do not eat, drink, or smoke until buccal medication has dissolved	*Male:* Jaundice, edema *Female:* Amenorrhea, virilization, hair growth, acne, change in **libido** (sex drive)
Antibacterials				
Miconazole (*Monistat 7*) Suppository, Cream	Local vaginal infections caused by *Candida* fungus	Fungicidal agent	1 suppository or applicator full of cream once daily at bedtime for 7 days; protect underclothing	Vaginal itching and burning
Metronidazole (*Flagyl*) Oral, IV	Trichomoniasis, amebiasis	Amebicide and trichomonacidal agent	2 g given as single dose or 250 mg TID for 7 consecutive days; male partner should also be treated	Nausea, vomiting, anorexia, headache, diarrhea; rarely, seizures, peripheral neuropathy
Antiretroviral				
Zidovudine (*AZT, ZDV, Retrovir*) Oral	Human immunodeficiency virus (HIV) infection	Blocks reverse transcriptase	200 mg PO TID or 100 mg PO 5 times a day; drug of choice to initiate treatment	Fatigue, headache, rash, nausea, seizures, severe bone marrow depression, confusion, agitation
Sildenafil citrate (*Viagra*) Oral	Impotence	Penile erection	25 mg, 50 mg, or 100 mg 1 hour before sexual activity; may interact with drugs containing nitrates such as nitroglycerin	Headache, diarrhea, flushing, indigestion, nasal congestion, increased sensitivity to light

[a] Trade names given in parentheses are examples only. Check current drug references for a complete listing of available products.

[b] Average adult doses are given. However, dosages are determined by a physician and vary with the purpose of the therapy and the particular patient. The doses presented in this text are for general information only.

■ **EQUIPMENT**

Medication orders for vaginal medications

Kardex, medicine cards, medication record, patient chart

Medicine tray or cart

Vaginal medications (practice with one or all four): suppository, ointment, cream, or jelly

Applicator for inserting medication

Disposable gloves

Tissues

Perineal pad (optional)

■ **PROCEDURE**

1. Assemble equipment.

2. Read the medication order and set up medications. Check for the "five rights."

3. Wash your hands.

4. Identify the patient. Explain what you are going to do. Have the patient void before beginning the procedure. Curtain off the area for privacy.

5. Assist the patient into a position for insertion. She should lie on her back, with the knees bent and legs spread apart to expose the perineum. Drape the patient for privacy and warmth.

6. Put on disposable gloves, unwrap the suppository, and lubricate rounded end with petroleum jelly. Suppositories are inserted by the dominant hand. Creams, ointments, and jellies are inserted with an applicator, using the dominant hand.

7. With the nondominant hand, gently retract the labial fold to expose the vaginal opening (refer to Figure 13.2 on page 252).

8. Insert medication.
   By hand: Insert rounded end of suppository along posterior wall of the vaginal canal, the length of index finger (approximately 3 to 4 inches).
   By applicator: Fill the applicator with cream and insert 2 to 3 inches into the vagina. Push down on applicator plunger to release medication into vagina, to allow equal distribution along vaginal wall (Figure 13.5).

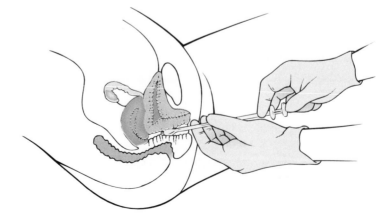

Figure 13.5
Inserting vaginal
medication with
an applicator.

Continued

9. Withdraw finger or applicator and wipe vaginal opening with tissue, if necessary, or let the patient do this.

10. Clean or discard applicator, and remove and discard gloves.

11. Assist the patient back into a comfortable position and give any needed instructions. Provide perineal pads to collect excess vaginal discharge and to avoid staining underclothes.

12. Wash your hands.

13. Chart the medication.

Demonstrate this procedure for your instructor.

Define each of the terms listed below.

1. Oxytocic _____

2. Dysmenorrhea _____

3. Engorgement _____

4. Endometrium _____

5. Abortifacients _____

6. HIV _____

7. AIDS _____

Complete the following statements by filling in the blanks.

8. Female sex cells, the ova, are produced by the _____.

9. Male sex cells, the sperm, are produced by the _____.

10. The tubular structure that serves as the birth canal is called the _____
_____.

11. The structure that holds the fertilized ovum while it develops inside the woman's body is the
_____.

12. Lactation occurs when the _____ glands in the breast go into production.

13. The ejaculatory duct passes through the _____ gland, where mucus and other fluids are added to the sperm.

14. Semen leaves the male body through a tube called the _____, which is shared with the urinary system.

Match the hormones to their function in regulating human reproduction.

_____ 15. Estrogen
a. stimulates sperm production and development of deep voice and chest and facial hair

_____ 16. Progesterone
b. acts in partnership with estrogen to regulate ovulation and prepare uterus for pregnancy

_____ 17. Testosterone
c. triggers the onset of labor

_____ 18. Oxytocin
d. stimulates development of breasts, shapeliness, and the feminine voice

Answer the following questions in the spaces provided.

19. List all the therapeutic uses you can think of for sex hormones (both male and female). _____

_____

_____

_____

_____

Continued

20. What are the possible side effects of estrogen therapy (including oral contraceptives)? _____

_____

_____

_____

_____

21. What are the possible side effects of testosterone therapy? _____

_____

_____

_____

_____

Place a t in the blank if the statement is true. Place an f in the blank if the statement is false.

_____ 22. Sexually transmitted diseases are all easily treated and cured with drugs.

_____ 23. Chlamydial infections are common but have no serious effects.

_____ 24. Dysuria refers to difficult or painful urination.

_____ 25. Endometriosis can be a factor in infertility.

_____ 26. Osteoporosis is caused by too much estrogen.

_____ 27. Oral contraceptives work by preventing ovulation.

_____ 28. Testosterone relieves the symptoms of breast cancer.

_____ 29. Androgens is another word for male sex hormones.

■ CASE STUDIES FOR CRITICAL THINKING

Choose the disorder that best matches each description below. Write the name of the disorder in the blank.

Cervicitis	Benign prostatic hyperplasia (BPH)	Genital herpes simplex
Endometriosis	Acquired immune deficiency syndrome (AIDS)	

30. Nancy Bullock had an unusual vaginal discharge that caused itching and burning, but she ignored it. Now the doctor says that the infection has spread to the opening of the uterus.

_____

31. Harry Jackson, age 62, is having more and more trouble urinating lately. The doctor thinks something may be blocking the urethra. Harry says this is the same condition that several friends his age have had.

_____

32. Akiko Niki has an inflammation of the uterine lining, and her doctor has placed her on progesterone therapy.

_____

33. John Sullivan, age 28, is experiencing night sweats, diarrhea, and a persistent fever. A physical examination revealed that he is an IV drug user.

_____

Continued

34. Sara Davis is diagnosed with a sexually transmitted viral disease and treated with acyclovir (*Zovirax*).

_____

■ APPLICATIONS

Obtain a current copy of a drug reference book or the PDR®. Use it to answer the following questions in a notebook or on file cards.

35. Use the *PDR®* to find another product name for each drug in the Representative Drug table on pages 260–261 of this text.

36. In Section 3 of the *PDR®*, Product Category Index, find Endometriosis Management. Make a list of all the drugs you see listed there.

InterNET CONNECTION

To learn more about diseases of the reproductive system, including sexually transmitted diseases, go to the Centers for Disease Control and Prevention at http://www.cdc.gov. Click on Health Information and click on the letter *S*. If you click on Sexually Transmitted Diseases, you will find a listing of the most common types as well as recent statistics.

Drugs for the Endocrine System

In this chapter you will learn about hormones and the glands that manufacture them. You will learn what goes wrong when the glands produce too much or too little of the hormones and how hormone therapy can help correct hormone imbalances. You will learn about the treatment of diabetes and the uses of corticosteroid hormones and hormonelike drugs.

OBJECTIVES

After studying this chapter, you should be able to

- name the hormones produced by the seven major glands.
- state the action of each of these hormones or hormonelike drugs: somatotropic hormone, thyroxine, parathyroid, corticosteroids, epinephrine (adrenaline) and norepinephrine, insulin, adrenocorticotropic hormone, and antidiuretic hormone.
- state which hormones are lacking in the condition of diabetes mellitus, diabetes insipidus, Addison's disease, and hypothyroidism, and give examples of drugs used for replacement in each case.
- use correct medical terms in referring to parts of the endocrine system and symptoms of hormone imbalances.
- list the types of insulin available for treatment of diabetes mellitus, and give examples of each group.
- give examples of oral hypoglycemics used for diabetes treatment and explain how they work.
- recognize the symptoms of hyperglycemia and hypoglycemia and explain how they are treated.
- state what factors affect the insulin needs of a patient with diabetes mellitus.
- list at least three uses of corticosteroids.
- name five possible side effects of long-term corticosteroid therapy.

KEY TERMS

adrenals: paired glands covering the superior surface of the kidneys; made up of the adrenal cortex, which secretes steroids, and the adrenal medulla, which secretes epinephrine and norepinephrine

antidiabetic agents: insulin and oral hypoglycemics

corticosteroids: hormones produced by the adrenal cortex; they have anti-inflammatory action and suppress the immune reaction

diabetes mellitus: most common pancreatic disorder, characterized by an inability to use carbohydrates;

insulin production is ineffective or not available

diabetic coma: unconsciousness caused by too little insulin accompanied by increased caloric intake, physical or emotional stress, or undiagnosed diabetes mellitus; also called diabetic ketoacidosis

gland: specialized epithelial tissue that secretes hormones

glucagon: hormone secreted by the pancreas that raises the level of blood sugar; counteracts effects of insulin

glucocorticoids: adrenal corticosteroids that regulate the metabolism of carbo-

hydrates and fats by body cells and have an anti-inflammatory effect

glycogen: form of glucose stored in the liver or muscles for release as the body needs it

glycosuria: glucose in the urine

hormone: chemical substance secreted by glands that regulates many body functions; each hormone has specific functions

hyperplasia: actual increase in the number of cells

hypoglycemia: low blood sugar; can be the result of administering too much insulin

hypothalamus: portion of the pituitary gland linked to the brain; controls many body functions such as temperature, sleep, and appetite

insulin: naturally occurring hormone secreted by the beta cells in the islets of Langerhans in the pancreas in response to increased blood glucose levels

iodine: mineral needed by the thyroid to produce thyroxine

islets of Langerhans: made up of beta cells that secrete insulin and alpha cells that secrete glucagon

ketoacidosis: acidosis caused by a surplus of fatty acids (ketones) in the bloodstream; a complication of diabetes mellitus

mineralocorticoid: hormone secreted by the adrenal cortex that maintains normal blood volume, and promotes sodium and water retention and urinary excretion of potassium

oral hypoglycemics: drugs that stimulate the beta cells of the pancreas to secrete insulin

parathyroid hormone: hormone secreted by the parathyroids; regulates the calcium content of the bloodstream

parathyroids: four glands located behind the thyroid; secrete parathormone

pituitary: gland at the base of the brain, known as the "master gland," that regulates many body activities and stimulates other glands to secrete their own hormones

polydipsia: excessive thirst

polyuria: excessive urination

somatotropin: growth hormone secreted by the pituitary gland

tetany: muscle spasms caused by lack of calcium in the bloodstream

thyroid: gland below the larynx that produces, stores, and releases thyroid hormone

thyroxine: hormone secreted by the thyroid gland; regulates the speed of metabolism in body cells

Type I, insulin-dependent diabetes mellitus (IDDM): disorder wherein there is an inability to metabolize carbohydrates as a result of insulin deficiency; insulin must be given for treatment

Type II, non-insulin-dependent diabetes mellitus (NIDDM): usually affects individuals who are obese and over the age of 35; insulin may be part of treatment

ENDOCRINE SYSTEM

The endocrine system is made up of **glands,** structures that secrete chemical substances called **hormones.** Hormones regulate many body functions. They are carried by the blood to sites where they exert their action. Hormones are the main regulators of metabolism, growth and development, reproduction, homeostasis, energy production, and immunity.

The endocrine glands include the hypothalamus, pituitary, thyroid, parathyroids, pineal, thymus, adrenal, pancreas, ovaries, and testes (Figure 14.1).

PITUITARY GLAND

The **pituitary,** a small gland about the size of a pea, is located at the base of the brain. The pituitary stalk connects the pituitary to the hypothalamus. Although the pituitary is one gland, it has two lobes: the anterior lobe and the posterior lobe. The anterior lobe is particularly important in sustaining life. One of the hormones it secretes is the growth hormone, **somatotropin,** which promotes skeletal, visceral, and general growth. If too much growth hormone is produced, the body grows too fast and becomes overly large. When this occurs in a child, it is called gigantism. In adulthood, it is called acromegaly. Too little of the hormone results in stunted growth or dwarfism.

Other pituitary hormones control the secretions of the sex glands, the thyroid gland, and the adrenal glands. Because it controls the hormone production of other glands, the pituitary is known as the master gland.

THYROID GLAND

The **thyroid** gland is wrapped around the trachea just below the larynx, or voice box. It secretes two thyroid hormones and thyrocalcitonin. The two thyroid hormones are **thyroxine** and triiodothyronine (T_4). These thyroid hormones control metabolism. Metabolism refers to the rate at which all cells produce energy (heat, muscle strength, etc.). When the thyroid produces extra thyroxine and triiodothyronine (hyperthyroidism), the metabolic rate is increased and there is an increase in temperature, respiration, heart rate, nervous and muscular activity, and a feeling of warmth. Too little thyroxine and triiodothyronine (hypothyroidism) causes cell metabolism to slow down.

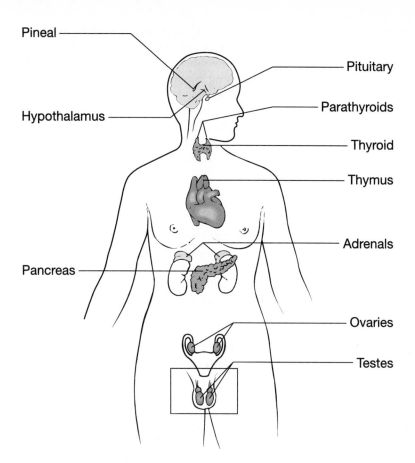

Figure 14.1
Glands of the endocrine system.

Signs of hypothyroidism include intolerance to cold, personality changes, fatigue, dry skin, brittle nails, slow speech, and weight gain.

To produce adequate thyroxine and triiodothyronine, the thyroid gland needs **iodine,** a mineral that is present in vegetables and seafood. The availability of iodized table salt helps people take in enough iodine to fulfill the needs of the thyroid. Thyrocalcitonin helps maintain a normal blood calcium level.

PARATHYROID GLANDS

The **parathyroids** are four small glands located behind the thyroid gland. The hormone they produce is called **parathyroid hormone (PTH).** The main function of this hormone is to maintain a normal blood calcium level. A certain amount of calcium is needed in the bloodstream for muscles to work properly. Extra calcium is stored in the bones. When the level of calcium in the blood is low, the parathyroid glands produce parathyroid hormone to release stored calcium from the bones. If too much parathyroid hormone is manufactured, too much calcium may be taken out of the bones. As a result, the bones may become soft and easy to bend. If too little parathyroid hormone is produced, the muscles may go into spasms, and convulsions and gradual paralysis may occur. This condition, which affects mainly the face and the hands, is called **tetany,** and can be fatal. The symptoms of tetany are relieved by administration of calcium.

ADRENAL GLANDS (SUPRARENALS)

The two **adrenal** glands sit on top of (superior to) the two kidneys. Each adrenal gland has two layers: the adrenal cortex and the adrenal medulla. The adrenal cortex is the largest portion of the adrenal gland and secretes two hormones called **corticosteroids. Glucocorticoids** regulate the metabolism of carbohydrates and fats and have an anti-inflammatory effect. **Mineralocorticoids** maintain normal blood volume and promote sodium and water retention and urinary excretion of potassium.

The adrenal medulla secretes epinephrine and norepinephrine. These hormones help the body meet stressful situations. Epinephrine and norepinephrine prepare the body to react to emergencies by stimulating the heartbeat, increasing blood pressure, and releasing extra sugar into the bloodstream. Epinephrine and norepinephrine are produced in the body but are also available as drugs to be administered. Epinephrine made in the body is also known as adrenaline. As a drug, it is used in the treatment of bronchial asthma, as described in Chapter 10. Norepinephrine is used in the emergency treatment of shock because of its ability to constrict blood vessels.

PANCREAS

As noted in Chapter 11, the pancreas secretes enzymes as part of the digestive system. It also contains a number of secreting structures that are part of the endocrine system. These structures are called the **islets of Langerhans.** They secrete two hormones: insulin and glucagon.

Insulin controls the cell's use of sugar. It also stimulates the liver to store extra sugar in the form of **glycogen.** When the pancreas fails to produce insulin, the cells cannot burn sugar. Instead, it remains in the bloodstream and is excreted in the urine. This condition is known as **diabetes mellitus.**

The hormone **glucagon** stimulates the liver to release stored sugar into the bloodstream. It is administered in emergencies when diabetic patients have received too much insulin.

OVARIES AND TESTES

These are the sex glands, or gonads. They are responsible for the different physical characteristics of males and females and for the manufacture of sex cells for reproduction. The female gonads are the ovaries. The male gonads are the testes.

The ovaries, located in the pelvis of the female, secrete the hormones estrogen and progesterone. The testes, located in the scrotum of the male, produce testosterone, the male hormone. However, both males and females have both types of hormones in their bodies. These hormones and their uses in drug therapy are described in Chapter 13.

HORMONE CONTROL SYSTEM

The level of hormones in the blood is constantly adjusted to meet the body's requirements. A large intake of carbohydrates, for example, stimulates the pancreas to release insulin to help reduce the blood sugar level. A complex chemical control system is required to ensure proper hormone levels. At the center of this control system is the pituitary gland, which stimulates other glands to produce hormones.

The pituitary, in turn, is linked to the brain's control system (the nervous system) by the **hypothalamus.** This is a portion of the brain stem that lies just behind the pituitary. It is connected to the pituitary by a stalk. The hypothalamus controls basic body functions such as sleep, appetite, and body temperature.

The hypothalamus and pituitary form a partnership in running the hormone chemical message system. The hypothalamus can stimulate or inhibit the pituitary according to conditions inside and outside the body. Because of this link, the endocrine system is influenced by the nervous system. Thus, emotions, fears, and moods have an impact on body processes through hormone stimulation as well as nerve stimulation.

The levels of circulating hormones provide feedback to the control system. As mentioned, hormones are distributed throughout the body via the bloodstream. When the proper hormone level is reached, the hypothalamus signals the pituitary to stop stimulating hormone production.

As an example, say the body needs extra sugar and fat for a heavy physical task. The pituitary excretes adrenocorticotropic hormone (ACTH), which is

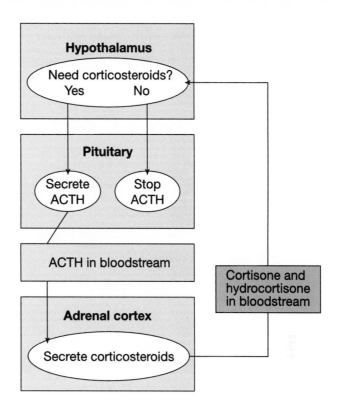

Figure 14.2
Hormone levels in the bloodstream determine when hormone secretion will occur.

swiftly transported by the bloodstream to the adrenal cortex. The ACTH then stimulates the adrenal cortex to produce corticosteroids. These help liberate extra sugar and fat for the body to burn for energy. When the hypothalamus senses that there are enough corticosteroids in the bloodstream, it signals the pituitary to "cancel the order" for ACTH. The adrenal cortex then stops secreting its hormones until they are needed again (see Figure 14.2).

DISORDERS OF THE ENDOCRINE SYSTEM

Hormones control body processes—growth, metabolism, kidney function, and so forth. Consequently, when there is a disturbance in the production of hormones, the body processes go out of control. If a child's pituitary produces too much growth hormone, it can result in a condition called gigantism; an adult develops diabetes mellitus because the pancreas fails to produce enough insulin to maintain sugar metabolism.

Symptoms of endocrine disorders are logically related to the specific hormones that are out of balance. That is, when a certain hormone is lacking, symptoms show that the body process it regulates is no longer working properly.

Endocrine disorders arise because a gland overproduces, underproduces, or produces its hormones too early or too late. Table 14.1 on page 272 lists examples of endocrine disorders and their symptoms. Note that the names of the various disorders usually tell you something about how hormone production has gone wrong. Recall that *hypo* means too little (less than normal) and *hyper* means too much (more than normal).

There are several reasons that a gland may secrete too much, too little, or too early. One is that the gland may be overdeveloped, a condition called **hyperplasia.** Or it may contain a tumor. Usually tumors and hyperplasia cause too much hormone production because there are far more secreting cells than normal. In these cases, surgery or radiation treatment may be needed to reduce the number of cells and thus restore normal hormone balance.

One form of radiation treatment is the radioactive "cocktail." The patient drinks a radioactive material that travels to the gland to destroy the tumor. In

TABLE 14.1: Selected Hormones and Their Disorders

HORMONE	FUNCTION	DISORDER	SYMPTOMS	TREATMENT
Pituitary				
Somatatropin	Regulates growth	Hypersecretion in adulthood—acromegaly	Enlargement of hands, feet, face, jaws, and cheeks	Radiation, surgery
		Hypersecretion in childhood—gigantism	Growth to an extreme height	Sex hormones
		Undersecretion—dwarfism	Failure to grow to normal height, remaining small and fragile	Somatatropin (growth hormone replacement)
Follicle-stimulating hormone (FSH)	Regulates development of sex characteristics by stimulating gonads (ovaries and testes) to secrete sex hormones	Too much, too early—overdevelopment	Development of adultlike sex characteristics as early as 5 years of age	Hormone replacement
		Too little—underdevelopment	Failure to develop sex characteristics during the teens	
Luteinizing hormone (LTH) (called ovulating hormone)	Stimulates ovulation	Too little—failure to ovulate	Menstrual irregularities	Hormone replacement
Antidiuretic hormone (ADH)	Regulates reabsorption of water in kidney tubules	Too little—diabetes insipidus	Polyuria, polydipsia	Hormone replacement, some diuretics
Thyroid				
Thyroxine and triiodothyronine (regulated by the thyroid-stimulating hormone [TSH] of the pituitary)	Regulates metabolism	Too much of either thyroxine or triiodothyronine—hyperthyroidism	Nervousness, weight loss, heat intolerance, tachycardia, elevated temperature, insomnia, bulging eyes, etc.	Surgery, radioactive iodine cocktail, antithyroid drugs such as Propylthiouracil and methimazole (*Tapazole*)
Calcitonin	Inhibits calcium reabsorption from bone, increases calcium storage in bone, increases renal excretion of calcium and phosphorus, lowers calcium level in blood	Too little—hypothyroidism (also cretinism and myxedema, depending on when deficiency occurs)	Slowed mental and physical processes, fatigue, hair loss, constipation, intolerance to cold, weight gain, dry skin, brittle nails	Synthetic oral thyroxine (*Synthroid, Levothroid, Noroxine*)
		Enlargement of thyroid gland—goiter	Enlargement of thyroid, swelling in neck	Thyroid hormone may prevent further enlargement; surgery for large goiters
Parathyroid				
Parathyroid hormone	Regulates blood level of calcium	Too much—hyperparathyroidism	Too much calcium taken out of bones, resulting in bone weakness, loss of appetite, increased need for sleep, short attention span, calcium stones in kidneys	Antihypercalcemic agents
		Too little—hypoparathyroidism	Muscle spasms (tetany), convulsions, gradual paralysis	IV calcium salts, vitamin D

TABLE 14.1: Selected Hormones and Their Disorders (continued)

HORMONE	FUNCTION	DISORDER	SYMPTOMS	TREATMENT
Pancreas				
Insulin	Permits body to burn sugar for energy, regulates storage of sugar in the liver	Too little—diabetes mellitus	Thirst, constant hunger, weight loss, fatigue, changes in vision, slow-healing cuts	Insulin replacement, oral hypoglycemics, management of diet, exercise
		Too much—hypoglycemia	Weakness, tachycardia, cold clammy skin, emotional changes	Sugar, food with high sugar content, glucagon
Adrenal Cortex				
Mineralocorticoids (aldosterone, desoxycorticosterone)	Regulates body's salt/water balance by stimulating kidneys to retain sodium and excrete potassium	Too much aldosterone—aldosteronism	Low serum potassium, alkalosis, high blood pressure, headache	Surgery, drugs
Glucocorticoids (cortisone, hydrocortisone)	Stimulates breakdown of protein molecules into carbohydrates	Too much—Cushing's disease	Weight gain, rounding of face, fat deposits on back of neck and on shoulders, hypertension	Surgery
		Too little of all adrenal cortex hormones—acute adrenal crisis, chronic Addison's disease	Shock symptoms in acute cases; in Addison's disease, weakness, tiredness, skin hyperpigmentation, anorexia, weight loss, gastrointestinal symptoms	Hydrocortisone
Androgenic steroids (small amounts of male and female hormones secreted in both males and females)	Thought to contribute to development of sex characteristics (but gonads secrete most of necessary hormones)	Too much of wrong sex hormone—feminization of males, virilization of females	Inappropriate sex characteristics (e.g., manliness, deep voice in females; loss of body hair, high voice in males)	Surgery

the case of a thyroid tumor, for example, the physician can take advantage of the fact that the thyroid traps circulating iodine to use in making thyroxine. A cocktail of radioactive isotopes of iodine can be given so that when they arrive at the thyroid, they destroy the offending cells.

Genetic factors are another reason for gland malfunctions. Some individuals are simply born with defective glands or are missing the necessary chemicals for producing certain hormones. People can inherit tendencies to develop some types of endocrine problems—for example, diabetes mellitus. Genetically caused problems can usually be treated with replacement hormones. Chances for cure are good if these conditions are discovered early enough, before growth and development are permanently affected.

Finally, there may be nothing wrong with a gland itself. The problem may be that the gland is receiving faulty messages from the pituitary. A small tumor on the pituitary, for example, can cause over- or underproduction of the hormones that direct the other glands. Underproduction is diagnosed by administering pituitary hormones to see if they successfully stimulate the other glands. If the problem lies with the pituitary, then either surgery, radiation, or appropriate hormone replacement is required.

Hormone replacement is the most common use of hormones in drug therapy. Replacement is necessary whenever hormones are missing because of either genetic defects in the glands, surgical removal of glands, or production of poor-quality hormones. Some hormones and hormonelike drugs are used because of actions that are not related to the endocrine system—for example, the anti-inflammatory action of the adrenal corticosteroids.

Most hormones used for drug therapy are taken from animals: hogs, cattle, sheep, and horses. A few hormones have been synthesized in the laboratory. Recombinant DNA technology will increase the availability of these important substances.

CAUTION: Hormone Doses

Hormones are powerful chemicals that have profound effects on the human body. They must be administered carefully, according to a doctor's orders. Often the doses are very small. They may be measured in micrograins (a micrograin is one-thousandth of a milligram). The exception is corticosteroids, which are given in large doses to combat allergic reactions and inflammation.

DRUG MANAGEMENT OF DIABETES MELLITUS

Diabetes mellitus is a condition in which the beta cells of the islets of Langerhans in the pancreas do not secrete enough of the hormone insulin. Alterations in insulin production result in abnormal metabolism of carbohydrates, fats, and proteins. As a result, sugar remains in the bloodstream and is excreted in the urine. Meanwhile, body cells "starve." To compensate, they burn protein and fat. The three classic symptoms of diabetes are hunger (polyphagia), thirst (**polydipsia**), and frequent urination (**polyuria**). Other symptoms include weight loss and weakness. Urine tests may reveal large quantities of sugar in the urine.

Diabetes can appear in childhood (**Type I, insulin-dependent diabetes mellitus [IDDM]**) or in adulthood (**Type II, non-insulin-dependent diabetes mellitus [NIDDM]**). Many older adults develop some degree of diabetes along with the changes of aging. Over time, diabetes causes damage to the tissues and organs, especially the heart, kidneys, and eyes. It always carries the danger of complications, such as diseases of the blood vessels and nervous system. Gestational diabetes is the onset of glucose intolerance during pregnancy.

Many mild cases of diabetes can be managed by controlling diet, maintaining normal body weight, and exercising enough to burn off excess blood sugar. Patients with diabetes are encouraged to eat small meals throughout the day rather than a few large meals. The purpose is to avoid large fluctuations in the amount of sugar in the blood. When these measures are not enough to control the diabetes, drug therapy is indicated.

Insulin. The major drug for Type I diabetes is insulin, which is administered by injection. Insulin must be administered by injection because it is destroyed by the gastric secretions. Several oral drugs are available to control blood sugar in Type II NIDDM. Insulin therapy replaces the missing hormone that enables the body to use sugar. More than one preparation of insulin is available, and doctors prescribe different preparations according to individual cases. Dosages are highly individualized and depend on many factors. Insulin preparations are grouped into three basic categories: fast-acting, intermediate-acting, and long-acting. They differ according to how quickly they take effect (onset of action), how soon they reach their peak effect, and how long their effect lasts (duration of action). Table 14.2 summarizes some of these differences.

TABLE 14.2: Types of Insulin

CATEGORY	TYPE	SOURCE	ONSET OF ACTION (HOURS)	PEAK EFFECT (HOURS)	DURATION OF ACTION (HOURS)
Fast-acting	Regular (*Humulin R*)	Beef, pork, human recombinant	$\frac{1}{2}$–1	2–4	5–7
	Semilente	Beef, pork	1–3	2–8	12–16
Intermediate-acting	NPH (*Humulin N*)	Beef, pork, human recombinant	3–4	6–12	18–28
	Lente	Beef, pork, human recombinant	1–3	8–12	18–28
	Novolin 70/30 (70% regular plus 30% NPH)		$\frac{1}{2}$	4–8	24
Long-acting	Ultralente	Beef, pork	4–6	18–24	36
	Protamine zinc	Beef, pork	4–6	18–24	36

Popular drugs for diabetes control are the intermediate-acting insulins: lente and NPH. They reach their peak effectiveness in about 7 hours and last up to 16 hours. They are thus convenient for once-a-day doses, usually administered $\frac{1}{2}$ hour before breakfast. Some doctors prefer to keep closer control over insulin dosages by using the fast-acting semilente and regular insulins. These are given several times during the day (e.g., $\frac{1}{2}$ hour before each meal), and dosages are varied on the basis of frequent urine tests.

Most insulin is derived from beef and pork pancreases. These insulins, especially that of pork, are similar to human insulin. Their use raises the risk of allergies, and they have become expensive. Biosynthetic insulin has come to be used almost exclusively. *Humulin N* or *Humulin R* are produced genetically by altering common bacteria or yeast using DNA technology. These insulins cause fewer allergic reactions, and their insulin activity is more predictable.

A diabetic person's need for insulin varies according to diet, amount of exercise, and emotions. All three factors must be kept under control for insulin-replacement therapy to be effective. Changes in these factors affect the dosage requirements for insulin and can lead to over- or underdoses. For this reason, health team members as well as patients must be thoroughly familiar with the symptoms of insulin overdose and underdose.

Too little insulin in the bloodstream, hyperglycemia, is serious and can be fatal if the situation is not caught early and corrected. The first signs are vomiting, excessive thirst, diarrhea, urine containing large amounts of sugar (**glycosuria**), and (occasionally) increased appetite and eating without weight gain. Later the patient becomes dazed (stuporous), respirations are deep, and the face is dry and flushed. There is a fruity acetone smell to the breath, signaling that the body is burning excessive amounts of fat. This is called **ketoacidosis.** If these symptoms go undiagnosed, the person becomes unconscious within a day or two, a condition referred to as **diabetic coma.** The treatment is to immediately administer insulin and replace fluid and electrolytes.

The opposite situation, too much insulin, is called **hypoglycemia.** Symptoms are increased appetite, nervousness, heart palpitations, cold sweating, shakiness, difficulty concentrating, and blurred vision. They occur as a result of strenuous physical effort, overly large doses of insulin, or eating too little food. These situations cause all the blood sugar to be burned off so that the level of sugar in the bloodstream is too low (hypoglycemia). A urine test reveals that there is no sugar in the urine, either. Treatment consists of giving sugar in some easily digestible form—120–180 ml of orange juice, 180–240 ml of regular soft drink, two packets of sugar, or 5 or 6 hard candies, for example—to increase the blood sugar level quickly. In extreme cases, glucose or glucagon may be given parenterally. You should look for signs of hypoglycemia anywhere from 5 minutes to several hours after a dose of insulin. Be especially watchful for these signs during the hours of peak effect. Keep in mind that the peak effect of any insulin varies according to the individual patient's physical condition and level of activity.

The term *hypoglycemia* means low blood sugar. **Oral hypoglycemics (antidiabetic agents)** purposely lower blood sugar levels to reduce diabetic symptoms. Overdoses of hypoglycemics or of insulin result in drug-induced hypoglycemia, a dangerous adverse reaction. There is another type of hypoglycemia, however, that is unrelated to diabetes. It is called reactive hypoglycemia and is extremely rare. The symptoms are similar to those of insulin-induced hypoglycemia. A definite diagnosis can be made only after a blood glucose level of less than 50 mg/dl. Treatment consists of frequent small meals balanced in carbohydrates and protein.

Insulin pumps have improved the metabolic state of IDDM patients who have not achieved adequate diabetic control after a combination of dietary restrictions and insulin injections. The insulin infusion system, worn on the belt or at the side, is battery-operated and connected to a small computer programmed to release small amounts of insulin each hour (Figure 14.3). The amount of insulin released is based on the individual's daily needs according to diet and physical exercise. The patient pushes a button to obtain a dose of insulin after eating. Although these pumps can be effective, they present potential problems in the way of battery failure and line leakage, and they are expensive.

Diabetic patients are largely responsible for administering their own insulin, so they and their families should be educated about all aspects of the disease and its treatment. They must learn new dietary habits and injection and testing procedures. You can help by reinforcing their attempts to moderate their diet and exercise and by encouraging them to stay on a regular schedule of medication. Caution them to read OTC medication labels, because many have high sugar content. They should also avoid alcoholic beverages.

Oral Hypoglycemics. These drugs are unrelated to insulin and are not oral insulins. They can be used only with certain types of diabetic patients.

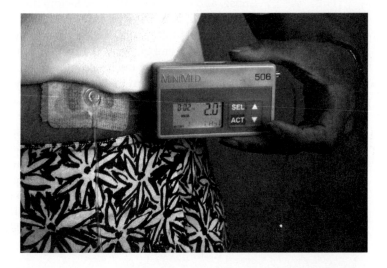

Figure 14.3
Insulin infusion
pump.

Generally the patient who responds best to oral hypoglycemic drugs is over the age of 40, has had diabetes less than 5 years, is normal weight or obese, has a consistent diet, has never received insulin, or has been controlled on 40 units or fewer of insulin a day. The major oral hypoglycemics are tolbutamide (*Orinase*), chlorpropamide (*Diabinese*), tolazamide (*Tolinase*), and acetohexamide (*Dymelor*), as well as the newer glipizide (*Glucotrol*), glyburide (*DiaBeta, Micronase*), and metformin (*Glucophage*). They are used in cases where the beta cells of the islets of Langerhans of the pancreas are already producing some insulin. Their effect is to stimulate these cells to secrete insulin in response to a rising blood glucose level. There is evidence that they may also make the body cells more receptive to the action of insulin. The second generation of oral hypoglycemic drugs has fewer side effects than the first generation. Those to watch for are nausea, diarrhea, and flatulence. Table 14.3 summarizes the timing of drug actions for the six major oral hypoglycemics.

TABLE 14.3: Oral Hypoglycemic Agents for NIDDM (Type II)

	ONSET OF ACTION (HOURS)	DURATION OF ACTION (HOURS)	DAILY DOSE RANGE	DAILY DOSES
First Generation				
Tolbutamide[a] (*Orinase*)	1	6–12	500 mg–2 g[b]	2–3
Tolazamide (*Tolinase*)	4–6	12–24	100–1000 mg	1–2
Acetohexamide (*Dymelor*)	1	12–24	250–1500 mg	2
Chlorpropamide (*Diabinese*)	1	36–60	100–500 mg	1
Second Generation				
Glipizide (*Glucotrol*)	1	10–24	Initial: 50 mg Maintenance: 5–40 mg	1
Glyburide (*DiaBeta, Micronase*)	2–4	24	Initial: 2.5–5 mg Maintenance: 2.5–20 mg	1
Metformin (*Glucophage*)	1	12–24	500–2550 mg	1

[a] Trade names given in parentheses are examples only. Check current drug references for a complete listing of available products.
[b] Dosages for the elderly and the debilitated are usually smaller. Average adult doses are given here. However, dosages are determined by a physician and vary with the purpose of the therapy and the particular patient. The doses presented in this text are for general information only.

Urine and Blood Tests. All diabetics must monitor their condition by one of two methods (urine or blood) for testing glucose levels. Urine testing is less common since the development of home-monitoring blood glucose devices. Urine testing should be done in people with IDDM who have unexplained hyperglycemia or during illness. Urine is tested for both glucose and ketones. Unfortunately, urine testing yields unpredictable results.

Tests for sugar in the urine include Clinitest, Diastix, and Testape. The urine must be a freshly voided specimen. Results are determined by matching the color of the test to the manufacturer's chart; the chart colors represent a range of sugar content. Precision QID is a glucose monitor marketed for home use.

Blood tests for sugar can be done with a glucose meter. This type of monitoring is more accurate than urine tests, but more expensive. Some types of blood glucose meters include Accucheck, Glucometer, and Ultra. The machines display the results digitally.

There are also methods for monitoring blood glucose by visual examination. A drop of blood placed on special strips induces a color change. Like the urine tests, the color change is compared to the manufacturer's color scale on the side of the container. Examples of visual blood glucose tests are Chemstrip bG and Dextrostix.

Results of these tests must be charted so the physician can properly adjust the drug doses.

DIABETES MELLITUS IN THE PEDIATRIC PATIENT

Diabetes mellitus in childhood is Type I or insulin-dependent diabetes mellitus. Glycosuria, polyuria, and a history of weight loss or failure to gain weight despite a hearty appetite are indications of diabetes. The management of the child with IDDM must be a multidisciplinary approach. The child, family, physician, diabetic nurse educator, nutritionist, and exercise physiologist must be included. Often psychological support is also needed because it is generally difficult for a child of any age to accept and comply with the treatment regimen. Communication is very important among all of the members of the health care team, the child, and the family, but must also extend to the child's teachers, school nurse, school guidance counselor, and coach. The treatment is insulin. However, insulin needs are affected by nutritional intake, activity, stress, illness, and puberty. Therefore, successful management includes both education and support. Initially, the parents are responsible for the care of the diabetic child, but the child should assume responsibility for self-management as soon as she or he is capable. Children at age 4 or 5 years can begin to check their blood glucose levels. Children at age 9 can begin to administer their own insulin (Figure 14.4).

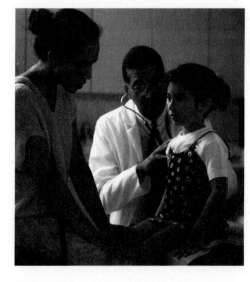

Figure 14.4 Communication is very important among the child, the parents, and members of the health care team to help the child comply with the diabetes treatment regimen.

COMPLICATIONS OF DIABETES

As the disease progresses, patients with diabetes are prone to urinary and vaginal infections and to blood vessel diseases that lead to vision problems, gangrene, foot and leg problems, and dental problems. These complications must be treated separately, keeping in mind that any added drugs may have an impact on the dosage of insulin. Many drugs interact with insulin and oral hypoglycemics, so any drug therapy for these secondary conditions must always be carefully planned (Table 14.4). As a member of the health care team, you can help the patient prevent infections by teaching good habits of skin, foot, and dental care.

TABLE 14.4: Drugs That Commonly Interact With Insulin

DRUGS THAT INCREASE GLUCOSE	DRUGS THAT DECREASE GLUCOSE
CNS stimulants	Alcohol
Corticosteroids	Salicylates
Diuretics	Sulfonamides
Estrogen	
Nicotine	

CORTICOSTEROIDS

Corticosteroids are a group of hormones secreted by the adrenal cortex. Insufficient production of corticosteroids (Addison's disease) can be fatal. There are two major groups of corticosteroids, each group having different functions: (1) the glucocorticoids (cortisone, hydrocortisone, and cortisol) affect fat and carbohydrate metabolism; and (2) the mineralocorticoids (aldosterone and desoxycorticosterone) regulate the salt/water balance.

The glucocorticoids often included in drug therapy are hydrocortisone (*Cortef, Hydrocortone*), cortisone (*Cortone*), triamcinolone (*Aristocort, Kenacort*), prednisone (*Deltasone*), prednisolone (*Delta-Cortef*), dexamethasone (*Decadron, Hexadrol*), and methylprednisolone (*Medrol, Solu-Medrol*). Fludrocortisone (*Florinef*) is used for its mineralocorticoid effects.

Corticosteroids have many uses. One important use is in hormone replacement therapy. The pituitary may not produce enough ACTH to stimulate corticosteroid production in the adrenal cortex. Or the adrenal cortex itself may not work properly (Addison's disease). In both cases, corticosteroids can be used to replace the missing hormones.

Large doses of corticosteroids are used with many conditions unrelated to adrenal functioning: allergic reactions, skin inflammations, some cancers, autoimmune reactions and suppression of immunity in organ transplants, and eye and respiratory diseases. The main reason for their use in these diseases is that corticosteroids suppress inflammation, which is the body's normal reaction to irritation or injury.

Recall that the inflammation reaction is signaled by redness, warmth to the touch, pain, and swelling. Corticosteroids change the tissue's response to irritation in such a way as to reduce these symptoms. They also reduce fever and itching. Because of their anti-inflammatory action, corticosteroids are often used in chronic inflammatory diseases such as rheumatoid arthritis; skin, gastrointestinal, and blood disorders; or in combination with other drugs for cancer, kidney, and eye disorders and respiratory diseases.

When used in small doses for a short time, corticosteroids show beneficial effects. In long-term use and in the large doses required for suppressing inflammation, however, there are many dangers. In general, long-term systemic use of steroids is not desirable. One problem with corticosteroids is that they mask infection and may cause it to spread. Inflammation is suppressed, but the irritation or injury remains. Tissue destruction can continue even though the symptoms are not obvious. There are other dangers, too: old infections can be reactivated and new infections can start, but the symptoms will be hidden because the drug suppresses them.

Another problem with long-term corticosteroid therapy is the side effects. Some of these are weight gain, sodium (salt) retention and edema, hypertension, facial rounding ("moon" face), diabetes, easy bruising, thinning of the skin, failure of wounds to heal, psychological changes, ulcers, osteoporosis, hyperglycemia, and many other effects. In addition, corticosteroid therapy interferes with the feedback between the adrenal glands and the pituitary. After withdrawal of corticosteroids, the chemical signal system between the glands takes several months to return to normal. Consequently, physicians order gradually smaller doses (tapering doses) of a corticosteroid before the patient discontinues it.

If steroids can be discontinued within 7 days of the time therapy is initiated, then tapering of doses is not necessary, because the drug has not yet inhibited normal feedback control. On the other hand, abrupt discontinuation of steroids after prolonged therapy can result in adrenal insufficiency. Signs of adrenal insufficiency are nausea, fatigue, shortness of breath, low blood pressure, hypoglycemia, and muscle and joint aches.

For all these reasons, doctors try to prescribe the smallest dose possible for the shortest time needed to achieve the desired therapeutic effect. This principle is important, of course, in all drug therapy, but especially when giving corticosteroids. Doses must be individualized according to each patient's response to the drugs. Those who administer medications must be watchful for the side effects mentioned previously.

OTHER HORMONES

Thyroid hormone replacement is not uncommon. It is done in cases where thyroid activity has been suppressed by radiation or surgery and in hypothyroid conditions such as goiter and myxedema. Natural hormones such as liotrix (*Euthroid*) and liothyronine sodium (*Cytomel*) are available, but synthetic thyroid hormones, such as levothyroxine sodium (*Synthroid, Levothroid*), are used more frequently.

The hormone corticotropin (ACTH, *Acthar*) may be given for diagnosing pituitary malfunction and also for stimulating the adrenals to produce glucocorticoids.

Vasopressin tannate (*Pitressin*) is the antidiuretic pituitary hormone (ADH) that regulates reabsorption of water in the kidneys. It is given to control diabetes insipidus, a disorder in which too much water is excreted in the urine. Vasopressin causes water to be reabsorbed so that the patient urinates normally.

DIAGNOSIS OF HORMONE DEFICIENCIES

Hormones can be used to find out whether a gland is failing to produce its hormone. Suppose, for example, that the body lacks a certain adrenal hormone. Is this the fault of the pituitary or of the adrenal glands? One way to find out is to administer the pituitary hormone ACTH. If this makes the adrenals secrete the missing hormone, we know the problem lies with the pituitary; the pituitary has not been secreting enough of its own ACTH to stimulate the adrenals. On the other hand, if the dose of ACTH does not stimulate the adrenals, we know that the adrenals are not working properly. In this situation, the patient will likely be put on a regular course of hormone therapy to replace the missing adrenal hormone.

Representative hormones and hormonelike drugs used for replacement therapy and inflammation are listed at the end of this chapter. Other uses of hormones—for example, in arthritis, cancer therapy, and contraception—are discussed in Chapters 13 and 15.

ADMINISTERING INSULIN

Insulin is given parenterally, and as a health care worker, you should not administer it unless you are trained and permitted by law to give medications by injection. General instructions for giving injections are provided in Chapter 19. The following are special instructions for giving insulin:

- Keep insulin at room temperature for up to four weeks, unless room temperature is above 85°.

- Check the expiration date on the package and discard any insulin that is out of date.
- When giving insulin suspensions (e.g., NPH, *Lente, Ultralente*), gently rotate the vial between the palms of your hands before drawing up into the syringe.
- Check insulin that is cloudy to be sure it can be administered; lente, ultralente, and NPH are suspensions and should be cloudy, whereas regular insulin should be clear.
- Do not shake the vial. If there are any signs of clumping in the vial after you have rotated it gently, discard it.
- Timing is important. The physician orders insulin to be given at the correct time so that it will reach its peak level when blood sugar is highest.
- Measure insulin carefully. The proper dose is crucial. To make sure you have the proper dose, use only an insulin syringe and use the correct syringe size for the strength of the insulin. Insulin strength is measured in units (U).

Insulin is most commonly given subcutaneously, although intramuscular (IM) or intravenous (IV) administration of regular insulin may only be used when rapid onset of action is needed. Rate of absorption depends on the site of injection. Rate of absorption is greatest in the abdomen, followed by the arm, thigh, and buttocks. Rotate injection sites in the same anatomical area because of the differences in absorption at the various sites. Follow a rotation plan as described in Chapter 19.

Be aware of the peak action time for the type of insulin you are giving. You can thus be alert for signs of hypoglycemia and have juice or sugar available if necessary. With long-acting insulin, hypoglycemia may occur during the night, signaled by restless sleep and sweating.

Two different types of insulin can be drawn up into the same syringe, as long as one type is regular insulin. The regular insulin should be drawn first.

REPRESENTATIVE HORMONES AND HORMONELIKE DRUGS[a]

CATEGORY, NAME[b], ROUTE	USES AND DISEASES	ACTIONS	USUAL DOSE[c] AND SPECIAL INSTRUCTIONS	SIDE EFFECTS AND ADVERSE REACTIONS
Hormones				
Glucagon SC, IM, IV	Severe insulin reaction; hypoglycemia	Raises blood sugar by stimulating liver to convert glycogen to glucose	0.5–1 mg; may be repeated 1 or 2 times as ordered	Nausea, vomiting, rash, dizziness
Levothyroxine sodium (*Synthroid, Levothroid*) Oral	Hypothyroid conditions such as cretinism, myxedema, goiter, mild hypothyroidism, surgical removal of thyroid gland	Replaces thyroid hormone, stimulates metabolism	Maintenance: 25–100 mcg PO daily in single dose, increase by 50–100 mcg PO every 1 to 4 weeks until desired response occurs	Headache, palpitations, sleeplessness, weight loss, nervousness, tachycardia, hypertension
Vasopressin tannate (*Pitressin*) SC, IM	Diabetes insipidus	Replaces ADH of pituitary, promotes reabsorption of water in kidneys	5–10 units IM or SC, 2–3 times a day	Tremor, dizziness, headache, bradycardia, abdominal cramps, nausea, vomiting
Somatropin (*Humatrope*) SC, IM	Growth failure due to growth hormone deficiency	Stimulates growth	Up to 0.06 mg/kg SQ, or IM three times a week with minimum 48 hours between doses	Pain at site of injection, headache, localized muscle pain, weakness, intolerance to cold, weight gain, dry skin and hair

REPRESENTATIVE HORMONES AND HORMONELIKE DRUGS[a] (continued)

CATEGORY, NAME[b], ROUTE	USES AND DISEASES	ACTIONS	USUAL DOSE[c] AND SPECIAL INSTRUCTIONS	SIDE EFFECTS AND ADVERSE REACTIONS
Corticosteroids				
Prednisone *(Deltasone)* Oral	Hormone replacement, inflammatory diseases (e.g., arthritis, dermatitis), lymphatic cancer, allergies, ulcerative colitis, kidney disease	Suppresses inflammation and immune response, stimulates bone marrow, influences protein, fat, and carbohydrate metabolism	2.5–15 mg PO two, three, or four times a day, depending on specific disease, adjusted to lowest effective maintenance level; never abruptly discontinue drug; maintenance dose may be given daily or every other day	Euphoria, insomnia, edema, hypokalemia, GI upset (peptic ulcer), rounded (moon) face, delayed wound healing, weight gain, muscle weakness
Dexamethasone *(Decadron)* Oral, IV, IM	Hormone replacement, inflammatory diseases (e.g., arthritis, dermatitis), lymphatic cancer, allergies, ulcerative colitis, kidney disease, cerebral edema	Suppresses inflammation and immune response, stimulates bone marrow, influences protein, fat, and carbohydrate metabolism	.25-4 mg PO two, three, or four times a day depending on specific disease; never abruptly discontinue	Euphoria, insomnia, edema, hypokalemia, GI upset (peptic ulcer), rounded (moon) face, delayed wound healing, weight gain, muscle weakness
Oral Hypoglycemics				
Glyburide *(DiaBeta, Micronase)* PO	Type II diabetes mellitus (NIDDM)	Stimulates release of insulin from beta cells in islets of Langerhans in pancreas	2.5-5 mg PO daily with breakfast	Nausea, vomiting, abdominal discomfort, flatulence, anorexia, diarrhea or constipation

[a] See also the hormones listed in Table 14.1.
[b] Trade names given in parentheses are examples only. Check current drug references for a complete listing of available products.
[c] Average adult doses are given. However, dosages are determined by a physician and vary with the purpose of the therapy and the particular patient. The doses presented in this text are for general information only.

Define each of the terms listed below.

1. Tetany _____

2. Glycosuria _____

3. Hypoglycemia _____

4. Insulin _____

5. Glucagon _____

6. Glycogen _____

Match these hormones to the jobs they do.

_____ 7. Somatotropin

_____ 8. Parathyroid hormone

_____ 9. Corticosteroids

_____ 10. Epinephrine and norepinephrine

_____ 11. ADH

a. prepare the body to cope with stress

b. keeps the kidneys from excreting too much urine

c. regulates growth

d. suppress inflammation

e. regulates the amount of calcium in the blood

Complete the following statements by filling in the blanks.

12. The gland that traps iodine while producing its hormone is the _____ gland.

13. The glands that sit on top of the kidneys are the _____ glands.

14. Diabetes mellitus is caused by a lack of the hormone _____.

15. Diabetes insipidus is caused by a lack of the _____ hormone.

16. Addison's disease is caused by a long-term lack of _____ hormones.

The following drugs are used in the management of diabetes mellitus. Next to each drug, place the letter that tells what drug group it belongs to, as follows:

L = long-acting insulin

I = intermediate-acting insulin

F = fast-acting insulin

O = oral hypoglycemic

_____ 17. *Ultralente*

_____ 18. NPH

_____ 19. *Diabinese*

_____ 20. Regular insulin

_____ 21. *Humulin N*

_____ 22. Tolbutamide

_____ 23. *Humulin R*

_____ 24. *Semilente*

Answer the following questions in the spaces provided.

25. What is the main action of the oral hypoglycemics? _____

_____

_____

26. What are three factors that bring about changes in the diabetic patient's need for insulin? _____

    _____

    _____

    _____

27. What is the difference between glucocorticoids and mineralocorticoids? _____

    _____

    _____

    _____

    _____

28. List all the uses you can think of for corticosteroids. _____

    _____

    _____

    _____

    _____

29. Now list the possible side effects of long-term use of corticosteroids. _____

    _____

    _____

    _____

    _____

    _____

Match these drugs to their uses.

_____ 30. ACTH

_____ 31. vasopressin tannate

_____ 32. *Solu-Medrol*, prednisone, *Florinef*

a. replacement of pituitary hormone that stimulates production of corticosteroids

b. inflammatory diseases, allergic reaction,
   replacement of corticosteroids

c. diabetes insipidus

■ CASE STUDIES FOR CRITICAL THINKING

Patients with diabetes who are on insulin must live with the risk of insulin overdose or underdose. Decide which of these two problems is signaled by each set of symptoms below. Give the usual treatment for each.

Symptoms	Problem	Give
33. Polydipsia, polyuria, polyphagia, fruity breath, confusion	_____	_____
34. Nervousness, shakiness, blurred vision, cold sweating, palpitations, increased appetite, difficulty concentrating	_____	_____

Continued

■ APPLICATIONS

Obtain a current copy of the PDR® from your school, nursing unit, or clinic. Use it to answer the following questions in a notebook or on file cards.

35. Use the *PDR*® to find another product name for each drug in the Representative Drug table on pages 281–282.

36. In Section 3 of the *PDR*®, Product Category Index, find Hypoglycemic Agents/Diabetes Agents. Make a list of all the oral hyperglycemic agents you see listed there.

 *Inter**NET** CONNECTION*

An interesting site to browse is http://www.diabetes.org. Under the heading Diabetes Info click on Take the Risk Test. This program asks you to enter information about yourself and then determines your likelihood for developing diabetes based on your answers. This area also contains clinical information regarding the care of the diabetic patient and insulin administration.

In this chapter you will review the various parts of the musculoskeletal system and the correct terms used to describe them. You will learn what disorders affect this system and what drugs are used to control them.

OBJECTIVES

After studying this chapter, you should be able to

- use correct medical terms to describe major parts, functions, and disorders of the musculoskeletal system.
- recognize descriptions of major disorders that affect the musculoskeletal system.
- explain the differences among gout, osteoarthritis, and rheumatoid arthritis.
- describe the actions of drug groups commonly used in the treatment of gout, osteoarthritis, and rheumatoid arthritis, and give examples.
- identify the side effects of the various drug categories used to treat musculoskeletal disorders.
- describe malfunctions of bone marrow and their effects on blood.
- describe the usual care of patients with musculoskeletal disorders.

KEY TERMS

antiarthritic: drug that suppresses inflammation in degenerative diseases of the joints

antihyperuricemic: drug that reduces formation of uric acid

antispasmotic: a drug that controls muscle spasms

arthritis: name for several disorders of the joints, each having different causes and treatments (e.g., gouty arthritis, osteoarthritis, rheumatoid arthritis)

atrophy: wasting away of body tissue (e.g., atrophy of a muscle from lack of use)

bone marrow depression: disorder of the blood-forming tissue that produces

erythrocytes (red blood cells), leukocytes (white blood cells), and platelets

bursa: small, fluid-filled sac that cushions places where bones and muscles rub together (plural, bursae)

contracture: abnormal, permanent shortening of a muscle caused by muscular atrophy

fascia: fibrous membrane that supports and covers muscles

ligaments: connective tissue fibers that attach one bone to another

muscle tone: normal, slightly contracted state of skeletal muscles that keeps them prepared for action

myalgia: muscle pain

osteomyelitis: infection inside a bone

skeletal muscles: muscles responsible for body movement

synovial capsule: enclosed space between a bone and a joint

tendons: connective tissue fibers that form a cord and connect muscles to bones

uricosuric: drug that prevents reabsorption and increases excretion of uric acid through the kidneys

The bones, muscles, joints, cartilage, ligaments, tendons, fascia, and bursae make up the musculoskeletal system. Like all body structures, the muscular and skeletal systems play a part in the body's achievement of its overall goal of survival. Its main functions are support, protection of vital organs, movement, blood cell production, and storage of minerals.

Bones form the body's supporting framework. Without this support, the body would be unable to move and would collapse. The bones and their connecting joints act like a series of levers. The muscles exert force on these levers, and the result is movement. Some of the major bones and muscles are shown in Figure 15.1.

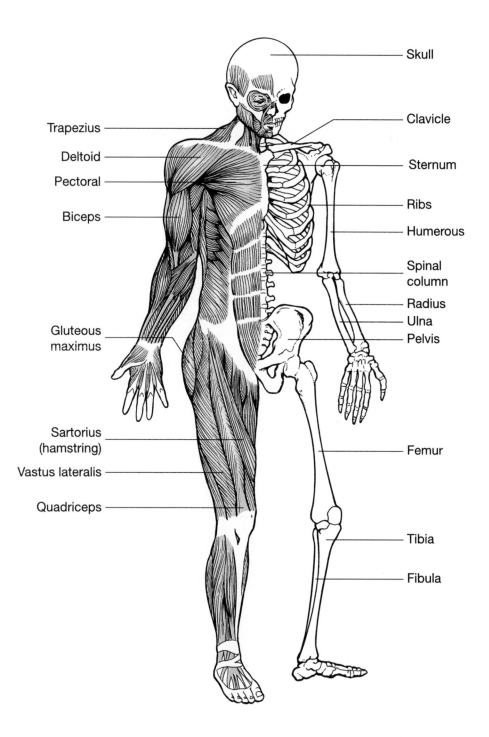

Skull

Clavicle

Sternum

Ribs

Humerous

Spinal column

Radius

Ulna

Pelvis

Femur

Tibia

Fibula

Trapezius

Deltoid

Pectoral

Biceps

Gluteous maximus

Sartorius (hamstring)

Vastus lateralis

Quadriceps

Figure 15.1
The musculo-skeletal system, showing major bones and muscles.

BONES

Bones are made up of both organic (collagen) and inorganic (calcium, phosphate) material. Even though they appear lifeless, bones are living tissue. The reason for their hardness is that the spaces between bone cells are filled with calcium. Bones start out relatively soft and pliable in babies. During childhood, calcium is deposited in the spaces between bone cells, so that the bones gradually harden. Because of their softness, young bones heal more easily than older ones. Throughout life there is constant replacement of older bone elements. This occurs because of the eating away (reabsorption) of bone in some areas along with the formation of new bone in other areas.

We think of bones mainly as a framework for the muscles, but they perform other important functions as well: they produce blood cells, act as a storage area for calcium, and protect delicate organs of the body. The skeleton is made up of 206 bones. They are classified by shape. The four classifications of bone are long, short, flat, and irregular. The femur, radius, and humerus are long bones. The carpals and tarsals are short bones. The ribs, scapula, skull, and sternum are classified as flat bones. Irregular bones include the vertebrae, sacrum, and mandible.

Inside most bones is a spongy type of tissue called bone marrow. Red bone marrow manufactures the three formed elements of the blood: all the red blood cells, certain white blood cells, and all the platelets. Yellow bone marrow, found only in the hollow parts of the long bones of the arms and legs, is a storage area for fat.

Cartilage is a rigid connective tissue that both provides support and allows joint movement. Unlike bone that has a rich blood supply, cartilage has no blood supply. Cartilage lines every joint and gives shape to the ears and nose.

JOINTS

The places where bones connect to each other are called joints (Figure 15.2). There are two types of joints: diarthroses and synarthroses. Diarthroses are joints in which there is a small space, the joint cavity, between the articulating surfaces of the two bones that form the joint. These joints are classified as freely movable. Examples of diarthrotic joints include saddle, hinge, pivot, ellipsoidal, ball and socket, and sliding joints. For example, the elbow joint is a freely movable joint. Synarthroses are joints that do not have a joint cavity, but instead have tissue (fibrous, cartilage, or bone) growing between their articulating surfaces and making them unable to move freely against each other.

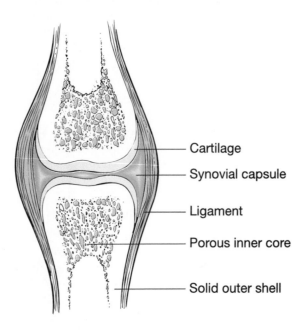

- Cartilage
- Synovial capsule
- Ligament
- Porous inner core
- Solid outer shell

Figure 15.2
Close-up of a joint.

These are joints that do not allow free movement, such as the four bones of the pelvis. Examples of synarthrotic joints include fibrous and cartilaginous joints.

The ends of bones are covered with cartilage. A capsule of connective tissue joins two bones to form a cavity lined with a synovial membrane. The membrane secretes synovial fluid, which functions as a lubricant and decreases friction in the joint. **Ligaments** are dense bands of connective tissues that connect bones to bones at joints such as the elbow joint. Ligaments provide movement while maintaining stability.

MUSCLES

The muscles that work together with bones to allow movement are called **skeletal muscles.** There are two other types of muscle tissue: smooth and cardiac. Smooth muscle tissue lines the gastrointestinal tract, urinary tract, blood vessels, airways, and uterus. Cardiac muscle tissue makes up the heart.

Skeletal muscles are made up of long, thin muscle fibers bundled together with sheets of connective tissue called **fascia.** The muscles are richly supplied with blood, because they need great quantities of oxygen to generate the energy needed for their heavy work. The more exercise these muscles get, the more blood vessels grow into them to supply the needed nutrients and carry away wastes.

Skeletal muscles are attached to the bones by cords of connective tissue called **tendons.** The muscles exert a force on the bones by contracting, which means that the muscles become shorter and thicker. When this effort is no longer needed, the muscles relax and assume their normal size.

Muscles that are well exercised are always slightly contracted, so that they will be ready for action as needed. This is referred to as **muscle tone.** Poor muscle tone is considered a sign of lack of use. If muscles are not used for a prolonged period, as in the case of bed rest, they become wasted and decrease in size (**atrophy**). Without physical therapy, **contractures,** or a shortening of the muscle or ligament, may result.

DRUG TREATMENT OF MUSCULOSKELETAL DISORDERS

PHYSICAL INJURIES

Muscles and bones and their accessory parts are subject to various injuries. Strains occur when a muscle is stretched. Sprains result from tearing of a ligament. The symptoms of sprains and strains are similar and generally include pain, edema, decrease in function, and bruising. Pain is worse with movement and use. A fracture is a break in the continuity of the structure of a bone. There are many different types of fractures. The type of fracture dictates the treatment. Fractures are usually accompanied by pain, decreased function, and inability to use.

OSTEOMYELITIS

Osteomyelitis is an infection inside a bone, with symptoms usually appearing near a joint. There is pain and tenderness, and fever is present. The infection destroys bone tissue, and pus may drain through the skin. Osteomyelitis is treated with antibiotics. Surgery may be necessary to drain abscesses inside the bone.

OSTEOPOROSIS

Osteoporosis is a decrease in total bone mass. It is a major cause of fractures in women past menopause. Osteoporosis is eight times more common in women because women have less bone mass than men because of their smaller size. Women also tend to have lower calcium intake throughout their lives. Pregnancy and breast feeding also deplete a woman's skeletal reserve. And finally, women live longer than men, which increases the likelihood of osteoporosis.

Osteoporosis is a condition in which the bones thin out, become abnormally porous, and are easily broken or fracture spontaneously. Osteoporosis most commonly occurs in the wrists, hips, and spine. Wedging and fractures of the vertebrae cause a gradual loss of height and a humped back and are often the cause of the stooped appearance of an elderly person. Osteoporosis can also result from an inadequate calcium intake, inactivity (as in bedridden patients), and diseases such as rheumatoid arthritis. Treatment consists of estrogen, calcium supplements, and a diet rich in calcium. Vitamin D is important to bone and calcium metabolism.

Alendronate (*Fosamax*) is used to prevent osteoporosis in postmenopausal women. It is the first nonestrogen, nonhormonal option for preventing bone loss in the early postmenopausal period. This drug can cause hypocalcemia and significant gastrointestinal upset. *Fosamax* may be taken orally. Calcitonin is also used to prevent osteoporosis in postmenopausal women. It is given only by injection, and also causes gastrointestinal upset, although research is being done to develop a nasal spray form of this costly drug. Another recent drug to appear on the market is *E-vista*, designed to prevent osteoporosis, and which also has properties that prevent cardiovascular disease.

Osteoporosis is a preventable disease; therefore, educating patients about it is essential.

PATIENT EDUCATION

Osteoporosis

- Premenopausal women should take 1000 mg of calcium per day.
- Postmenopausal women should take 1500 mg of calcium per day.
- Regular exercise is important to keep bones strong.

- Foods that are high in calcium include milk, yogurt, cottage cheese, ice cream, sardines, spinach, and turnip greens (Figure 15.3).
- Women whose diets are low in calcium should consult their physician about possible estrogen replacement therapy or calcium supplementation.

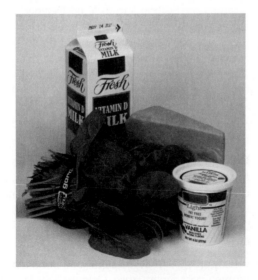

Figure 15.3 Foods high in calcium include dairy products and leafy green vegetables such as spinach.

BURSITIS, MYOSITIS, AND SYNOVITIS

Various inflammations arise because of repeated physical stress on joints or muscles. Bursitis involves the **bursae,** which are small, fluid-filled pouches located between bones and ligaments and between bones and muscles. The bursae are designed to keep these parts from rubbing against each other when they move. Myositis is an inflammation of the muscles. Synovitis is an inflammation of the cavity surrounding a joint (the **synovial capsule**). All these inflammations produce symptoms of pain, stiffness, redness, and swelling. Often the only needed treatment is rest. Other treatment is with oral anti-inflammatory agents, such as indomethacin (*Indocin*) and naproxen (*Naprosyn*). Sometimes hydrocortisone (a corticosteroid) is injected directly into the inflamed area. The injection reduces inflammation in the local area while avoiding the systemic effects of an oral corticosteroid.

GOUT

Arthritis is the name for several disorders of the joints, each having different causes and treatments—gouty arthritis, osteoarthritis, and rheumatoid arthritis. Gout, or "gouty arthritis," is an inflammation of the joints that starts when there is an excess of uric acid in the bloodstream. Uric acid is a normal waste product of cell metabolism. In gout, either the kidneys do not excrete uric acid efficiently or there is some reason (genetic, chemotherapy, etc.) that makes the body produce larger than normal amounts of uric acid. Because the uric acid is not completely excreted, crystals of the acid are deposited in the cartilage around the joints such as those of the big toe, ankle, knee, and elbow. The deposits cause the joints to become red, hot, swollen, and painful. The condition can flare up or become worse with heavy alcohol drinking, prolonged fasting, trauma, surgery, or infection. Uric acid crystals can also form in the urine, causing "gravel" or urate stones in the bladder and kidneys.

Chronic gout may be treated with **uricosuric** drugs. These are drugs that promote excretion of uric acid, such as sulfinpyrazone (*Anturane*). Alternately, chronic gout may be treated with **antihyperuricemic** drugs, such as allopurinol (*Zyloprim*), which decrease the amount of uric acid the body produces. These drugs are particularly beneficial for patients with uric acid stones or renal impairment.

The most common drugs for acute attacks of gout are colchicine, anti-inflammatory drugs, and corticosteroids. Colchicine produces dramatic relief of pain within 24 to 48 hours. Its exact mechanism of action is unknown. It may also reduce the frequency of gouty attacks. Caution should be used when administering colchicine to elderly patients because they are more likely to have cumulative toxic effects of the cardiac, renal, or gastrointestinal systems.

Patients being treated for gout must drink large amounts of fluids to help wash away the uric acid crystals. Eight glasses of water a day are recommended. Future attacks of gout are prevented by a maintenance dose of colchicine, weight reduction if necessary, avoidance of alcohol, drugs to reduce the serum uric acid, and a low purine diet. Uric acid is the major end product of the catabolism of purines. High purine foods include sardines, meat soups, chicken, salmon, crab, veal, bacon, pork, beef, and ham. Some vegetables that contain a moderate purine content include asparagus, shell beans, lentils, mushrooms, peas, and spinach.

OSTEOARTHRITIS

Osteoarthritis is also called degenerative joint disease. It is a progressive disorder that slowly destroys the mobile joints. It affects mainly the weight-bearing joints—the spine, hip, and knee. Most people over the age of 50 have some form of it, but not all show symptoms. As people grow older, the cartilage that cushions joints begins to thin out and wear away. As a result, bones rub against each other when the joints are moved. With continual rubbing and scraping, these bones thicken and become knobby or lumpy. Movement becomes painful, stiff, and limited. Symptoms are especially noticed toward evening, after a full day's wear and tear on the joints. There is pain and stiffness, but usually no inflammation. Treatment consists of relieving the pain, protecting the joints from additional injury, and restoring joint function. **Antiarthritic** drugs, which suppress inflammation in the joints, are commonly used in treatment of arthritis. Aspirin is the drug of choice and is used for pain control and inflammation, if present. Nonsteroidal anti-inflammatory drugs are used for patients who cannot tolerate aspirin. Corticosteroids may be injected into the joint during an acute flareup. Nonpharmacological treatment consists of application of heat or cold and range of motion exercises.

RHEUMATOID ARTHRITIS

Rheumatoid arthritis is a chronic inflammatory disease that affects the mobile joints. Unlike osteoarthritis, rheumatoid arthritis is systemic, involving other organs. It is characterized by periods of remissions and exacerbations. It also is a significant national health problem, particularly in women. The symptoms are pain in the joints (especially of the wrists, fingers, ankles, and other peripheral joints, such as the elbows, shoulders, knees, and hips) and stiffness. The stiffness occurs mainly in the morning and tends to improve throughout the day. There may also be fever, anorexia, weight loss, weakness, easy tiring, and aching muscles. The inflamed joints may feel warm to the touch. As the disease progresses, cartilage is slowly destroyed and the bones may even fuse together, causing loss of movement and sometimes deformity.

The cause of rheumatoid arthritis is unknown and there is no specific cure. Some researchers think the cause may be genetic, perhaps from an infection, or a form of autoimmune response, in which the body reacts to its own tissues as if they were foreign invaders like allergens and microorganisms. Treatment for rheumatoid arthritis consists of making patients as comfortable as possible, using drugs and a variety of physical measures. Nonpharmacological treatment measures include the application of ice during an acute flareup and the application of heat for daily chronic stiffness. Alternating periods of rest and activity are scheduled both to protect the joints and to prevent further joint immobility. A procedure called arthroplasty may be a last resort. It is a surgical procedure involving reconstruction or replacement of a joint.

The drugs used to treat mild rheumatoid arthritis have changed significantly in recent years. Whereas in the past high doses of aspirin and nonsteroidal anti-inflammatory drugs were used, now drugs called disease-modifying agents are used because they decrease the permanent effects of the disease, specifically joint immobility. The most common disease-modifying drug is hydroxychloroquine (*Plaquenil*). The most common side effects are nausea, abdominal discomfort, and rash.

Corticosteroids may be given either alone or in combination with *Plaquenil*. Corticosteroids have a wide range of side effects, such as euphoria, insomnia, GI upset, muscle weakness, delayed wound healing, weakening of the bone, and hypertension, so the smallest possible dose is administered for the shortest possible time.

The drug of choice for moderate to severe rheumatoid arthritis is methotrexate. It is used for its rapid anti-inflammatory action. It reduces the symptoms of rheumatoid arthritis in days. Gold therapy is reserved for those patients who do not respond to methotrexate. The action of gold therapy is unknown and poses side effects such as diarrhea, rash, and mouth sores. Azathioprine (*Imuran*) and penicillamine (*Depen*) may be used if both methotrexate and gold therapy fail to relieve the patient's symptoms. Both carry a high incidence of serious side effects, such as disorders of the blood. Along with these new drug regimens, aspirin and nonsteroidal anti-inflammatory drugs are still used. The nonsteroidal anti-inflammatory drugs may be used for patients who have an intolerance to aspirin.

MUSCLE PAIN

There are many reasons for pain in the skeletal muscles **(myalgia):** overexercise, inflammation, sprains, degenerative osteoarthritis, multiple sclerosis, herniated vertebral disc, or other conditions causing spasms. Skeletal muscle relaxants may be prescribed for patients with these conditions. The exact action of skeletal muscle relaxants is unknown, but they do depress the central nervous system, which results in relaxation of the muscle spasm. The most common muscle relaxants used for spasticity **(antispasmotics)** are baclofen (*Lioresal*), diazepam (*Valium*), and dantrolene (*Dantrium*). Other skeletal muscle relaxants used are methocarbamol (*Robaxin*), carisoprodol (*Soma*), chlorzoxazone (*Paraflex;* with acetaminophen in *Parafon Forte*), and cyclobenzaprine hydrochloride (*Flexeril*). Side effects are primarily fatigue, lethargy, and sedation.

BONE MARROW DISORDERS

Because red bone marrow produces most of the important components of the blood, any disorder that affects the bone marrow can create serious problems. Failure of the bone marrow to produce enough of all three components of the blood is called aplastic anemia. Overproduction of white blood cells is called leukemia.

Bone marrow depression is a serious adverse reaction linked to many drugs, especially certain antihistamines, tranquilizers, chloramphenicol, phenylbutazone, sulfonamides, antineoplastics, thyroid medications, antidepressants, and diuretics. For this reason, you should be aware of symptoms that indicate that a drug may be affecting the bone marrow:

- Lack of red blood cells—weakness, pale skin (pallor), dyspnea
- Lack of white blood cells—agranulocytosis, soreness of mucous membranes in the mouth and throat, fever, chills, extreme fatigue, urinary and vaginal infections
- Lack of platelets—bleeding from the gums, nose, or gastrointestinal tract; signs of hemorrhage under the skin such as purpura, petechiae, and ecchymoses

Like any unusual symptoms, these should be charted so that the physician can prescribe alternative drugs or treatments. Treatment of bone marrow depression involves:

- Transfusing red blood cells or platelets
- Discontinuing the offending drug(s)
- Providing antibiotics until the white blood cell count is restored
- Treating non-drug-induced cases, such as bone marrow infections or cancer
- Considering erythropoietin to increase the red blood cell count and colony-stimulating factor

CARE OF PATIENTS WITH MUSCULOSKELETAL DISORDERS

Patients with arthritis and other musculoskeletal disorders must live with pain. Sometimes every movement causes discomfort. Analgesics and anti-inflammatory drugs relieve this pain, but not completely. A person who is in pain can easily become impatient with those who are trying to help. Keep this in mind when caring for your patients. They hurt, and they may be angry that they must depend on others for routine care such as dressing and eating. There are several things you can do to make things easier for them:

- Give pain medications on time. This ensures that patients do not have to endure unnecessary pain while waiting for their next dose of medication.
- Handle patients with care. Do not bump against the bed as you prepare to administer medications. If you need to move patients for any reason, do it slowly and support their body parts. Avoid sudden, jarring movements that could cause pain.
- After moving a patient, reposition body parts in their natural alignment to reduce strain on joints and muscles.
- Attend to psychological needs. Be calm and reassuring. Explain procedures clearly beforehand. Help patients "talk out" the depression and frustration that may come with restricted movement and constant pain.
- Let your actions show that you are aware of the patient's fears and needs. You will be able to do your job better, and the patient will appreciate your help.

REPRESENTATIVE DRUGS FOR THE MUSCULOSKELETAL SYSTEM

CATEGORY, NAME[a], AND ROUTE	USES AND DISEASES	ACTIONS	USUAL DOSE[b] AND SPECIAL INSTRUCTIONS	SIDE EFFECTS AND ADVERSE REACTIONS
Anti-inflammatory Agents (Antiarthritics)				
Aspirin Oral, suppository	Mild to moderate pain, inflammatory diseases (e.g., osteoarthritis)	Reduces pain (analgesic), inflammation (anti-inflammatory), and fever (antipyretic); inhibits prostaglandin synthesis	*Mild pain:* 325–650 mg every 4 hours PRN *Rheumatoid arthritis:* 3.6–5.4 g daily in divided doses Give oral forms with food, milk, or full glass of water to avoid stomach irritation unless enteric coated	Nausea, stomach pain, indigestion, gastrointestinal bleeding, overdose (tinnitis, rapid breathing, dizziness, severe headache)
Nonsteroidal Anti-inflammatory Agents				
Ibuprofen (*Motrin*, prescription; *Nuprin*, *Advil*, OTC) Oral	Rheumatoid arthritis, osteoarthritis, mild to moderate pain	Reduces pain, inflammation, fever; inhibits prostaglandin synthesis	200–800 mg PO TID or QID, adjusted individually; give with milk or food if stomach irritation occurs; takes up to 2 weeks to show effects; if no relief in 2 weeks, consult physician	Epigastric distress, nausea, headache, dizziness, tinnitus, rash, visual disturbances, gastrointestinal bleeding, renal impairment
Indomethacin (*Indocin*) Oral	Moderate to severe rheumatoid arthritis including acute flares of chronic disease, moderate to severe ankylosing spondylitis, moderate to severe osteoarthritis, bursitis, tendonitis, acute gouty arthritis	Inhibits prostaglandin synthesis; anti-inflammatory agent with ability to relieve pain, swelling, fever of arthritis	25–50 mg BID–TID; may increase by 25 mg daily; do not exceed 200 mg daily	Nausea, vomiting, indigestion, dizziness, headache, fatigue, tinnitis, renal impairment, gastrointestinal bleeding
Naproxen (*Naprosyn*) Oral	Rheumatoid arthritis, osteoarthritis, ankylosing spondylitis, tendonitis, bursitis, acute gout	Inhibits prostaglandin synthesis; anti-inflammatory agent with antipyretic and analgesic effects	250 to 500 mg BID in morning and evening for rheumatoid arthritis, osteoarthritis, ankylosing spondylitis; for gout: 750 mg, then 250 mg every 8 hours until attack subsides	Gastrointestinal bleeding, heartburn, nausea, headache, dizziness, itching, tinnitis, edema

REPRESENTATIVE DRUGS FOR THE MUSCULOSKELETAL SYSTEM

CATEGORY, NAME[a] AND ROUTE	USES AND DISEASES	ACTIONS	USUAL DOSE[b] AND SPECIAL INSTRUCTIONS	SIDE EFFECTS AND ADVERSE REACTIONS
Gold				
Auranofin (*Ridaura*) Oral	Rheumatoid arthritis; synovitis in early stage	Unknown; anti-inflammatory effects caused by inhibition of cellular metabolism	6 mg PO BID, increased to 9 mg after 6 months if response is inadequate	Diarrhea, pruritus, rash, alopecia, nausea, vomiting, conjunctivitis, proteinuria, anemia, leukopenia, eosinophilia, thrombocytopenia, stomatitis
Antihyperuricemics				
Allopurinol (*Zyloprim*) Oral	Gout, excess uric acid, prevention of hyperuricemia associated with cancer chemotherapy	Suppresses formation of uric acid	100 mg PO daily; take with meals and drink 10–12 glasses of fluid daily	Drowsiness, vomiting, rash, headache
Sulfinpyrazone (*Anturane*) Oral	Chronic and intermittent gouty arthritis	Blocks renal tubular reabsorption of uric acid and increases renal excretion of uric acid	100–200 mg PO BID first week, then 200–400 mg PO BID, maximum dose 800 mg, with meals or milk, individualized	Upper gastrointestinal disturbances, nausea, rash
Colchicine Oral, IV	Acute gout	Inhibits inflammatory response	Oral: 0.5–0.6 mg PO daily, then 1 tab every hour until pain relief occurs or adverse gastrointestinal effects develop	Diarrhea, nausea, vomiting, bone marrow depression, neuritis, aplastic anemia
Muscle Relaxants				
Carisoprodol (*Soma*) Oral	Acute, painful musculoskeletal conditions	Unknown; blocks interneuronal activity in descending reticular formation and spinal cord	350 mg QID	Drowsiness, dizziness, vertigo, skin rash, fever, tachycardia, nausea, hypotension, leukopenia, gastrointestinal upset
Methocarbamol (*Robaxin*) Oral, IV, IM	Acute, painful musculoskeletal conditions	Unknown; central nervous system depression	Initial: 1500 mg QID; maintenance: 1000 mg QID	Lightheadedness, dizziness, drowsiness, nausea, rash, pruritus, and other allergic manifestations; avoid alcohol
Baclofen (*Lioresal*) Oral	Muscle spasm	Reduces transmission of impulses from spinal cord to skeletal muscle	5 mg tid; increase dose slowly; do not exceed 80 mg/day; do not discontinue abruptly; give with meals to decrease GI distress	Drowsiness, confusion, dizziness, nausea, constipation; avoid alcohol
Antineoplastic Agent				
Methotrexate Oral, IV	Severe rheumatoid arthritis	Binds with folic acid to inhibit synthesis of DNA and RNA	7.5 mg weekly, either as initially single dose or divided doses	Blood disorders, GI bleeding, nausea, vomiting, liver toxicity

[a]Trade names given in parentheses are examples only. Check current drug references for a complete listing of available products.
[b]Average adult doses are given. However, dosages are determined by a physician and vary with the purpose of the therapy and the particular patient. The doses presented in this text are for general information only.

Define each of the terms listed below.

1. Antihyperuricemic _____

2. Antispasmodic _____

3. Atrophy _____

4. Strain _____

5. Sprain _____

6. Bursa _____

Complete the following statements by filling in the blanks.

7. The musculoskeletal system supports the body and gives it the ability to _____ _____.

8. Bones are connected to each other by means of _____.

9. Bones are living tissue. They get their hardness from deposits of the mineral _____.

10. Bundles of tissue that connect muscles to bones are called _____.

11. The spongy part of the bone where blood cells are produced and fat is stored is called the bone _____.

12. The skull, spinal column, sternum, ribs, and pelvis _____ the vital organs of the head, chest, and abdomen.

13. Smooth muscles allow movement in the gastrointestinal tract and blood vessels, while _____ _____ muscles allow movement of the bones.

14. Healthy muscles are slightly contracted at all times. This is called muscle _____.

15. Strains are injuries to muscles and tendons, whereas _____ are injuries to ligaments.

Match these drugs to their categories or uses.

_____ 16. *Ecotrin*

_____ 17. *Anturane, Zyloprim,* colchicine

_____ 18. Hydrocortisone

_____ 19. *Robaxin, Flexeril, Soma, Parafon Forte*

a. drugs that reduce the formation of uric acid crystals in the joints

b. muscle relaxants

c. corticosteroid sometimes injected into the synovial capsule to reduce joint inflammation

d. enteric-coated aspirin

Place a T in the blank if the statement is true. Place an F in the blank if the statement is false.

_____ 20. After middle age, calcium is no longer deposited in the bones, causing the development of osteoporosis.

_____ 21. Myalgia is pain in the skeletal muscles.

_____ 22. Aplastic anemia is a bone marrow disorder.

Continued

_____ 23. Gout is a condition that results from too little uric acid in the bloodstream.

_____ 24. Surgery is frequently used to treat osteoporosis.

_____ 25. Lack of estrogen is a factor in the development of osteoporosis.

_____ 26. Ligaments are strong bands of connective tissue that hold bones together.

_____ 27. An inflammation of the synovial capsule is known as synovitis.

_____ 28. Crystals of uric acid deposited in the cartilage around joints can cause the joints to become red, hot, swollen, and painful.

_____ 29. Rheumatoid arthritis is caused by wear and tear on the joints.

■ CASE STUDIES FOR CRITICAL THINKING

Answer the following question in the spaces provided.

30. When administering medications to patients with painful musculoskeletal conditions, what can you do to help make them comfortable?

_____

_____

_____

_____

Choose the disorder that best matches each description below. Write the name of the disorder in the blank.

Osteomyelitis   Osteoporosis   Bursitis   Gout

31. An elderly patient must eat a diet rich in calcium, and she is taking small doses of hormones. This is because her bones have become very porous and fracture easily.

_____

32. A patient has developed an infection in the leg bone near the knee joint. He is taking antibiotics, and surgery is planned to drain the infected material from the bone.

_____

33. A small, fluid-filled pouch in a patient's shoulder joint is inflamed. This is causing swelling, pain, and stiffness. The doctor plans to inject hydrocortisone directly into the joint to reduce the inflammation.

_____

34. Increasing levels of uric acid in a patient are causing crystals to form in the cartilage around the joints. A dose of colchicine relieves the pain in his joints within a few hours.

_____

Continued

■ APPLICATIONS

Obtain a current copy of the PDR® from your school, nursing unit, or clinic. Use it to answer the following questions in a notebook or on file cards.

35. Find another product name for each of the muscle relaxants listed in the Representative Drugs table on pages 294–295 of this text.

36. In Section 3 of the *PDR®*, Product Category Index, find the Arthritis Medications. Then find the subheading NSAIDs. Make a list of all NSAIDs (Nonsteroidal Anti-Inflammatory Drugs) you see listed there.

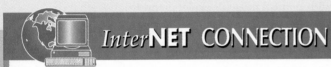

*Inter*NET CONNECTION

To learn more about some of the more recent drugs used to treat arthritis, go to http://www.arthritis.org and click on The New Drugs: The Latest Information. This gives information about recent drug therapies and treatments.

16

Drugs for the Nervous and Sensory Systems

In this chapter you will learn how the nervous system coordinates all systems of the body and responds to changes inside and outside the body. You will become familiar with the disorders that affect the nervous and sensory systems, the types of drugs used to treat them, and how to administer the drugs properly.

OBJECTIVES

After studying this chapter, you should be able to

- name the two main divisions of the nervous system and their parts.
- state the basic functions of the autonomic nervous system.
- give the correct medical terms for symptoms of nervous system disorders.
- recognize descriptions of the major nervous system disorders for which medications are given.
- teach patients about preventing strokes.
- teach patients about the effects of caffeine.
- describe the actions and give examples of the following drug groups: central nervous system stimulants, analgesics, anticonvulsants, and antiparkinsonian drugs.
- follow general instructions for administering pain medications, long-term medications, stimulants, and emergency drugs.

KEY TERMS

adrenergic blocking agent (sympatholytic): drug that blocks the effects of impulses transmitted by the sympathetic nervous system

analgesic: drug that relieves pain

anticholinergic: drug that inhibits the impulses transmitted by the parasympathetic nervous system; also known as parasympatholytic

anticonvulsant: drug that prevents, treats, and halts seizures

autonomic nervous system (ANS): part of nervous system that regulates involuntary vital functions of cardiac and smooth muscles and glands

bradykinesia: slowness of movement

central nervous system (CNS): composed of the brain and spinal cord

cerebral: pertaining to the brain

cerebrovascular accident (CVA): hemorrhage or thromboembolism in the brain; also called stroke

cholinomimetic: a drug that simulates the release of acetylcholine (a neurotransmitter)

convulsion: periodic, sudden attack of involuntary muscular contractions and relaxations

cranial: pertaining to the skull

dopaminergic: taking part in the activity of a neurotransmitter (dopamine)

extrapyramidal: referring to a group of clinical disorders characterized by abnormal involuntary movements of the muscles (e.g., Parkinson's disease)

impulse: electrochemical message transmitted by nerve cells

insomnia: sleeplessness, or inability to fall asleep or stay asleep

myelin sheath: insulating covering of the nerve cells

narcotics: group of potent analgesic drugs whose use can lead to physical dependence

neurons: primary functional units of the nervous system

neurotransmitter: a chemical substance released from nerve endings transmitting across synapses to other nerves, muscles, and gland impulses; can be inside or outside the nervous system

paralysis: inability to move the muscles

parasympathetic nervous system: part of the autonomic nervous system that functions mainly to conserve energy and restore the body; the system of rest and digestion

parasympatholytic: a drug that opposes the action of substances released by the parasympathetic nervous system; also known as anticholinergic

parasympathomimetic: drug that simulates the action of substances released by the parasympathetic nervous system

patient-controlled analgesia (PCA): system by which patients control the administration of their own pain medication from machines filled with analgesics

peripheral nervous system: the thoracolumbar (sympathetic) and craniosacral (parasympathetic) divisions of the autonomic nervous system, as well as the sensory and motor nervous systems and all the nerves of the body that come and go to the brain and spinal cord

rigidity: stiffness

seizure: temporary loss of consciousness during which there is overactivity of part of the brain, often resulting in uncontrolled body movements

spasticity: abnormal increase in muscle tone

spinal cord: part of the central nervous system; carries messages between the brain and the peripheral nerves

stroke: a loss in the supply of blood to any part of the brain; also called cerebrovascular accident (CVA)

stupor: state of mental dullness, confusion, or being in a daze

sympathetic nervous system: part of the autonomic nervous system that

involves expenditure of energy and increases the blood sugar, heart activity, and blood pressure; the "fight or flight" system

sympatholytic: also known as adrenergic blocking agent

sympathomimetic: a drug that simulates the action of substances released by the sympathetic nervous system

synapse: gap between neurons

transient isclemic attacks (TIAs): transient periods of neurologic deficit

tremor: trembling, shaking

vertigo: dizziness, whirling feeling in the head

THE NERVOUS AND SENSORY SYSTEMS

The brain, the spinal cord, and the nerves make up the nervous system, which is a highly specialized system (Figure 16.1). The function of the nervous system is to control and integrate many of the body's activities. The brain interprets messages from nerves and sense organs and decides on an appropriate

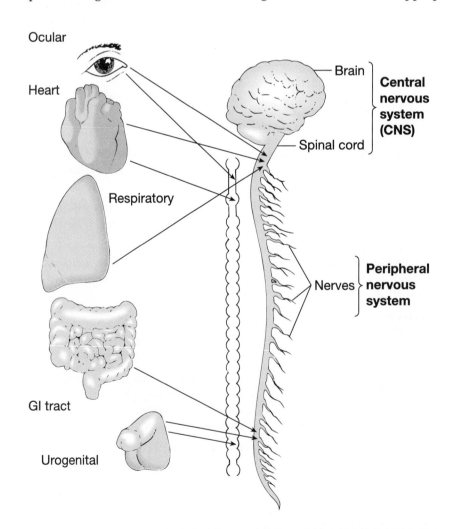

Figure 16.1
The central nervous system and the peripheral nervous system control all the body's systems.

set of actions. The brain then sends out "action messages," which are relayed by the nerves to various parts of the body. The brain's messages can involve voluntary actions (walking, talking, etc.), feelings (fear, anger, love, etc.), or automatic actions (breathing, heartbeat, blood vessel contraction, etc.). In this way, the body is able to respond to constantly changing conditions, both within and without the body.

The nervous system has two main parts: the **central nervous system (CNS)** and the **peripheral nervous system**. The CNS consists of the brain and the spinal cord. The peripheral nervous system consists of the cranial and spinal nerves and peripheral components of the autonomic nervous system (ANS).

THE NERVES

The nervous system is made up of two types of cells, neurons and neurolgia. N**eurons** are the primary functional units and have many different shapes and sizes. Neurons consist of a cell body, an axon, and several dendrites. The axon is the metabolic center of the neuron and contains the nucleus and cytoplasm. The axon carries the nerve impulses to other neurons and the dendrites receive the impulses from the axons and send the impulses to the cell body (Figure 16.2).

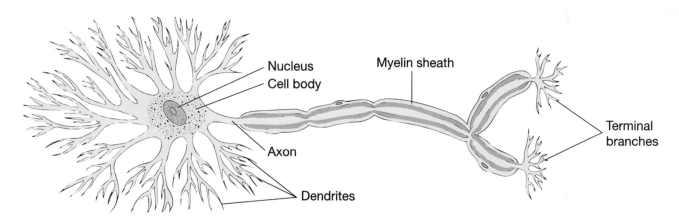

Figure 16.2
Nerve cell.

The neurolgia are greater in number, and they serve to support, protect, and nourish the neurons.

Neurons have the ability to initiate, receive, and process messages or **impulses.** This is done by means of special chemicals (acetylcholine, norepinephrine) in the ends of neurons and in the gaps **(synapse)** between them. Many drugs that affect the nervous system are designed to increase or decrease the concentration of these chemicals.

Nerve impulses travel along the nerve pathways at all times so that the brain and body parts are in constant communication. Some neurons are specialized for transmitting messages to the CNS; others are specialized for carrying messages away from the CNS to various tissues and organs of the body.

BRAIN AND SPINAL CORD (CNS)

The brain is the control center for all body functions. It consists of the cerebral cortex (**cerebral** means pertaining to the brain), the cerebellum, and the brain stem. As Figure 16.3 on page 302 shows, different parts of the brain have special functions to carry out. Most of our conscious thought processes—plus speech, hearing, and sight—are controlled by the cerebrum. Unconscious brain activity, balance, muscle coordination, and gland stimulation are regulated in the brain stem and the cerebellum.

The **spinal cord** is attached to the brain stem and passes from the neck down to the lower back. It acts as a reflex center and as a pathway for impulses to and from the brain.

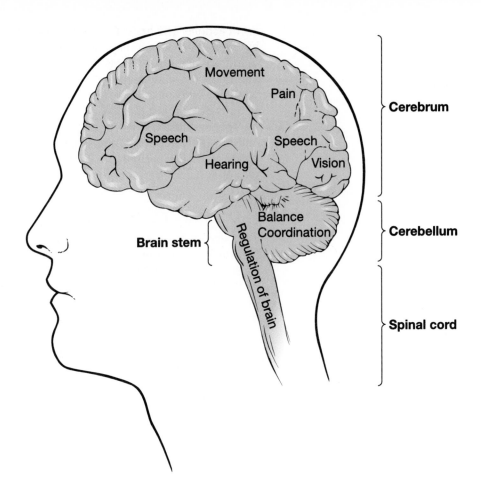

Figure 16.3
Conscious brain activity is controlled by the cerebrum, and unconscious activity by the brain stem and cerebellum.

PERIPHERAL AND AUTONOMIC NERVOUS SYSTEM

The peripheral nervous system consists of all structures that lie outside the central nervous system. These include the **cranial** (pertaining to the skull) and spinal nerves and portions of the autonomic nervous system. The primary function of the **autonomic nervous system (ANS)** is to regulate the functions of the cardiac and smooth muscles.

The ANS includes six visceral systems: digestive, respiratory, urinary, genital, endocrine, and vascular. It is made up of the peripheral system and the central control centers. The peripheral system is composed of the thoracolumbar (sympathetic) and craniosacral (parasympathetic) divisions.

Sympathetic or Thoracolumbar Division. The **sympathetic nervous system** is concerned with the use of energy. Under conditions of stress, it prepares the body to meet an emergency by producing epinephrine. This agent speeds up the heart rate and raises the blood pressure. The bronchial tubes dilate to allow more oxygen to enter the body, and the digestive system is slowed by the inhibition of peristalsis. With these changes, the body is ready for action. For this reason, the sympathetic portion of the ANS is called the "flight or fight" system.

Parasympathetic or Craniosacral Division. The **parasympathetic nervous system** restores and conserves body energy and brings the body back to normal conditions. It works the opposite way of the sympathetic division.

THE SENSES

Our ability to feel, see, hear, taste, and smell things around us is due to special nerve cells called sense receptors. They are specialized to pick up only specific sensory messages. For example, some pick up color, some react to feelings of pressure, and others respond only to odors. It is up to the brain to figure out what the messages mean according to which receptors sent the messages.

We are used to thinking of only five senses—sight, hearing, smell, taste, and touch. But there are other senses as well, including pressure, pain, temperature, body position, thirst, and hunger. Some types of sensory receptors are found in only certain parts of the body or in specialized organs such as the eyes and the ears. Other types of sensory receptors are spread throughout the body.

The Nose. The upper part of the nasal cavity is lined with olfactory cells that perform the function of smelling. These cells are connected to the olfactory nerve leading to the brain. The brain interprets messages from the olfactory cells as odors.

The Tongue. The tongue contains taste-sensitive cells inside oval-shaped taste buds. Dissolved foods and liquids stimulate the taste buds to send messages to the brain by way of the glossopharyngeal nerves and facial nerves. Taste buds on different parts of the tongue detect different tastes: sweet, sour, salty, and bitter. The olfactory cells of the nose also assist in the sense of taste because the aroma of foods is an important part of taste. A person who cannot smell properly also cannot taste properly.

Other Sense Receptors. Receptors for hunger are located in the stomach ("hunger pangs" come from these receptors). Receptors for thirst seem to be centered in the mouth, nose, and throat. A number of other sense receptors are widely spread throughout the body. These are the receptors that feel pressure, touch, heat and cold, pain, and body position.

AGING OF THE NERVOUS SYSTEM

For healthful living, there must be functional nerve pathways and responsive receptors within the CNS and the peripheral nervous system. But, unfortunately, aging brings structural and functional changes to the human nervous system. Changes occur, and some nerve cells may die. Therefore, there are decreases in reception and conduction and reflex reaction. Reflexes first may become sluggish and then may disappear completely. These changes result in varying degrees of muscular incoordination, paralysis, and asthenia (weakness). Sensory receptors are less reactive unless the stimulus is much stronger.

NERVOUS SYSTEM DISORDERS

Almost any disease or injury is likely to affect the nervous system in some way. There are many signs that show that the nervous system is being affected. The signs do not always mean that the nervous system itself is malfunctioning or diseased. They can signal a drug overdose or side effects, a psychological disorder, or a problem elsewhere in the body. Pain, for example, is a danger signal picked up by sensory receptors to alert the brain to a possible injury.

Some other signs that the nervous system is being affected by disease or drugs are: trembling **(tremor); spasticity;** dizziness **(vertigo);** loss of muscle control; dry mouth; blurred vision; inability to move **(paralysis);** unusual postures and body movements; convulsions; deep sleep from which a person cannot be roused (coma); being "in a daze" **(stupor);** irritability, excitation, agitation, restlessness, and/or sleeplessness **(insomnia);** nausea; headache; speech difficulties; and changes in pulse, respiration, and pupil size.

PARKINSON'S DISEASE

Parkinson's disease is a syndrome characterized by slowing of movement **(bradykinesia),** stiffness **(rigidity),** tremor, and impaired postural reflexes. Tremor makes it hard to do simple tasks like eating and writing. Rigidity can lead to bent posture, difficulty walking, deformities of the hands and feet, and poor equilibrium.

The exact cause of Parkinson's disease is unknown. There is a degeneration of dopamine-producing neurons. Dopamine is a **neurotransmitter** necessary for normal functioning of the **extrapyramidal** motor system, which includes control of posture, physical support, and voluntary movement.

There is no cure for Parkinson's disease, so treatment is aimed at relieving symptoms. There are treatments in the form of special medicines (antiparkinsonian agents) and physical therapy. The drug of choice is often carbidopa/levodopa (*Sinemet*). The levodopa is converted to dopamine and functions as a neurotransmitter. The carbidopa prevents destruction of the levodopa. Physical therapy is important to keep the muscles functioning despite their stiffness. Massage, stretching, and overall exercise can help keep the disease from completely crippling the patient. The only other treatment is for severe unilateral tremor. It is most effective in young patients. The role of surgical intervention is varied. Transplantation of adrenal tissue into the brain to provide dopamine-producing cells has proved unsuccessful. Experimentation with transplanting fetal tissue for the same purpose holds more promise.

MYASTHENIA GRAVIS

Myasthenia gravis is a disease of the neuromuscular junction characterized by a fluctuating weakness in certain skeletal muscle groups. It is caused by an autoimmune process that affects acetylcholine and prevents muscle contraction. Anticholinesterase drugs are used in the treatment of myasthenia gravis. The most commonly used anticholinesterase drugs are neostigmine (*Prostigmin*) and pyridostigmine (*Mestinon*).

MULTIPLE SCLEROSIS

Multiple sclerosis (MS) is a chronic, progressive, degenerative disease that attacks the outer covering (**myelin sheath**) of the nerves. Once the myelin sheath is gone, the nerves are unable to conduct impulses. Multiple sclerosis can attack any part of the body: brain, spinal cord, or peripheral nerves. Symptoms depend on which nerves are damaged and are usually intermittent, with lengthy remissions. They include paralysis, blurring of vision, speech problems, unsteady walk, and numbness. The cause and cure of MS remain unknown. Treatment is aimed at relieving the symptoms.

Adrenocorticotropic hormone (ACTH) and prednisone are helpful during acute exacerbations of the disease. They decrease edema and inflammation at the site of myelin destruction. Immunosuppressive drugs such as azathioprine (*Imuran*) and cyclophosphamide (*Cytoxan*) have also been used in patients with relapsing multiple sclerosis. Beta-interferon (*Betaseron*) has proven successful in controlling the disease in patients who are managed at home.

EPILEPSY

Epilepsy is a set of disorders that cause periodic **seizures.** Seizures are temporary losses of consciousness caused by overactivity of the nerve signals in part of the brain. Epilepsy commonly appears in the first 6 months of life as a result of birth defects or infections. Causes of epilepsy in childhood and young adulthood include trauma, brain tumors, and infections. Epilepsy after the age of 50 is usually the result of a cerebrovascular accident (CVA) or malignant brain tumor. Seizures occurring in childhood and young adulthood are called petit mal seizures. In this type of seizure, the patient stares into space for a few seconds and the seizure often goes unnoticed.

During tonic-clonic seizures, formerly called "grand mal" seizures (the most common generalized seizure), the epileptic patient suffers **convulsions** with loss of consciousness. With convulsions, the large muscles tighten and twitch uncontrollably. Most epilepsy is controllable with medications that prevent seizures (**anticonvulsants**) such as phenytoin (*Dilantin*), carbamazepine (*Tegretol*), phenobarbital, primidone (*Mysoline*), and divalproex (*Depakote*).

Epileptic patients must take their medications regularly and on time. A missed or late dose may result in a seizure. Teaching the patient the importance of regularity is part of your responsibility as a giver of medications.

Pediatric Concerns on Epilepsy. Typical absence seizures or petit mal seizures generally occur only in children and rarely continue past adolescence. As the child grows up, they may cease altogether or evolve into another type of seizure. During a petit mal seizure, the child has a brief staring spell that may go unnoticed. A brief loss of consciousness can occur. If left untreated, there can be up to 100 seizures per day. Seizures that begin before age 4 tend to result in some degree of mental retardation and behavior and learning problems. The treatment consists of antiepileptic drugs and helping the child live as normal a life as possible. When the child has been seizure-free for two years and has a normal EEG (electroencephalogram), the antiepileptic treatment may be discontinued.

CEREBROVASCULAR ACCIDENT (CVA)

A **cerebrovascular accident (CVA),** commonly known as **stroke,** is the sudden onset of a neurological deficit resulting from disease of the blood vessels that supply the brain. Strokes may happen with or without a warning. Patients who have had a **transient isclemic attack (TIA)** have a greater incidence of having a stroke. A TIA is a transient period of neurologic deficit. Strokes are currently the third leading cause of death in the United States and are a significant health problem, especially in the elderly population. Therefore, it is especially important for the health care provider to educate the older adult population on stroke prevention.

PATIENT EDUCATION

Stroke Prevention

- Have regular blood pressure checks.
- Take blood pressure medication as prescribed.
- Reduce dietary salt intake.
- Stop smoking.
- Reduce and control weight within a normal range.
- Decrease intake of foods high in saturated fats and cholesterol.
- Avoid drinking alcohol.
- Be monitored by a physician if taking oral contraceptives.
- Increase daily activity.
- Increase fruits and vegetables in the diet.

The cause of stroke can be a cerebral thrombus or embolus or a hemorrhage in part of the brain. Symptoms depend on the location of the interruption in the blood supply to the brain and can range from minor impairment to total incapacitation.

> ## CAUTION: Signs of Stroke
>
> - Memory loss
> - Dizziness (vertigo)
> - Headache
> - Fainting
> - Weakness
> - Blurred vision
> - Speech difficulty
> - Partial paralysis

The treatment of a patient after a stroke depends on the type of stroke and the extent of injury. The goal is prevention of strokes, and measures have proven successful in decreasing the number of strokes. These measures include administration of aspirin, dipyridamole (*Persantine*), or ticlopidine hydrochloride (*Ticlid*), which prevents the formation of a thrombus or embolus.

Once a stroke has occurred, the goal is to preserve life and decrease and prevent further disability. Anticoagulants such as heparin sodium (*Heparin*) and enoxaparin sodium (*Lovenox*) may be used to prevent further clotting when a stroke is in progress. Long-term anticoagulation therapy is accomplished with warfarin sodium (*Coumadin*). The physician may prescribe acetylsalicylic acid (aspirin) or ticlodipine (*Ticlid*) to treat symptoms of a progressing stroke.

TUMORS

Any abnormal growth in the brain is dangerous, even though it may not be cancerous (malignant). The danger arises because the brain is encased in a hard covering, the skull. Any growth or swelling that presses on the healthy parts of the brain may cause damage or malfunctions. Surgery, antineoplastics, and radiation are three possible treatments for brain tumors. Diuretics and corticosteroids may be used to reduce edema.

INFECTIONS AND INFLAMMATIONS

Infections and inflammations have specific names, depending on which part of the nervous system they attack. Inflammation of the brain is called encephalitis. Inflammation of the linings of the brain and the spinal cord (meninges) is called meningitis. Nerve inflammations are called neuritis and are characterized by weakness, abnormal sensations, temporary paralysis, and loss of reflexes. Neuralgia is a painful condition of the nerves caused by inflammation or irritation. These conditions are treated with pain relievers (analgesics) and with antibiotics if the infection can be identified as not viral.

DRUGS THAT AFFECT THE CNS

Because they act on the body's control systems, nervous system drugs often affect the whole body. How they work is not well understood. They appear to influence the chemical changes that allow nerve impulses to be transmitted between nerve cells.

We will focus on drugs that affect mainly the CNS. These are divided into two major categories: CNS stimulants and CNS depressants. Stimulants speed up the cell processes and make it easier for nerve cells to transmit messages. Depressants slow cell activity and inhibit the passing of nerve impulses. Within these two broad categories are many specific types of drugs.

Some drugs affect the peripheral ANS and the automatic regulation of internal organs. These drugs (e.g., epinephrine and atropine) are described in other chapters (e.g., Chapters 9 and 10) because they are used to treat disorders affecting other body systems. You will see these drugs referred to in drug references as **sympathomimetic, sympatholytic (adrenergic blocking agent), parasympathomimetic** or **cholinomimetic,** and **parasympatholytic** or **anticholinergic.** The names of the drug categories may be confusing; just keep in mind that they all affect the unconscious, automatic processes that keep the body functioning.

CNS STIMULANTS

Central nervous system stimulants have been commonly used for a variety of purposes. They were formerly used to treat obesity and to counteract overdoses of CNS depressant drugs. Today, however, they are essentially obsolete. Their use is limited in practice to attention deficit disorder and episodes of excessive drowsiness and uncontrolled sleep attacks during the day (narcolepsy). Indiscriminate use of CNS stimulants may result in cardiac dysrhythmias, hypertension, convulsions, or violent behavior. Examples of CNS stimulants used for attention deficit disorder and narcolepsy are methylphenidade hydrochloride (*Ritalin*) and phenmetrazine hydrochloride (*Preludin*). Because of the high risk of toxicity, CNS stimulants are controlled substances (Schedule II). Although caffeine is not often thought of as a drug, it is a CNS stimulant, and health care providers should educate patients about the effects of caffeine.

PATIENT EDUCATION

Caffeine

- Know which foods and beverages contain caffeine, such as chocolate, cocoa, coffee, tea, and soft drinks.
- Eliminate caffeinated beverages from your diet and replace them with decaffeinated beverages.
- Some medications, such as cold preparations, contain caffeine. Discuss their use with your physician.

- Avoid drinking caffeinated beverages, eating chocolate, or taking medications containing caffeine at bedtime.
- Avoid or limit caffeine consumption if you are pregnant, because of the potential for birth defects.
- Avoid caffeine if you are breast feeding, because it is passed into the breast milk and causes the baby to be jittery.
- Drinking two or more cups of coffee may result in nervousness, irritability, or headache.

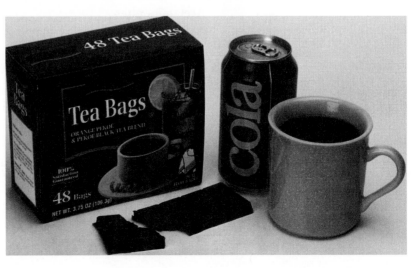

Figure 16.4 Caffeine is a CNS stimulant. The health care worker should educate the patient about products that contain caffeine.

Some CNS stimulants, such as doxapram (*Dopram*), are used in the treatment of respiratory depression induced by drug overdose. It is often administered intravenously, since immediate effect is needed in such emergencies.

CNS DEPRESSANTS

Drugs in this category can either depress the whole CNS (e.g., sedatives) or selectively depress only parts of the nervous system (e.g., analgesics, tranquilizers, anticonvulsants). CNS depressants are used in the treatment of both physical and psychological problems. Like CNS stimulants, the depressants have high potential for abuse. In addition, many of them can cause physical dependence. (Sedatives and tranquilizers will be discussed in Chapter 17.)

Analgesics. **Analgesics** are pain-relieving drugs. They relieve pain either by affecting the brain itself or by interfering with the ability of pain receptors around the body to send pain messages to the brain. One large group of analgesics is the **narcotics.** Along with pain relief, these drugs bring euphoria and a sense of calm; therefore, they are often abused. Examples of narcotic analgesics are morphine, codeine, oxycodone (one ingredient in *Percodan*), meperidine (*Demerol*), methadone, and pentazocine (*Talwin*).

A common group of nonnarcotic analgesics has the ability to reduce fever (antipyretic) as well as relieve pain. This group includes the familiar drugs aspirin and acetaminophen (*Tylenol*). They reduce fever by eliminating heat through vasodilation and increased respiration. Aspirin also has anti-inflammatory effects, which are put to use in treating musculoskeletal disorders. Analgesic antipyretics are often combined with narcotic analgesics or sedatives in prescription pain relievers—for example, *Tylenol* with Codeine, *Empirin* Compound with Codeine, and *Fiorinal* (butalbital with aspirin and codeine). Ibuprofen, a nonsteroidal anti-inflammatory drug (e.g., *Motrin, Nuprin,* and *Advil*), are both prescription and nonprescription products. Ibuprofen acts by inhibiting the release of prostaglandin, a substance involved with pain. Ibuprofen is one of the three major pain-relieving drugs available without prescription: aspirin, acetaminophen, and ibuprofen. Each has analgesic and antipyretic activity, and aspirin and ibuprofen also have anti-inflammatory activity.

CAUTION: Nonprescription Pain Relievers

Aspirin
- May cause gastrointestinal upset and bleeding
- Possible allergies (shortness of breath, rash, swelling, hives, asthma, or shock)

Acetaminophen
- Risk of overdose greater than from either aspirin or ibuprofen
- Individuals who have alcoholism, cirrhosis, or other serious liver diseases should consult their physician before taking acetaminophen

Ibuprofen
- Should not be taken by individuals who have had a severe allergic reaction to aspirin
- May cause renal failure
- May cause gastrointestinal upset and bleeding

Anticonvulsants. Anticonvulsants are used to control or prevent seizures. Aside from cases of epilepsy, seizures may occur as reactions to high fever, to drug overdose, to injury, and for unexplained reasons.

Although the exact mechanism of action of anticonvulsants is unknown, it is thought to stabilize the cell membrane by altering sodium, potassium, and calcium across the membrane. Anticonvulsants often cause drowsiness and may be toxic to the liver. Because there is a small difference between enough drug to be effective and too much drug (causing serious side effects), anticonvulsant doses must be finely adjusted. This is done by monitoring drug concentrations in the blood. Phenytoin (*Dilantin*) is the major drug prescribed. Others include primidone (*Mysoline*), ethosuximide (*Zarontin*), valproic acid (*Depakene*), and carbamazepine (*Tegretol*).

Antiparkinsonian Agents. Several types of drugs are used to treat Parkinson's disease. Some of them control tremors by interrupting the nerve messages that cause them. Others are used for relaxing rigid muscles. Gentle stimulants help to counteract slowness. Levodopa (*Dopar, Larodopa*) appears to work by replacing missing chemicals that transmit messages between nerve cells. A combination of levodopa and carbidopa, *Sinemet* is widely used because it can be given in smaller doses, with fewer side effects than levodopa alone. Other drugs for Parkinson's disease are benztropine (*Cogentin*), trihexyphenidyl (*Artane*), procyclidine (*Kemadrin*), bromocriptine (*Parlodel*), selegiline (*Eldepryl*), and amantadine (*Symmetrel*).

Dizziness, drowsiness, and blurred vision are common side effects of antiparkinsonian agents. Those that have an anticholinergic effect can cause dry mouth. This is relieved by giving the patient hard candy or gum or by rinsing the mouth with water.

GIVING MEDICATIONS FOR THE NERVOUS AND SENSORY SYSTEMS

To give medications that affect the nervous system, you will need to know how to administer drugs efficiently and courteously by all the usual routes. In addition, there are specific principles to follow in administering certain types of drugs.

LONG-TERM MEDICATIONS

Patients on long-term drug therapy to control seizures and Parkinson's disease must be watched carefully for signs of toxicity (drug poisoning). Your observations may suggest that the patient needs blood and urine studies, and this may help avoid serious overmedication. Patients need to be educated as to the importance of taking their medicines regularly over a long period of time, even after symptoms disappear. Patients with Parkinson's disease may have tremors that make it difficult for them to care for themselves and even to take their medicines. You should stress the importance of continued drug treatment despite their difficulties.

DRUGS FOR PAIN

Unfortunately, the reality of actual clinical patient care is that there is often a long delay between the time when a patient feels pain severe enough to alert the nurse and the time when the pain medicine provides relief.

To be effective, analgesics must be given on time. The objective is to keep the patient as comfortable as possible. If you wait too long to give the next dose of analgesic, the last dose will have worn off, the patient will suffer needlessly, and the pain will be much harder to control. In an effort to reduce this time difference, **patient-controlled analgesia (PCA)** pumps may be used. As the name implies, PCA pumps are machines filled with analgesics (often IV morphine or meperidine) that patients themselves control. When pain is felt, the patient simply pushes a button, and a dose of analgesia is given. The immediate response puts patients at ease, and they may actually end up using lower total daily doses of their narcotic. Pumps have a built-in safety mechanism to prevent overdosing.

Let patients know that the medication you are giving is for pain. The psychological effect of telling them their medication will decrease pain may help the drug work better (this is the placebo effect).

If the pain reliever is a narcotic, remember to discard the unused portion (chart this properly!) and the equipment used to administer it. There should be no chance of anyone else's using the leftover medication.

Some analgesics have antipyretic (fever-reducing) effects. With these drugs, take the patient's temperature as ordered, give extra liquids, and chart these procedures so the doctor can review the patient's progress.

Pain medications ordered before surgery must be given on time so that they take effect before the procedure begins. Insist on undisturbed bed rest for the patient after giving a preoperative medication. This will help the medication take effect. Encourage the family to cooperate with your instructions. After surgery, check on the patient often and administer pain medications as needed. An anesthetic does not eliminate the pain of surgery. It only makes the patient drift in and out of consciousness. During conscious moments, the patient may feel pain.

STIMULANTS

Dryness in the mouth is a side effect of some stimulants and other CNS drugs. To counteract dryness, suggest the use of hard candy or sugarless gum or rinsing the mouth with water.

EMERGENCY DRUGS

Many medical emergencies are treated with drugs that affect the nervous system. Emergency drugs are powerful, and errors in dosage can be extremely hazardous. Be certain to check the dosage strength and the route before administering them. As a matter of routine, the supply of emergency drugs should be reviewed often to be sure all medications are in good condition and not discolored or expired.

Explain the possible effects of emergency nervous system drugs to the patient to avoid fear and worry when new symptoms appear. Support the patient's family in emergency situations.

Emergency patients often receive IV infusions. Be careful when moving these patients to avoid letting the fluids pass into surrounding body tissues. Check often to be sure the needle is in the vein.

REPRESENTATIVE DRUGS FOR THE NERVOUS SYSTEM

CATEGORY, NAME[a], AND ROUTE	USES AND DISEASES	ACTIONS	USUAL DOSE[b] AND SPECIAL INSTRUCTIONS	SIDE EFFECTS AND ADVERSE REACTIONS
Stimulants				
Methylphenidate (*Ritalin*) Oral	Attention deficit disorder in children, narcolepsy	Cerebral stimulant	20–30 mg/day in divided doses for adults; 10 mg/day for children; adjusted individually	Nervousness, insomnia, seizures, hypersensitivity, palpitations

REPRESENTATIVE DRUGS FOR THE NERVOUS SYSTEM

CATEGORY, NAME[a], AND ROUTE	USES AND DISEASES	ACTIONS	USUAL DOSE[b] AND SPECIAL INSTRUCTIONS	SIDE EFFECTS AND ADVERSE REACTIONS
Analgesics				
Oxycodone and aspirin (*Percodan*) PO	Moderate to severe pain	Relieves pain, sedates, reduces fever	One tablet every 6 hours PRN; give with food or with a full glass of water or milk	Dependence, respiratory depression (esp. in elderly), dizziness, drowsiness, gastrointestinal upset, constipation
Pentazocine (*Talwin*) PO, IM, SC, IV	Moderate to severe pain; preparation for surgery	Relieves pain, sedates	50–100 mg every 3–4 hours PO; 30 mg IM; caution patient to avoid alcohol and OTC drugs	Dependence, dizziness, drowsiness, euphoria, nausea, dyspnea, hypotension, dry mouth, urinary retention
Meperidine (*Demerol*) IM, SC, IV, PO	Moderate to severe pain; preparation for surgery	Relieves pain, sedates	50–100 mg every 3–4 hours PRN orally or parenterally; may cause drowsiness; caution patient to avoid alcohol	Dependence, dizziness, drowsiness, nausea, flushing, sweating, dry mouth, orthostatic hypotension, seizures
Anticonvulsants				
Phenytoin sodium (*Dilantin*) Oral, IV	Grand mal epilepsy; psychomotor seizures	Controls seizures	300 mg/day divided every 8 hours for liquid oral and IV administration; one dose for kapseals	Back-and-forth eye movements (nystagmus); diplopia (double vision); swollen, tender gums; staggering walk (ataxia); slurred speech; constipation; dizziness; nausea and vomiting; rashes, anemia, sedation
Carbamazepine (*Tegretol*) Oral	Tonic-clonic seizures; other seizure types	Prophylactic treatment of seizures	200 mg BID increased to 800–1200 mg/day; should not be used by pregnant women or nursing mothers	Dizziness, drowsiness, nausea, vomiting; ataxia; mouth sores
Antiparkinsonian Agents				
Carbidopa and levodopa (*Sinemet*) Oral	Parkinson's disease or Parkinsonlike symptoms	Reduces rigidity of head and limbs, **dopaminergic** (involving activity of a neurotransmitter)	Initial dose 1 tablet (10 mg carbidopa/100 mg levodopa or 25/100) tid; maintenance dose 1 or 2 tablets (25/250) tid, individually adjusted; watch for symptoms of depression; give with food; may cause drowsiness	Mood changes; unusual, uncontrolled body movements; palpitations; difficult urination; dry mouth; nausea; vomiting; orthostatic hypotension
Benztropine mesylate (*Cogentin*) Oral, IM	Parkinson's disease adjunct	Anticholinergic	0.5–6 mg/day	Dry mouth, blurred vision, constipation, palpitations

[a]Trade names given in parentheses are examples only. Check current drug references for a complete listing of available products.
[b]Average adult doses are given. However, dosages are determined by a physician and vary with the purpose of the therapy and the particular patient. The doses presented in this text are for general information only.

Define each of the terms listed below.

1. Tremor _____

2. Vertigo _____

3. Paralysis _____

4. Coma _____

5. Stupor _____

6. Insomnia _____

7. Bradykinesia _____

8. Seizure _____

Fill in the blank with the word or phrase that best completes the statement.

9. The two main divisions of the nervous system are the _____ nervous system and the _____ nervous system.

10. The _____ carries messages from the peripheral nerves to the brain.

11. The organs of the chest and the abdomen are regulated automatically by a part of the peripheral nervous system called the _____ nervous system.

12. Neurons carry _____ to and from the CNS.

Tell what these types of drugs do; for example, cerebral stimulants speed up brain activity, which speeds up the whole body.

13. Analgesics _____

14. Antipyretics _____

15. Anticonvulsants _____

Match drug names to drug categories.

_____ 16. Caffeine, methamphetamine, *Ritalin*   a. analgesic antipyretics

_____ 17. *Demerol, Percodan*, morphine   b. anticonvulsants

_____ 18. Aspirin, acetaminophen   c. cerebral stimulants

_____ 19. *Dilantin*, valproic acid, phenobarbital   d. narcotic analgesics

_____ 20. Levodopa, *Artane*, benztropine   e. antiparkinsonian agents

Fill in the blanks with the word or phrase that best completes the statement.

21. Patients on long-term drug therapy should be encouraged to _____ .

22. They should also be watched for any signs of drug _____ .

23. To keep the patient as comfortable as possible, analgesics must be given _____ .

24. Always _____ any leftover narcotic and the equipment used to administer it.

25. With analgesic antipyretics, take the patient's _____ .

Continued

26. To soothe a dry mouth caused by stimulants or antiparkinsonian agents, give the patient _____ _____ or rinse the mouth with water.

■ CASE STUDIES FOR CRITICAL THINKING

Select the disorder that best matches the description. Write the name of the disorder in the blank.

Epilepsy	Stroke or CVA	Meningitis
Parkinson's disease	Multiple sclerosis (MS)	

27. Mr. Brown has trouble getting dressed in the morning because his hands shake so badly. When he walks, he moves very slowly and has trouble keeping his balance.

_____

28. Dick Fox has blurred vision in his left eye, and his left leg is paralyzed. The doctor says it is because the disease has destroyed some of the myelin sheath that covers the nerves.

_____

29. Mrs. Poston has a sudden hemorrhage in a part of the brain. This causes her to feel dizzy and have difficulty speaking.

_____

30. Joan Weiss is taking *Dilantin* regularly. If she were to skip a dose, she knows she might have a seizure.

_____

31. George Thompson has a serious inflammation of the covering of the brain and the spinal cord.

_____

■ APPLICATIONS

Obtain a current copy of the PDR® from your school, nursing unit, or clinic. Use it to answer the following questions in a notebook or on file cards.

32. In Section 4 of the *PDR®*, Generic and Chemical Index, find another product name for each of the drugs on the Representative Drugs table on pages 310–311.

33. In Section 3 of the *PDR®*, Product Category Index, find the subheading Serotonin Uptake Inhibitors. List all the drugs in this category.

*Inter*NET CONNECTION

The National Institue of Neurological Disorders and Stroke at http://www.ninds.nih.gov contains a database of public information on a wide range of neurological disorders. Click on Health Information. Here you will find an alphabetic guide to neurological disorders. Click on Attention Deficit Disorder to get more information on treatment, prognosis, and research.

Psychotropic Drugs

In this chapter you will learn how the central nervous system and biochemical mechanisms relate to emotions. You will become familiar with the major mental disorders and the drugs used to treat them, how to properly administer them, and how to prevent unwanted side effects.

OBJECTIVES

After studying this chapter, you should be able to

- describe the biochemical mechanisms of the central nervous system that affect emotions.
- define the correct medical terms for symptoms of mental disorders.
- recognize descriptions of the major mental disorders.
- differentiate between when a sedative is recommended and when a hypnotic is recommended.
- describe the actions and give examples of the following drug groups: antidepressants, sedatives/hypnotics, antipsychotics, antianxiety drugs, and antimanics.
- teach the patient about the appropriate administration of lithium.
- follow general instructions for administering sedatives/hypnotics, antidepressants, antianxiety drugs, antipsychotics, and antimanics.
- identify drugs that are often involved in drug abuse.

KEY TERMS

akathisia: usually occurs within 5 to 30 days (up to 90 days) of starting an antipsychotic drug; characterized by motor restlessness, inability to sit or stand still; individual feels the need to pace, rock, or tap foot

antimanics: group of drugs used to treat the mania episode of manic depressive illness

antipsychotic: group of drugs used to treat serious mental illnesses, such as being out of touch with reality; they produce a state of tranquility and work on abnormally functioning nerves; same as neuroleptic and major tranquilizer

anxiety: state of feeling apprehensive, uneasy, uncertain, or in fear of an unknown or recognized threat

anxiolytics: same as antianxiety drugs

atypical depression: depression with features that include hypersomnia, weight gain, mood reactivity, and sensitivity in interpersonal relationships

barbiturates: drugs that suppress the central nervous system; largely replaced by benzodiazepines

benzodiazepines: drugs that do not exert a general central nervous system depressant effect; act as a muscle relaxant, antianxiety, anticonvulsant, and hypnotic

catatonic: state of psychologically induced immobilization at times interrupted by episodes of extreme agitation

delusions: false beliefs that are resistant to reasoning

depression: disorder characterized by a sense of worthlessness or hopelessness

and often resulting in inability to carry out normal activities

dystonia: muscle spasms of the face, tongue, neck, or back; tongue may protrude, and facial grimaces usually occur after large doses of antipsychotic drugs

endogenous depression: characterized by the absence of external causes for depression; may be caused by genetic determination and biochemical alterations

exogenous depression: response to a loss or disappointment; referred to as "the blues" or normal depression, which generally remits in several months without the use of antidepressant medications; also known as reactive depression

extrapyramidal: refers to a group of symptoms that are usually related to the close and prolonged administration of antipsychotic drugs

hallucination: impairment of the special senses (auditory, visual, tactile, olfactory) by which the individual perceives in response to his or her own inner stimulation; that is, beliefs, delusions, feelings, unfulfilled wishes, and needs

hypnotic: drug that produces sleep by depressing the central nervous system

insomnia: sleeplessness, or inability to fall asleep or stay asleep

major tranquilizer: drug that is given in psychotic disorders in which an individual is out of touch with reality; same as antipsychotic and neuroleptic

mania: a mood disorder characterized by grandiose behavior, flight of ideas, hyperactivity, poor judgment, and aggressiveness

minor tranquilizer: drug that is given to calm anxious or agitated individuals

neuroleptics: same as antipsychotics and major tranquilizers

psychosis: mental disorder in which the patient loses touch with reality

schizophrenia: mental illness in which psychosis is the classic feature; characterized by hallucinations, delusions, disorganized speech, and disorganized behavior

sedative: drug that calms without producing sleep

tardive dyskinesia: potentially irreversible neurological side effects of antipsychotic drugs in which there are involuntary repetitious movements of the face, limbs, and trunk

THE NERVOUS SYSTEM AND EMOTIONS

Knowledge of how the nervous system functions is essential to understanding the actions of psychotherapeutic drugs. You have already learned how the central nervous system controls bodily functions such as heart rate, blood pressure, respiration, temperature, and gastric secretions (Chapter 16). Now you will learn how the central nervous system is responsible for behavior, memory, learning, consciousness, imagination, and abstract thinking.

BIOCHEMICAL MECHANISMS

The functions of the central nervous system are dependent on the actions of neurohormonal agents in the brain. The neurohormones stimulate transmission of reactions. During activity, acetylcholine is released from nervous system tissue to the cerebrospinal fluid. Norepinephrine is also present in the central nervous system. Tryosine and dopamine are normal constituents of the brain. Both norepinephrine and dopamine function as transmitters. They have both inhibitory and excitatory effects on functions such as sleep, arousal, and memory. Serotonin is another transmitter substance found in the central nervous system. Alterations in the level of serotonin are associated with changes in behavior. Other neurotransmitters include histamine, amino acids, and prostaglandin. There is strong evidence that dopamine, serotonin, and histamines play an important role in maintaining mental health. The role dopamine plays in psychotic disorders has received much attention over the years. Drugs such as the phenothiazines block the effect of dopamine.

MENTAL DISORDERS

DEPRESSION

There are two types of **depression. Exogenous depression** is also called reactive depression. It is depression in response to a loss, such as the loss of a loved one, or a disappointment, such as not meeting one's expectations. This type of depression is usually referred to as "the blues" or normal depression. The second type of depression is **endogenous depression**. It is characterized by the absence of external causes for depression. It may be caused by genetics or biochemical alterations. It is for this type of depression that antidepressants are useful.

PSYCHOSIS

Psychosis is an impaired ability to recognize reality, demonstration of bizarre behaviors, and inability to deal with life's demands. It is characterized by **hallucinations,** a disorder of perception involving one of the five senses, and **delusions,** false beliefs that are resistant to reasoning. **Schizophrenia** is a mental illness in which psychosis is the classic feature. In addition to hallucinations and delusions, disorganized speech and grossly disorganized or **catatonic** behavior may be present. Patients with schizophrenia may benefit from antipsychotic drugs.

PSYCHOLOGICAL DISORDERS

Disorders of the thought processes and emotions account for many uses of drugs that affect the nervous system. Psychological disorders range from mild depression or anxiety to severe changes in behavior. Drugs that energize, tranquilize, and control mood swings are among the types used for these conditions. They act by stimulating or depressing the CNS or specific parts of the brain. Mild tranquilizers, sedatives, and antidepressants are prescribed for people with temporary emotional problems or anxiety. For example, patients who are worried about upcoming surgery or about an illness might be given a mild sedative to help them sleep.

Much more powerful antipsychotic drugs are used to control symptoms in patients with severe behavior changes. These changes include psychotic depression, manic-depressive psychosis, and schizophrenia, which keep the patient from functioning in daily life.

PEDIATRIC CONCERNS

Attention deficit hyperactivity disorder (ADHD) and learning disability (LD) affect every aspect of a child's life but are most obvious in the classroom. Attention deficit hyperactivity disorder refers to developmentally inappropriate degrees of inattention, impulsiveness, and hyperactivity. The symptoms are present before the age of 7 years. Learning disability refers to a group of disorders manifested by difficulties in listening, speaking, reading, writing, reasoning, mathematic abilities, or social skills. The most frequently prescribed medications are dextroamphetamine (*Dexedrine*) and methylphenidate (*Ritalin*). Not all children benefit from these medications. Side effects include nervousness, **insomnia** (sleeplessness), decreased appetite, and weight loss. Long-term use of *Dexedrine* may cause suppressed growth.

SELECTION AND USE OF PSYCHOTROPIC DRUGS

Drug therapy plays a major role in contemporary approaches to psychiatric care. The administration of drugs alleviates a patient's symptoms, such as disturbances in mood and behavior, and facilitates compliance with other forms of treatment, such as psychotherapy. Although the drugs exert changes in mood and behavior, the changes are only temporary. It is through psychotherapy that permanent changes in mood and behavior occur. The appropriate selection of psychotherapeutic drugs is made by a physician on the basis of the patient's diagnosis. The physician matches the patient's symptoms to a particular drug's therapeutic effects.

ANTIDEPRESSANTS

These drugs intervene in the chemical processes in the brain. In so doing, they relieve deep depression. They work to normalize the chemical imbalance.

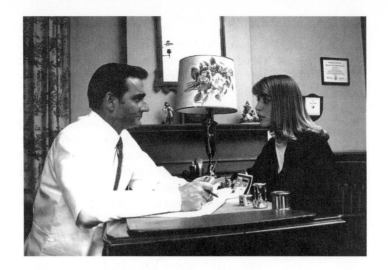

Figure 17.1
A combination of psychotherapy and drug therapy can benefit the patient and allow for permanent changes in mood and behavior.

One group of antidepressants is called monoamine oxidase (MAO) inhibitors. These drugs prevent an enzyme, monoamine oxidase, from metabolizing certain chemicals needed for nerve impulses to pass between neurons. By blocking the destruction of these chemicals, they aid the passage of nerve impulses, which appears to counteract depression. These drugs are used in **atypical depression,** depression with features that include hypersomnia, weight gain, mood swings, and sensitivity in interpersonal relationships. They have also been used with success in anxiety disorders, eating disorders, and for migraine headaches. The major side effects of these drugs are orthostatic hypotension, dry mouth, blurred vision, urinary retention, constipation, and weight gain. These drugs may have dangerous side effects, mainly hypertensive crisis, when mixed with certain drugs (e.g., antiasthmatics, antihypertensives, allergy and cold medications) and foods (e.g., cheese, liver, alcohol). Examples of MAO inhibitors are tranylcypromine (*Parnate*), isocarboxazid (*Marplan*), and phenelzine (*Nardil*).

Another chemical group of antidepressants, the tricyclic antidepressants (TCAs), increase the concentration of impulse-transmitting chemicals between neurons. Examples of TCAs are sinequan, amoxapine (*Asendin*), desipramine (*Norpramin*), nortriptyline (*Pamelor*), and imipramine (*Tofranil*). Unfortunately, TCAs have frequent side effects, such as dry mouth, blurred vision, constipation, sedation, and orthostatic hypotension.

Other antidepressants classified as serotonin selective reuptake inhibitors (SSRIs) act to block the reuptake of serotonin. Serotonin is a potent vasoconstrictor that is important in sleep and sensory perception.

Examples of SSRIs include clomipramine (*Anafranil*) and venlafaxine (*Effexor*). *Anafranil* is commonly used in the treatment of obsessive-compulsive disorder. Its effectiveness in the treatment of depression is still under investigation. The side effects are the same as with the tricyclic antidepressants. *Effexor* is the first of a new class of antidepressants that significantly block the reuptake of serotonin and norepinephrine. Side effects include headache, dizziness, nervousness, hypertension, blurred vision, constipation, dry mouth, and diaphoresis. Examples include fluoxetine (*Prozac*), sertraline (*Zoloft*), maprotiline (*Ludiomil*), trazodone (*Desyrel*), and buproprion (*Wellbutrin*). These serotonin inhibitors have fewer side effects and are better tolerated than TCAs. Their side effects include nausea, drowsiness, dizziness, headache, sweating, insomnia, and anorexia.

Patients should be educated to avoid alcohol, OTC drugs, and restricted foods while on antidepressants. Close watch must be kept for serious side effects, especially changes in blood pressure, and dosages must be carefully individualized. The physician increases the patient's dose slowly while the body becomes accustomed to the drug.

ANTIANXIETY, SEDATIVE, AND HYPNOTIC DRUGS

Antianxiety drugs, also called **anxiolytics,** are **minor tranquilizers.** Generally **anxiety** is a normal physiological and psychological mechanism that protects an individual from a threatening situation. This protective mechanism triggers the "fight or flight" reaction.

Sedatives and hypnotics are central nervous system depressants. The major difference between a sedative and a hypnotic is the degree of central nervous system depression. **Sedatives** produce a calming effect and decrease nervousness and excitability. **Hypnotics** are used to produce sleep. In the past, **barbiturates** were used as sedatives and hypnotics, but because of their many side effects, they have been replaced by benzodiazepines. **Benzodiazepines** do not cause a generalized central nervous system depressant effect. They have muscle relaxant, antianxiety, anticonvulsant, and hypnotic properties. The most frequent side effects are drowsiness and decreased coordination. Examples of benzodiazepines are alprazolam (*Xanax*), chlordiazepoxide (*Librium, Libritabs*), lorazepam (*Ativan*), diazepam (*Valium*), halazepam (*Paxipam*), oxazepam (*Serax*), prazepam (*Centrax*), midazolam (*Versed*), estrazolam (*ProSom*), flurazepam (*Dalmane*), temazepam (*Restoril*), and triazolam (*Halcion*). These drugs may cause drowsiness, so the patient must avoid tasks that require alertness. Flumazenil (*Mazicon*) is an antidote for benzodiazepine-induced sedation or benzodiazepine overdose.

There are many other drugs in the sedative/hypnotic category. Some of the better-known drugs are chloral hydrate (*Noctec*), ethchlorvynol (*Placidyl*), buspirone (*BuSpar*), and hydroxyzine (*Atarax, Vistaril*).

ANTIPSYCHOTICS

Antipsychotics are also known as **neuroleptics,** or **major tranquilizers.** They are used in patients with a psychotic disorder, in which there is an inability to recognize reality and bizarre behaviors are exhibited. Schizophrenia is a psychotic disorder in which antipsychotics are beneficial. Antipsychotics are dopamine receptor blockers. Examples of antipsychotics are mesoridazine (*Serentil*), perphenazine (*Trilafon*), thiothixene (*Navane*), molindone (*Moban*), loxapine (*Loxitane*), haloperidol (*Haldol*), clozapine (*Clozaril*), thioridazine (*Melleril*), trifluoperazine (*Stelazine*), fluphenazine (*Prolixin*), chlorpromazine (*Thorazine*), and risperidone (*Risperdal*).

The main side effects of antipsychotics are sedation, blurred vision, orthostatic hypotension, dry mouth, tachycardia, urinary retention, constipation, disorientation, and **extrapyramidal** symptoms (EPS). The major extrapyramidal symptoms include **dystonia** (muscle spasms of the face, tongue, neck, jaw, or back), **akathisia** (motor restlessness), **tardive dyskinesia** (abnormal involuntary muscle movements around the mouth, lips, and tongue), and parkinsonismlike symptoms such as shuffling gait, drooling, tremors, and increased rigidity. Prevention of tardive dyskinesia is essential because there is no effective treatment. Patients should be closely monitored for these side effects. The side effects are relatively predictable, and their likelihood increases with the size of the dose. The parkinsonismlike symptoms may be prevented by simultaneously using either benztropin (*Cogentin*) or diphenhydramine (*Benadryl*). Patients who take tranquilizers must not drink alcoholic beverages because alcohol potentiates these drugs and the results could be fatal.

Lithium is used as a mood stabilizer primarily in the treatment of bipolar disorder (manic-depressive illness). Lithium blood concentrations must be monitored closely. Signs of lithium toxicity vary from flulike symptoms to behavior changes and can even involve seizures, hypotension, and arrhythmias. Lithium is similar to sodium, and patients should be advised to avoid bingeing on salty foods. Sodium in the cells may increase as much as 200 percent in manic patients. Lithium and sodium are both actively transported across cell membranes, but lithium cannot be as effectively pumped out of the cell as sodium. Therefore, lithium may stabilize cell membranes. As a precaution, patients must follow a normal diet because lithium decreases sodium reabsorption by renal tubules, which may produce sodium depletion. Avoidance of salty foods should help minimize great fluctuations in lithium blood levels.

ANTIMANICS

Antimanic drugs are used in the treatment of bipolar disorders. The most common is manic depression. The drug of choice is lithium carbonate (*Eskalith, Lithane*). Its exact mechanism of action is unknown. It is thought to alter the chemical transmitters in the brain. The most common side effects include tremors of the hands, thirst, nausea, increased urination, and diarrhea. Many of the side effects are dose-related, so the patient should be monitored closely. Serum lithium levels should be done once or twice a week during the manic phase of the disorder and until the client stabilizes. Once the client is stabilized, serum lithium levels should be done on a continual basis every 2 to 3 months. Patient education is essential for compliance and effective drug therapy.

 PATIENT EDUCATION

Lithium

- Compliance, cooperation, and commitment are essential for stabilization of manic depressive disorder.
- Signs of drug toxicity include diarrhea, vomiting, tremors, lack of coordination, drowsiness, and muscular weakness.
- Notify the physician immediately if any signs of toxicity appear.
- Lithium may produce sodium depletion, so the patient must follow a normal diet with a consistent sodium level.
- A daily fluid intake of 2500 to 3000 ml is required.
- Avoid fluids such as coffee, tea, and cola because of their diuretic effects.
- Avoid exercise, saunas, and hot weather, which results in diaphoresis.
- Weigh yourself daily and notify the physician of any weight gain.
- Notify the doctor when ill and experiencing vomiting, diarrhea, or sweating.
- Report for all appointments to check blood lithium levels.
- Carry a medical identification card.

GIVING MEDICATIONS

To give medications that affect the nervous system, you will need to know how to administer drugs efficiently and courteously by all the usual routes. In addition, there are specific principles to follow in administering certain types of drugs.

SEDATIVES/HYPNOTICS

When prescribing these drugs, the physician's concern is to order the right amount so that the patient is quieted and comfortable, but not so much that he or she is in a daze and unable to function normally.

You can make sedatives more effective if you do the following:

- Reduce the noise level in the patient's room. Avoid loud talking. Turn down the television or radio.
- Relax the patient by giving a warm bath or a back rub.
- Listen to the patient's concerns and fears with sympathetic understanding.
- Make sure the patient gets enough exercise. Napping and lack of physical or mental exercise during the day can cause sleep problems at night. You may reduce the need for hypnotics simply by keeping the patient as active as he or she is able to be.

When sedatives are ordered PRN, be sure to ask the patient for the reason when he or she requests a sedative. If the reason is pain, sedatives will not help. The patient will need an analgesic to relieve the pain that is interfering with sleep.

Do not be too concerned about the possibility of drug dependence with sedatives/hypnotics if a patient is hospitalized for an illness. This is a period of great concern and tension. The patient's worries may be greater because of the unfamiliar surroundings of the hospital. Do not withhold PRN medications unless you have carefully studied the situation. Withholding PRN medications when they are really needed is as bad as giving them too often.

On the other hand, avoid overuse of sedatives. Do not give sedatives just to avoid having to listen to the patient's complaints and worries. Sedatives are no substitute for good care. Also, do not leave sedatives at the bedside to take as needed. If the patient takes the drugs too often or all at one time, overdose is possible.

Be observant of patients who are taking CNS depressants. Check their vital signs (pulse, blood pressure, respirations, etc.) often and report any notable changes. The dosage must be changed if a medication depresses the nervous system too much. Drugs such as the narcotics and barbiturates that depress the whole CNS tend to cause respiratory depression (very slow breathing) when an overdose is taken or given.

Look for idiosyncratic responses and drug interactions. Elderly people often become confused while under sedation. Depressant drugs given during the day may unexpectedly potentiate a sedative given at night.

Allow the proper amount of time for drugs to show their effects. Long-acting sedatives/hypnotics, such as phenobarbital, may take 30 to 60 minutes to give the desired results.

If patients are confined to bed and are taking sedatives, help protect them from complications. Their medication will keep them from moving about. You will need to change their positions often to prevent bedsores and pneumonia. The medications may also dry mucous membranes. Lubricate the eyes, the mouth, and the nose to prevent sores caused by dryness. Sugarless chewing gum and rinsing the mouth with water also help to relieve dryness.

GIVING DRUGS TO ALCOHOLICS

Be conscientious about giving medications to alcoholic patients. The medications are prescribed for their nutritional and psychological needs, so that they can recover from their alcoholism. Be sure to explain what drugs you are giving and what they are supposed to do. This will calm the patients' fears and gain their support for treatment.

PSYCHIATRIC PATIENTS

The care of psychiatric patients requires special training and knowledge. Medication handlers must fully understand the actions and the long-term side effects of antipsychotic drugs. Along with drug therapy, these patients often receive psychological therapy. As they begin to respond to drug therapy, there is sometimes a danger that they may attempt to commit suicide. You must be sure they do not manage to "pocket" their medications inside their cheeks and then spit them out when you are not looking. They may try to save pills in this way so as to take a fatal overdose later. Stay with patients until they swallow their oral medications, and watch carefully for signs of toxicity. Never forget to treat these patients kindly and with respect, despite any strange behaviors they may show.

DRUG ABUSE

Nervous system drugs are prone to abuse. This is true of aspirin as well as of narcotics, sedatives/hypnotics, and stimulants. Help to educate patients about the dangers of drug overuse. Support their efforts to understand and cope with their disease so that they do not depend on drugs for their support. Be aware, too, of opportunities for the misuse of alcohol and amphetamines. These are the most commonly abused drugs:

- Hallucinogens (psychedelics)—LSD, marijuana (aka "grass," "pot," "dope"), mescaline
- Narcotics—heroin, methadone, morphine, opium, *Demerol*
- Sedatives and tranquilizers—alcohol, barbiturates (aka "barbs," "phennies," "sleepees"), *Nembutal, Seconal*
- Stimulants—glue, cocaine ("crack,") or methamphetamines ("ice")

REPRESENTATIVE DRUGS FOR THE NERVOUS AND SENSORY SYSTEMS

CATEGORY, NAME[a], AND ROUTE	USES AND DISEASES	ACTIONS	USUAL DOSE[b] AND SPECIAL INSTRUCTIONS	SIDE EFFECTS AND ADVERSE REACTIONS
Antidepressants				
Fluoxetine (*Prozac*) Oral	Depression	Atypical antidepressant, inhibits serotonin reuptake	20–80 mg/day, given once or twice daily in divided doses	Anxiety, insomnia, weight loss, sexual dysfunction, nausea, headache, diarrhea, dry mouth
Imipramine (*Tofranil*) Oral, IV	Depression	Tricyclic antidepressant, inhibits serotonin reuptake	75–100 mg/day in divided doses or in a single dose at bedtime; up to 300 mg given to hospitalized patients; caution patient to avoid alcohol, OTC drugs, prolonged exposure to sunlight, and hazardous activities that require alertness	Drowsiness, dry mouth, blurred vision, urine retention, constipation, weight gain, tachycardia, photosensitivity
Sertraline (*Zoloft*) Oral	Depression, obsessive-compulsive disorders	Inhibits serotonin reuptake	Begin with 50 mg PO and gradually increase every few weeks; range 50–200 mg	Headaches, nausea, diarrhea, insomnia, male sexual dysfunction
Paroxetine (*Paxil*) Oral	Depression, obsessive-compulsive disorders	Inhibits serotonin reuptake	20–50 mg/day PO in divided doses	Headache, sedation, nausea, dry mouth

(continued)

CATEGORY, NAME[a], AND ROUTE	USES AND DISEASES	ACTIONS	USUAL DOSE[b] AND SPECIAL INSTRUCTIONS	SIDE EFFECTS AND ADVERSE REACTIONS
Antianxiety Agents and Sedative/Hypnotics				
Diazepam (*Valium*) Oral, IM, IV	Anxiety, tension before surgical procedures, muscle spasms, adjunct in seizure disorders	Benzodiazepine, depresses the central nervous system	2–10 mg TID to QID PO, adjusted individually to the lowest effective maintenance dose; caution patient to avoid alcohol; give with food to avoid upset stomach	Drowsiness, slurred speech, blurred vision, pain at injection site, unusual fatigue, dependence
Chlordiazepoxide (*Librium*) Oral, IM, IV	Anxiety, tension before surgical procedures, alcohol withdrawal	Depresses the central nervous system	5–25 mg 3 or 4 times daily PO; up to 100 mg IM or IV	Drowsiness, dizziness, confusion, lethargy, thrombophlebitis
Lorazepam (*Ativan*) PO, IM, IV	Anxiety, tension, insomnia, agitation, premedication before operative procedure	Depresses the central nervous system	2–6 mg daily in divided doses; caution patient to avoid alcohol; may cause drowsiness; 2–4 mg IM	Drowsiness, lethargy; dependence
Alprazolam (*Xanax*) Oral	Anxiety and tension	Benzodiazepine, depresses the central nervous system	0.25–0.5 mg TID	Drowsiness, lightheadedness, suicidal tendencies
Chloral hydrate (*Noctec*) Oral, Rectal	Insomnia, sedation	Unknown but has sedative effect	250–1000 mg TID or H.S. for hypnotic effect; give with full glass of liquid; caution patient to avoid alcohol and activities that require alertness	Nausea, vomiting, stomach pain, headache, drowsiness
Flurazepam (*Dalmane*) Oral	Insomnia	Acts on the central nervous system to produce hypnotic effects	15–30 mg H.S. for hypnotic effect; may take 2 or 3 nights for medication to reach full effectiveness; caution patient to avoid alcohol and activities that require alertness	Dizziness, daytime sedation, headache, lack of coordination
Triazolam (*Halcion*) Oral	Insomnia	Acts on the central nervous system to produce hypnotic effects	0.125–0.5 mg at bedtime	Headache, nausea, dizziness, lightheadedness
Antipsychotic Agents				
Chlorpromazine (*Thorazine*) Oral, IM, Rectal	Psychotic disorders, schizophrenia, severe agitation, severe nausea and vomiting, intractable hiccups	Blocks dopamine receptors in the brain	30–75 mg TID or QID and increased as necessary	Extrapyramidal reactions, sedation, tardive dyskinesia, dry mouth, constipation, urine retention, orthostatic hypotension

CATEGORY, NAME[a], AND ROUTE	USES AND DISEASES	ACTIONS	USUAL DOSE[b] AND SPECIAL INSTRUCTIONS	SIDE EFFECTS AND ADVERSE REACTIONS
Antipsychotic Agents (continued)				
Fluphenazine (*Prolixin*) Oral, IM	Psychotic disorders	Blocks dopamine receptors in the brain	0.5–10 mg PO daily in divided doses	Extrapyramidal reactions, tardive dyskinesia, dry mouth, constipation, urinary retention, orthostatic hypotension
Trifluoperazine (*Stelazine*) Oral, IM	Anxiety disorders, schizophrenia, other psychotic disorders	Blocks dopamine receptors in the brain	1–2 mg BID	Extrapyramidal reactions, tardive dyskinesia, dry mouth, constipation, urine retention, blurred vision
Haloperidol (*Haldol*) Oral, IM	Psychotic disorders	Blocks dopamine receptors in the brain	0.5–5 mg BID or TID; may cause drowsiness	Severe extrapyramidal reactions, tardive dyskinesia, blurred vision, urine retention
Antimanics				
Lithium carbonate (*Eskalith, Lithane*) Oral	Prevention or control of **mania** (mood disorder)	Alters chemical transmitters in the brain	300–600 mg PO up to QID	Arrhythmias, polyuria, elevated white blood cell count, tremors, drowsiness

[a]Trade names given in parentheses are examples only. Check current drug references for a complete listing of available products.
[b]Average adult doses are given. However, dosages are determined by a physician and vary with the purpose of the therapy and the particular patient. The doses presented in this text are for general information only.

Match the terms to their definitions.

_____ 1. False belief that is resistant to reasoning   a. akathisia

_____ 2. Muscle spasms of face, tongue, neck, or back   b. hallucination

_____ 3. Disorder of perception involving one of the five senses   c. dystonia

_____ 4. Motor restlessness   d. delusion

Define each of the terms listed below.

5. Anxiety _____

6. Depression _____

7. Mania _____

8. Schizophrenia _____

Fill in the blank with the word or phrase that best completes the statement.

9. The two neurohormones present in the central nervous system that affect emotions are _____ _____ and _____ .

10. _____ stimulate transmission of reactions.

11. Both norepinephrine and dopamine have _____ and _____ effects on the functions of sleep, arousal, and memory.

Tell what these types of drugs do; for example, cerebral stimulants speed up brain activity, which speeds up the whole body.

12. Antimanics _____

13. Antidepressants _____

14. Hypnotics _____

15. Antianxiety agents _____

16. Antipsychotics _____

17. Neuroleptics _____

Match drug names to drug categories.

_____ 18. *Placidyl, Dalmane, Noctec*   a. antidepressants

_____ 19. *Elavil*, imipramine   b. sedative/hypnotics

_____ 20. *Prolixin, Stelazine, Mellaril*   c. antianxiety agents

_____ 21. Alprazolam, oxazepam, prazepam   d. benzodiazepines

_____ 22. Lithium   e. antimanic

_____ 23. *Meprobamate, Librium, Valium*   f. antipsychotic agents (neuroleptics)

Continued

Fill in the blanks with the word or phrase that best completes the statement.

24. Patients on long-term antipsychotic therapy should be monitored for _____.

25. Patients taking tranquilizers should be cautioned not to drink _____.

26. To keep the serum lithium level stable, patients should have a consistent _____ _____ intake.

Answer the following questions in the spaces provided.

27. List at least three things you can do to make sedative/hypnotics more effective.

_____

_____

_____

28. List as many drugs as you can that are prone to abuse.

_____

_____

_____

_____

29. List at least two foods a patient taking a monoamine inhibitor (MAO) should avoid.

_____

_____

■ CASE STUDIES FOR CRITICAL THINKING

Select the disorder that best matches the description. Write the name of the disorder in the blank.

Anxiety   Psychosis   Depression

30. Sandy Peters is feeling threatened at work and experiencing the "fight or flight" reaction.

_____

31. Karen Jones is out of touch with reality and experiencing hallucinations and delusions.

_____

32. Alma West has a psychological disorder that keeps her from fully living her life. Without medication, she sits with her head buried in her hands most of the day. But when she takes amitriptyline (e.g., *Elavil*), she is able to function almost normally.

_____

Continued

■ APPLICATIONS

Obtain a current copy of the PDR® from your school, nursing unit, or clinic. Use it to answer the following questions in a notebook or on file cards.

33. In Section 4 of the *PDR*®, Generic and Chemical Index, find another product name for each of the drugs on the Representative Drugs table on pages 321–323.

34. In Section 3 of the *PDR*®, Product Category Index, find the subheading Serotonin Reuptake Inhibitors. List all the drugs in this category.

 *Inter***NET** CONNECTION

To learn more about mental health, go to http://mentalhelp.net. This site is organized into three separate section—Disorders and Treatments, Professional Resources, and The Reading Room. Click on Disorders and Treatments. This gives a listing of many mental health issues and disorders. Click on Medications to access references and databases on most of the commonly used medications for mental heath disorders.

CHAPTER 18

Antineoplastic Drugs

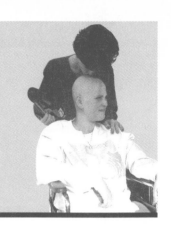

In this chapter you will learn basic facts about cells, tissues, organs, and systems. You will then learn about cancer. You will learn how cancers affect the body and how drugs are used to treat them.

OBJECTIVES

After studying this chapter, you should be able to

- use proper terms for discussing cells, tissues, organs, and body systems.
- name the four types of body cells.
- name the three characteristics of all cancers.
- explain how chemotherapy works.
- list common antineoplastic drugs and their effects on the cell cycle.
- list the side effects to look for when working with patients on chemotherapy.
- name at least three groups of antineoplastic drugs and give examples.

KEY TERMS

alopecia: hair loss

antineoplastic: drug that interferes with malignant cell replication or reproduction

benign: referring to a well-defined tumor that is contained and will not spread to other parts of the body

cell: the basic unit of structure of all living things

chemotherapy: drug therapy for cancer symptoms

cytoplasm: the part of the cell that contains water, protein, lipids, carbohydrates, and inorganic solutes

cytostatic: able to suppress cell growth and replication

cytotoxic: poisonous to cells

extravasation: discharge of blood or other substances into tissues

leukocytes: white blood cells that destroy germ cells

leukopenia: reduction in the number of leukocytes in the blood (4000 per cc mm or less)

malignant: cancerous; able to spread to other parts of the body or to invade locally

metastasis: spreading of malignant cells from one site to other parts of the body

neoplasm: new or abnormal growth of tissue; tumor

organ: two or more tissue types that perform a specific function

pathogens: harmful microorganisms

remission: period during which disease symptoms disappear

tissue: group of cells of the same type, working together to perform some function

tissue fluid: fluid found in spaces between cells; also called intercellular fluid

tumor: abnormal lump or mass of tissue

BODY SYSTEMS

CELLS

Cells are the basic unit of structure of all living things. There are millions of them in every human body. Each cell carries out certain routine functions to keep itself alive—absorbing food; creating energy for heat, growth, or movement; excreting waste products; and reproducing itself when conditions are right. But each cell works with other cells, too, to carry out more complex activities that keep the whole body working smoothly.

Epithelial cells
Linings of body tubes and cavities
Glands
Skin

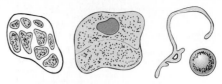

Connective cells
Bones, ligaments, cartilage
Scar tissue

Nerve cells
Brain
Spinal cord
Sense receptors
Nerves

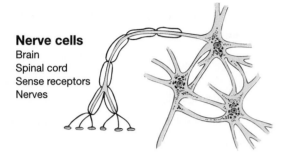

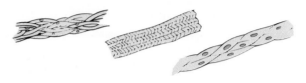

Muscle cells
Muscles that move bones
Smooth muscles in internal organs
Heart muscle

Figure 18.1
The four types of cells, with some of the body parts they make up.

For efficiency, cells are specialized to do certain jobs. Some are designed to form protective coatings and linings for body parts. Some specialize in producing chemicals that control body processes. Others are specialized for connecting body parts or creating body movement. Still others have the job of sending messages to and from the body's main control center, the brain. The four types of cells in the human body, each with its own special job, are epithelial cells, connective cells, muscle cells, and nerve cells (Figure 18.1).

Cells have the ability to divide into two when they reach a certain size. This is called cell reproduction. The two cells that result from division are exactly alike. They will do the same job in the body as the original cell. Cell reproduction enables living things to grow. As cells divide and redivide, the body grows larger. At some point the growth process stops: the human body reaches its full adult size. From then on, cells reproduce themselves only to replace worn-out or damaged cells.

During disease and trauma, many cells may be damaged. But because cells can reproduce themselves, the body can often replace damaged cells. This is called healing.

As the body grows older, the process of cell division begins to slow. Cells are not able to replace themselves as easily as they did during youth. Consequently, the body takes longer to heal after an accident or illness. The routine processes of digesting, producing energy, and excreting waste all slow down, too. The slowing down of body processes is why older people have special medical needs and why drug doses must be adjusted for age.

TISSUES, ORGANS, AND SYSTEMS

Cells are specialized to do certain jobs, but they do not do their jobs alone. They work together with other cells that have the same specialty. These groups of cells that together perform a certain function are called **tissues.**

Four basic types of tissues, corresponding to the four types of cells, make up all the body parts: epithelial tissue, connective tissue, muscle tissue, and nerve tissue. Each type of tissue has a different structure and function.

After cells and tissues, organs are the next most complex structures in the human body. **Organs** are made up of two or more types of tissue, organized to carry out a particular function. The heart, the liver, the stomach, the kidneys, and the skin are organs.

The important functions that keep the body alive—breathing, eating and digesting, elimination, thinking, and regulating the body processes—are performed by well-organized groups of organs and tissues called body systems. Of the body's 10 major systems, each is responsible for one important body function.

NECESSARY SUBSTANCES

The body is built of living cells, and it can manufacture many substances that it needs. However, there are some materials that the body must take in.

Water is the most important of these substances. In fact, about 66 percent of the body is composed of water. Water is the largest component of the fluid inside cells, or **cytoplasm.**

Water also surrounds the cells, bathing every tissue in fluid. This is important because water is the medium through which most of the body's chemical activities take place. Gases, liquids, and solids are dissolved in water before traveling through the body. The processes of absorption, distribution, biotransformation, and excretion all involve water. The water that surrounds the cells is known as **tissue fluid.**

Other substances that the body depends on for its life processes are minerals such as salt (tissue fluid is slightly salty) and calcium (for the hardness in bones and teeth), vitamins, fats, carbohydrates, and proteins. A well-balanced diet ensures that the body takes in a good supply of these necessary substances.

IMMUNITY

THE IMMUNE SYSTEM

The immune system has two parts: external and internal.

External. The external immune system gives protection from infection because of normal functioning defenses. The most important defense is the skin. It provides a tough physical barrier to the entry of **pathogens,** or harmful microorganisms. When the skin barrier is damaged, as when cut or burned, many pathogens can enter the body and cause infection.

Internal. The internal immune system is made up of microscopic substances whose specialized function is to fight infection.

Certain cells, called neutrophils, surround and digest the pathogens. **Leukocytes,** also called white blood cells, produce antibodies, which are proteins that help destroy pathogens as they enter the body.

Antibodies. Antibodies are proteins that either destroy or stop the growth of certain types of pathogens. Antibodies are carried in the bloodstream and can readily move to the site of entry.

Specific antibodies act against specific pathogens. When an unfamiliar pathogen enters the body, proteins in the blood are stimulated to produce a special antibody to act against it. The next time the same pathogen enters the body, the antibody "remembers" it and proceeds to destroy it. Antibodies make the body immune to a great many infections.

Immunity can be either temporary or permanent, depending on the type of antibody. People who, for some reason, cannot form antibodies are at risk because they cannot defend themselves against the pathogens to which we are all constantly exposed.

Cancer is not one disease but several hundred. The course of the disease and its treatment vary with the part of the body that is affected. The drugs used to treat cancer are best understood by looking at processes that take place at the cell level. All cancers have several features in common.

- *Rapid cell growth and reproduction.* Rapid growth is caused by a change in the genetic code (or "messages") governing normal cell reproduction. These changes cause cancer cells to reproduce at a much faster rate than normal cells.
- *Effects on adjacent cells.* Cancer cells can invade nearby tissues as they grow, causing destruction.
- *Seeding.* Cancer cells can "seed" (implant) themselves in other parts of the body and start new growths there. This is called **metastasis.** We say that a cancer has metastasized to another part of the body.

Rapid cell growth may give rise to **tumors,** which are lumps or masses of tissue. Not all tumors are cancerous, however. Noncancerous tumors are called **benign** tumors. They involve rapid cell growth, but the cells do not invade nearby tissues or spread to other parts of the body.

Cancerous tumors are called **malignant** tumors. As they grow, they put pressure on surrounding healthy tissues and organs and also invade them, causing destruction. Some cancers affect whole systems, such as the blood and lymph-forming organs, rather than causing a local tumor. In such cases, the cancer cells circulate throughout the body.

Early detection of cancer gives the best chance of curing the disease. The methods of treatment most often used first are surgery and radiation. Surgery is employed to remove tumors and nearby lymph glands, where cancer cells that have spread from the tumor may be trapped. Radiation may be focused on a specific spot to kill cancer cells. It may also be implanted in nearby tissue or swallowed in a substance that is attracted to the site of the cancer.

DRUGS FOR CHEMOTHERAPY

Drug treatment of cancer is called **chemotherapy.** Drugs can cure a few rare types of cancer, but they are more often used to control cancer symptoms in combination with surgery and/or radiation or after surgery and radiation have failed to bring about a cure. They are also used in systemwide invasions of cancer cells, such as leukemia and Hodgkin's disease.

The drugs used for chemotherapy are powerful and have strong effects on healthy cells as well as cancer cells. They are dangerous drugs whose use must be carefully planned and supervised by a physician. Some of the drugs are specifically attracted to cells that are multiplying rapidly. Thus they rush to the scene of a tumorous growth, killing cancer cells.

But at the same time, they are attracted to the blood-forming centers of the body because there the cells are also multiplying rapidly. When the drugs kill blood cells, they weaken the body and destroy some of its defenses. Patients receiving chemotherapy often bruise easily because many platelets (parts of the blood that help stop bleeding) have been destroyed. They may be especially prone to infection because of the destruction of white blood cells. Their bones may break easily and heal slowly because the cancer drugs weaken the bone tissue where blood cells are produced.

Other areas of the body that have rapidly multiplying cells are the skin and the linings of the mouth, throat, stomach, and intestines because they are near blood vessels and the lymph canal, allowing easy penetration by the invading organism. These areas, too, are affected by chemotherapy. Side effects such as nausea, vomiting, and hair loss are common.

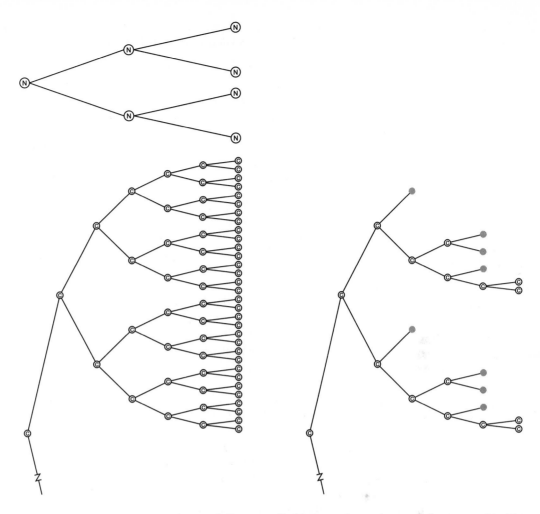

Figure 18.2
Compare the reproduction of cancer cells and normal cells. Chemotherapy slows reproduction by destroying some of the abnormal cells.

Doses must be carefully controlled because large doses can be toxic to healthy cells. Chemotherapeutic agents cannot differentiate between normal cells and cancer cells. Often some toxic effects are necessary to achieve the benefit of a drug's cancer-suppressing ability. Rather than giving a low dose continuously over a long period, cancer drugs are sometimes given in cycles—intensive treatment followed by a recovery period of 4 to 6 weeks, followed by another intensive treatment, and so on. This cyclical approach gives the body time to recover from the toxic effects and to build blood counts back up to normal levels.

No drug is able to kill all cancer cells at one time. But each successive dose kills a few more, so that the population is kept down to a level where the symptoms are under control. The effect of chemotherapy is shown in Figure 18.2, which depicts the reproductive life of a cancer cell. Without chemotherapy, after six generations this cell would have produced 64 cancer cells. With two waves of chemotherapy, it produced only six. During the same amount of time, a normal cell might have reproduced itself only one or two times.

Remission means the disappearance of symptoms (not just of cancer, but of any disease). The object of cancer chemotherapy is to bring about remission and to keep the symptoms from recurring. Chemotherapy is not guaranteed to cure cancer, but it can give a patient many years of useful life.

Drugs used against cancer are called **antineoplastics.** The prefix *anti-* means against, and *neoplasm* means tumor. Antineoplastics slow down or kill growing cells by interfering with chemical processes or by substituting for nutrients in the cells so the cells "starve" to death. Other terms used for anticancer drugs are **cytostatic,** which means that they stop all growth, and **cytotoxic,** which means poisonous to cells.

Alkylating Agents (Nitrogen Mustards). Alkylating agents are drugs that cross-link strands of cellular DNA and interfere with RNA, causing an imbalance of growth. This imbalance results in cell destruction. Nitrogen mustards are related to mustard gas, first used in World War I as a chemical weapon. In 1942, nitrogen mustard was first used to treat lymphosarcoma.

When nitrogen mustard is applied to the skin, the patient showers and thoroughly dries before each application and does not shower until before the next treatment. You should wear plastic gloves and avoid contact with the eyes, nose, and mouth. When given IV, reconstitute with sterile water or sodium chloride and administer within 15 minutes. Flush the vein with running IV solution for 2 to 5 minutes to clear the tubing of any remaining drug.

Alkylating agents function as cancer drugs by stopping the growth of many cancer cells. They also have toxic effects on the blood-building organs, the gastrointestinal system, and the sex glands. An immediate side effect is usually vomiting and nausea. But after a while, the patient's daily blood counts reveal that fewer lymph cells are being produced in the bone marrow, signaling remission. Examples of alkylating agents are mechlorethamine hydrochloride (*Mustargen*), chlorambucil (*Leukeran*), and cyclophosphamide (*Cytoxan*).

An alkylatorlike drug classified as a nitrosoureas is cisplatin (*Platinol*). Although the exact action of *Platinol* is unknown, it appears to act similarly to the alkylating agents. It is used in the treatment of bladder, testicular, and ovarian cancer.

Antimetabolites. Antimetabolites are structurally similar to a building block necessary in the formation of DNA. The cell accepts this substance; however, since it is an imposter, it interferes with the normal production of DNA, resulting in cell death. Examples of antimetabolites are fluorouracil (*5-FU*), mercaptopurine (*Purinethol*), cytarabine (*Cytosar-U*), and methotrexate (*Mexate*). The major side effects include nausea, vomiting, and **alopecia,** hair loss. These drugs may cause a decrease in the white blood cell count and must be monitored carefully.

Antibiotic Antitumor Drugs. Antibiotic antitumor drugs are both antineoplastic and antibiotic agents that bind DNA and inhibit RNA synthesis. Some antibiotics stop the growth of cancer cells and so are used in chemotherapy. Examples are dactinomycin (*Cosmegen*), bleomycin (*Blenoxane*), doxorubicin (*Adriamycin*), and plicamycin (*Mithracin*).

Miotic Inhibitors. Miotic inhibitors are plant alkaloids that block cell division in the metaphase. Vinblastine (*Velban*) and vincristine (*Oncovin*) are examples. Patients receiving these drugs should be watched closely for neuromuscular side effects such as numbness, tingling, headache, muscle pain, loss of deep tendon reflexes, and double vision. These symptoms may indicate early signs of neurotoxicity.

Hormones. Hormones may be used in the treatment of neoplasms that are sensitive to the body's hormonal growth. Their exact mechanism of action is unknown. They are thought to interfere with growth-stimulating receptor proteins at the cellular membrane. Estrogens are used to treat postmenopausal cancer. Progestins are used with cancer of the kidney. Androgens are used to treat breast cancer in menopausal women. Tamoxifen (*Nolvadex*) is a synthetic antiestrogen drug used in metastatic breast cancer in women. It has proved beneficial in preventing the recurrence of breast cancer in postmenopausal women.

Miscellaneous Antineoplastic Agents. Miscellaneous antineoplastic agents cannot be grouped by their action into any of the previously mentioned categories. Estramustine (*Emcyt*) is a combinaton of estradiol and nitrogen mustard. It is used in metastatic prostate cancer. Flutamide (*Eulexin*) was the first oral antiandrogen available. It is also used to treat metastatic prostate cancer. Interferon alfa-2a (*Roferon A*) and interferon alfa-2b (*Intron A*) have antiviral, antiproliferative, and immune properties. They appear to kill cancer cells and stimulate the immune system. They are used in certain types of leukemia and AIDS-related Kaposi's sarcoma.

Immunomodulating Agents. Immunomodulating agents activate the immune defenses or modify a biological response to an unwanted stimulus such as a tumor. Interferon beta-1b is an example.

Lymphokines. Lymphokines are involved in the regulation of immune system functions. Some of these products are interleukin-1 and -2 and colony-stimulating factor (CSF). CSFs are proteins normally produced by the body that trigger production of more blood cells. G-CFS (*Neupogen*) or GM-CSF (*Leukine* or *Prokine*) can be given to cancer patients with low blood counts caused by chemotherapy. These drugs, given by injection only, are extremely expensive.

Vomiting is a problem resulting from cancer chemotherapy. It can be such a serious problem that the doses of chemotherapy may have to be limited. Antiemetics are more effective in preventing vomiting than they are in treating it. They should be administered prophylactically before administering a chemotherapy drug. Frequently several antiemetic agents with different actions are administered together to increase their effectiveness. Examples are metoclopramide (*Reglan*) and lorazepam (*Ativan*), metoclopramide (*Reglan*) and dexamethasone, or prochloperazine (*Compazine*) and dexamethasone. Ondansetron (*Zofran*) is the first in a new class of serotonin antagonists approved for use in the prevention of nausea and vomiting associated with the use of antineoplastic drugs. It may cause a headache, which can be relieved by an analgesic. Granisetron (*Kytril*) is an injection for the prevention of nausea and vomiting associated with chemotherapy. It provides 24-hour antiemetic coverage. Its most common side effects are headache, sedation, diarrhea, or constipation. Dronabinol (*Marinol*) and nabilone (*Cesamet*) are antiemetics used when other antiemetics have proved ineffective.

CARE OF THE CANCER PATIENT

Patients undergoing chemotherapy need special care and emotional support from you. They must deal not only with the threat of cancer itself, but also with the unpleasant, often dangerous side effects of chemotherapy. Many of the drugs given for cancer therapy must be administered parenterally by specially trained nurses or by physicians. You may, however, be involved in giving some of the routine drugs for pain and nausea. You can provide emotional support by listening to your patients' fears and needs and by doing what you can to help make them comfortable. You should also observe them carefully for physical signs of drug side effects and disease effects, especially:

- nausea and vomiting
- irritation of the mucous membranes of the mouth and throat
- signs of developing infections, especially around the eyes, nose, and rectum
- pain caused by the disease that could be treated with analgesics (pain relievers)
- fluid retention
- **leukopenia** (reduction in the number of leukocytes in the blood—4000 per cc mm or less)
- diarrhea
- fever

Chart these observations and follow the physician's orders.

Because antineoplastics irritate the gastrointestinal tract, from the mouth through the rectum, eating is uncomfortable. Patients may develop a painful inflammation of the mucous membranes of the mouth, called stomatitis. Encourage them to eat by providing a pleasant atmosphere and letting them select their own foods. Avoid foods with strong odors and poorly tolerated foods such as red meats. A glass of wine with meals may help a patient's appetite. Help with their oral hygiene by rinsing their mouths often with water or mouthwashes. Clean the teeth and gums gently with a soft brush.

Finally, take special care not to infect chemotherapy patients with pathogens from other patients. It is most important to wash your hands after each contact with each patient. Remember, patients' natural defenses against infection may be seriously weakened by the antineoplastics they are taking.

REPRESENTATIVE ANTINEOPLASTICS

CATEGORY AND NAME[a]	USES AND DISEASES	ACTIONS	USUAL DOSE[b] AND SPECIAL INSTRUCTIONS	SIDE EFFECTS AND ADVERSE REACTIONS
Alkylating Agents				
Mechlorethamine (*Mustargen*)	Hodgkin's disease, lymphosarcoma	Inhibits rapidly growing cells	IV dosage according to body weight, adjusted to highest nontoxic dose; assist patient with oral hygiene; give adequate fluid; follow physician's orders carefully; note length of time for IV infusion; watch for pain at infusion site	Nausea, vomiting, anorexia, bleeding, bruising, metallic taste
Carmustine (*BiCNU*)	Brain tumor, Hodgkin's disease, lymphomas, melanoma	Inhibits rapidly growing cells	IV dosage according to surface area, pain at injection site common	Blood and liver problems, nausea, vomiting, diarrhea
Antimetabolites				
Fluorouracil (*Adrucil*)	Cancer of the breast, colon, rectum, stomach, pancreas, cervix, and bladder	Inhibits DNA synthesis	IV dosage according to body weight; avoid **extravasation** (discharge of blood or other substances into tissues)	Anorexia, nausea, vomiting, stomatitis, diarrhea, weakness, dermatitis
Mercaptopurine (*Purinethol*)	Leukemias	Inhibits DNA synthesis	Oral dosage according to body weight, adjusted to highest nontoxic dose	Blood and liver problems, anorexia, nausea, vomiting
Antibiotic Antitumor				
Dactinomycin (*Cosmegen*)	Cancer of the testes and uterus, Wilms' tumor	Inhibits cell reproduction	IV dosage according to body weight, adjusted to highest nontoxic dose. Drug is corrosive; avoid contact with skin; avoid extravasation	Nausea, vomiting, stomatitis, blood problems, bruising, loss of hair
Miscellaneous Antineoplastic Agents				
Tamoxifen (*Nolvadex*)	Cancer of the breast	Acts as estrogen antagonist	10 mg PO BID to TID	Nausea, vomiting, anorexia, rash, vaginal discharge

[a]Trade names given in parentheses are examples only. Check current drug references for a complete listing of available products.
[b]Average adult doses are given. However, dosages are determined by a physician and vary with the purpose of the therapy and the particular patient. The doses presented here are for general information only.

Define each of the terms listed below.

1. Leukopenia _____

2. Cell _____

3. Cytotoxic _____

4. Tumor _____

5. Chemotherapy _____

6. Metastasis _____

7. Malignant _____

8. Alopecia _____

9. Benign _____

10. Neoplasm _____

Match the characteristic or description to the appropriate term.

_____ 11. Basic unit of structure of all living things   a. tissues

_____ 12. Groups of cells working together   b. water

_____ 13. Substance that makes up two-thirds of the body   c. cells

_____ 14. Groups of organs and tissues working together   d. systems

_____ 15. Fluid found inside cells   e. cytoplasm

_____ 16. Fluid surrounding cells   f. tissue fluid

Answer the following questions in the spaces provided.

17. Name three characteristics of cancer cells. _____

_____

_____

_____

18. Antineoplastics harm healthy cells as well as cancer cells. Which parts of the body are especially affected by chemotherapy?

_____

_____

_____

Match drug names to drug categories.

_____ 19. *Mustargen, Leukeran, Cytoxan*   a. Antimetabolites

_____ 20. *5-FU*, methotrexate   b. Immunomodulating agents

_____ 21. *Adriamycin*, dactinomycin, *Mithracin*   c. Alkylating agents

_____ 22. Interferon beta-1b   d. Antiobiotic antitumor drugs

Continued

■ CASE STUDY FOR CRITICAL THINKING

Answer the following question in the spaces provided.

23. What signs should you look for when giving medications to cancer patients?

_____

_____

_____

■ APPLICATIONS

Obtain a current copy of the PDR® from your school, nursing unit, or clinic. Use it to answer the following questions in a notebook or on index cards.

24. Use the *PDR®*, Section 4, Generic and Chemical Name Index, to find another product name for each drug listed in the Representative Antineoplastics table on page 334 of this chapter.

25. In Section 3, Product Category Index, of the *PDR®*, find the subheading antimetabolites. List all the drugs named.

26. Section 3, Product Category Index, of the *PDR®* gives a page number for some drugs shown in Section 5, Product Identification Section. Using these page numbers, identify the pictures of those drugs shown as antimetabolites.

27. Notice the different forms Section 5 displays for two products. If solid, state the form. If liquid, how is it administered?

28. For the same two drugs you identified in the previous question, name the manufacturer. In Section 1 of the *PDR®*, Manufacturer's Index, find the address of the manufacturer.

29. In Section 2 of the *PDR®*, Product Name Index, identify the pages that give detailed information about these two drugs. Read about these two drugs in Section 6, Product Information.

30. In Section 6 of the *PDR®*, under Dosage and Administration, locate the information referring to children and the elderly and write it out.

31. In Section 7 of the *PDR®*, Diagnostic Product Information, find the name of the manufacturer that produced the two drugs you identified in Question 27.

32. List the diagnostic drugs produced by one of the manufacturers you identified in the previous question.

If you have a problem answering any of the above questions, look in the back of the *PDR®* under Discontinued Products to see if any of the drugs are listed there.

 *Inter***NET** CONNECTION

There are numerous Web sites that contain information on cancer. One of particular interest is OncoLink from the University of Pennsylvania Cancer Center. You can find it at http://www.oncolink.upenn.edu. Through OncoLink you can get information about specific types of cancer, updates on cancer treatments, and news about research advances. Click on About OncoLink and take the guided tour.

19 Administering Parenteral Medications

In this chapter you will learn how to give medications accurately and safely by the parenteral route and to protect yourself using Standard Precautions. You will also learn how to handle injection equipment and how to prepare medications for injection. In addition, you will learn to locate the proper sites of injections and follow specific injection procedures.

OBJECTIVES

After studying this chapter, you should be able to

- apply Standard Precautions.
- name and describe the major routes of parenteral administration.
- identify the parts of a needle and syringe.
- list the appropriate sizes of needles and syringes for different types and sites of injection.
- accurately identify dosages in calibrated syringes.
- dispose of injection equipment properly.
- draw up medications from ampules and vials, using aseptic technique.
- follow instructions for reconstituting and storing parenteral medications.
- locate the most common injection sites for intradermal, subcutaneous, and intramuscular administration.
- describe and follow proper procedures for carrying out intradermal, subcutaneous, and intramuscular injections.
- explain what to do when blood is aspirated during an injection.

KEY TERMS

abscess: localization of pus in any part of the body

acromion process: an extension of the shoulder blade that can be felt at the point where the upper arm meets the shoulder; a landmark for locating the deltoid injection site

aqueous: thin and watery

aspirate: to draw by suction; the process of pulling back on a syringe plunger to check for entry into a blood vessel during an injection

barrel: hollow cylinder with graduated markings on it that makes up the body of a syringe

flange: flared part of a syringe barrel; used to steady the syringe while pulling or pushing the plunger

gauge (G): diameter (width) of the lumen of a needle; the smaller the gauge number, the wider the lumen; selection of gauge depends on the viscosity of the solution to be injected

gluteal arteries: large arteries that supply the muscles of the buttock area

greater trochanter: knob on the upper leg bone (femur) that can be felt where the leg joins the hip; one of the landmarks used for locating the dorsogluteal injection site

hub: broad part of an injection needle that attaches to the syringe

iliac crest: highest point on the hip bone; one landmark used to locate the ventrogluteal injection site

induration: hardening of a tissue caused by inflammation or edema

lumen: hollow part of a needle through which medication flows

necrosis: death of tissue in a living body

needle cover: protective cover on a disposable injection needle; never put it back on the needle after administration

plunger: solid rod of a syringe that fits inside the barrel and pushes medication out under pressure

precipitate: solid particles that separate out from a solution as a result of a chemical reaction

reconstituting: the process of adding the recommended amount of fluid to dissolve; usually with a powdered drug

sciatic nerve: largest nerve in the body that pierces the buttocks and runs down the back of the thigh

shaft: the long portion of a needle that extends from the point to the hub and through which the medication passes

site rotation: the practice of injecting into different locations so as to avoid damaging tissue by repeated injections

sloughing: shedding of dead tissue from a wound or sore

Standard Precautions: recommended blood and body fluid precautions for use with all patients

syringe: used to inject or withdraw fluids from the body; consists of a plunger, barrel, and hub

tracking: backing up of medication in the channel through which a needle enters tissue

viscous: thick and sticky

Z-track: method of injection that minimizes tissue irritation by sealing the drug within muscle tissues

ORIENTATION TO THE PARENTERAL ROUTE

Parenteral administration is the method of giving drugs by injection using a needle and syringe. It is used when other routes would be ineffective or impractical. Because injection puts medication into direct contact with body tissues that contain many blood vessels and capillaries, absorption is more rapid by this route than by the oral, rectal, or topical routes. It is thus a valuable route in emergencies. Certain drugs that can be destroyed by digestive enzymes are given by the parenteral route so that they remain effective. Injections are also given when patients cannot take oral medications because of difficulty swallowing, nausea or vomiting, intestinal obstructions, or unconsciousness.

The parenteral route involves breaking through the skin's protective covering, which increases the risk of infection. The rapid absorption that occurs with injection means that the dose must be exact; reactions to an overdose can set in very rapidly and may require emergency treatment. Injections that are done improperly can stretch and injure tissues or hit bones, nerves, and blood vessels, causing pain and possibly serious damage.

Because of the dangers of injury, underdose, overdose, and infection, special training and certification are required for people who give medications parenterally. State laws regulate which categories of health care workers are permitted to give injections and what type of certification they must have. If you are not permitted to give injections, never administer drugs parenterally. The law protects your patients from injury and you from legal problems.

STANDARD PRECAUTIONS

Under **Standard Precautions,** all patients are considered potentially infectious with blood-borne pathogens. Examples are HBV (hepatitis B virus) and HIV (human immunodeficiency virus), the virus that causes AIDS (acquired immune deficiency syndrome). Healthcare workers are exposed to these pathogens primarily through mucous membranes, nonintact skin, and needlesticks. Standard Precautions apply to infections caused by blood, body fluids, nonintact skin, and mucous membranes. Standard Precautions combine the features of both Universal Precautions and Body Substance Isolation.

Blood is the most important vehicle for transmission of pathogens. Other body fluids that can be involved are cerebrospinal (CSF), synovial, pleural, peritoneal and amniotic fluids, semen, vaginal secretions, and human breast milk. Gloves should be worn for all contact with body fluids, mucous membranes, and nonintact skin that may be contaminated with blood. Use extreme caution in handling contaminated needles and other sharp instruments. To prevent needlesticks, needles should not be recapped, bent, broken, or removed from disposable syringes. Table 19.1 lists the universal blood and body fluid precautions.

TABLE 19.1: Universal Blood and Body Fluid Precautions

EMPLOYER: PROTECT HEALTH CARE WORKER.	WORKER: USE APPROPRIATE BARRIER PRECAUTIONS.	WORKER: PREVENT NEEDLESTICK INJURIES.
Explain activities that expose workers to blood-borne pathogens.	Wear gloves to reduce blood contamination of skin surface.	Do not break, bend, or remove needles by hand from syringes.
Develop standard operating procedures to prevent worker exposure.	Wash hands/skin immediately when exposed.	Do not recap needles.
Provide initial and ongoing education on Universal Precautions.	Change and discard punctured or torn gloves.	Place uncapped disposable needles in a rigid puncture-resistant container.
Follow up on worker compliance with guidelines.	Wear masks, gowns, and eye/face shields to protect mucous membranes when there is a risk of exposure with blood or body fluid.	Place these containers as close to the work area as possible.
Redesign the workplace and modify the workplace environment.	Do not work if you have dermatitis or exudative lesions.	Transport contaminated equipment to the appropriate waste area.
	If you are pregnant, *do not* risk exposing the fetus to blood-borne pathogens by lack of caution.	

EQUIPMENT

Four types of **syringes** (Figure 19.1) are used for injecting medications:

- the standard hypodermic syringe
- the insulin syringe
- the tuberculin syringe
- the Tubex syringe

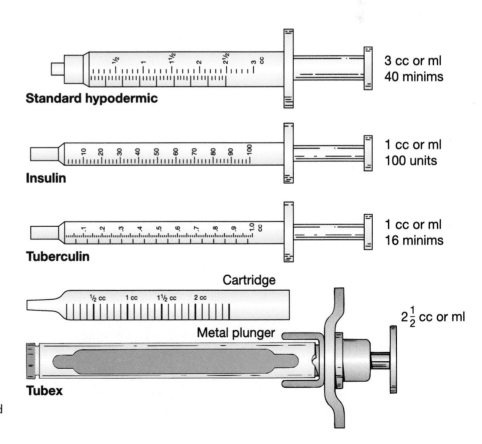

Figure 19.1
Standard hypodermic, insulin, tuberculin, and Tubex syringes and their capacities.

Standard hypodermic — 3 cc or ml / 40 minims

Insulin — 1 cc or ml / 100 units

Tuberculin — 1 cc or ml / 16 minims

Tubex — Cartridge — Metal plunger — $2\frac{1}{2}$ cc or ml

The standard hypodermic syringe is the most common type and is used with a variety of routes and medications. It is calibrated (marked) in cubic centimeters (cc) and in minims.

The insulin syringe, as its name implies, is used for subcutaneous injection of insulin and is calibrated in units. Most insulin is available as U100, indicating that each milliliter contains U100 of insulin. A U100 syringe must be used for U100 insulin. When a patient takes a smaller dose, insulin syringes with larger black lines are marked for 25, 30, or 50 U and are also used for U100 insulin.

The tuberculin syringe is designed for intradermal injection of very small amounts of substances in tests for tuberculosis and allergies. It is calibrated in hundredths of cubic centimeters and in minims.

Syringes are sized according to the volume of liquid they can hold. The most common size of the standard syringe is 2½–3 cc or milliliters (ml). Larger syringes of 5–50 cc are also available. These are not usually used for injections, but rather for adding fluids to intravenous flasks, for irrigating wounds, and for removing fluids from body cavities.

Syringes are made of disposable plastic or glass. They are packaged either separately or together with needles of appropriate sizes. Syringes and needles are packaged in peel-open paper wrappers. Syringes may be empty or prefilled with specific doses of medication. Prefilled glass cartridges are available for use with a special metal or plastic holder and plunger called a Tubex syringe.

The two main parts of a syringe are the **barrel** and the **plunger.** The barrel is a hollow cylinder that holds the medication. The plunger fits snugly in this cylinder and is used to change the pressure within. Pulling the plunger back lowers the air pressure inside the barrel, allowing air or medication to be pulled in from outside. Pushing in the plunger increases the pressure inside the barrel and forces air or medication out.

The barrel, plunger, and other parts of a syringe are identified in Figure 19.2. Obtain sample syringes from your instructor and locate these parts.

NEEDLES

Needles for injection are made of stainless steel and are available in various sizes for different purposes. They come packaged with a protective **needle cover** or sheath that keeps them from becoming contaminated. To understand how needle size is measured, study the parts of the needle diagrammed in Figure 19.2.

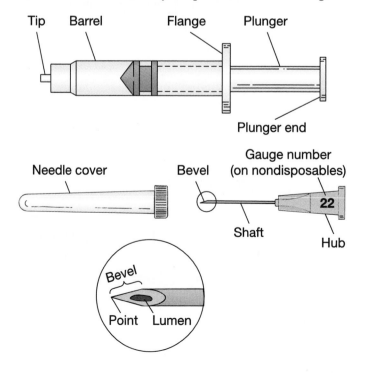

Figure 19.2
Parts of a needle and the syringe.

The tip of the needle, the point, breaks through the skin layers. The bevel or slanted portion of the needle tip spreads the tissues apart so the needle can enter smoothly. The longer the bevel, the sharper the needle and the more easily it passes through tissues, which minimizes the discomfort of subcutaneous and intramuscular injections. The **shaft** (stem or cannula) is the long part of the needle. It is embedded in the **hub,** which attaches to the syringe.

Needles are sized according to their length and gauge. The length of a needle is the distance from the point to the hub—in other words, the length of the shaft. The **gauge** (G) is the diameter of the **lumen,** the hollow part inside the needle through which medication passes. Needle lengths vary from ¼ inch to 5 inches. In general, the shorter lengths (¼ to ⅝-inch) are used for subcutaneous and intradermal injections and the longer lengths (1 to 1½ inches) for intramuscular injections. The longest needles (e.g., 5 inches) are usually used for other purposes, such as withdrawing fluids from body cavities.

The choice of needle length depends in part on the patient's age and body fat. Babies and small children require shorter needles to reach the proper tissues. People with heavy fat deposits require longer needles to reach their muscles (e.g., 2 inches). If a patient is obese or very thin and you are unsure what needle size to use, check with your supervisor.

The most common needles used are 19, 20, 21, 23, and 25 gauge. The smaller the gauge, the larger the needle diameter. Which gauge to use depends on how thick the medication is. Liquids that are thin and watery are described as **aqueous,** and those that are thick and sticky are described as **viscous.** Penicillin and other oil-based solutions are viscous, whereas most other medications are aqueous. Ordinary gauges (22–25G) are used for aqueous medications, but lower-numbered gauges (18–20G) must be used with viscous medications, which could easily clog a thinner needle. Package inserts for viscous medications may suggest the proper gauge to use.

The paper packages on disposable needles are labeled by both length and gauge. Always be certain you are using the proper length and gauge of needle for the route and medication.

KEEPING INJECTION EQUIPMENT STERILE

Because an injection breaks the skin that protects the body from microbes, it is vital to maintain asepsis when handling needles, syringes, and injectable medications. The parts of a needle and syringe that must be protected from contamination are the inside of the needle cover, the needle point and shaft, the inside and outside of the hub, the syringe tip, the inside of the syringe barrel, and the plunger. The only parts you may safely touch with your hands are the outside of the needle cover, the outside of the barrel, the **flange** (the flared part of the barrel), and the plunger end.

Disposable needles and syringes are presterilized and packaged in paper wrappers or plastic containers. To open these, peel back the paper or remove the cover and slide out the contents from that end. If the needle and syringe are packaged separately, attach them as follows: hold the needle cover and twist or press the hub onto the syringe tip, depending on the type of connection. After use, disposable equipment must be discarded in special puncture-resistant containers located within the working area. Contaminated materials should be disposed of properly.

DRAWING UP MEDICATIONS

When you are ready to fill a syringe with medication, attach the proper needle, if necessary, and remove the needle cover by pulling it straight off. The proper method for filling a syringe depends on whether the medication is contained in an ampule or a vial. Recall that an ampule is a single-dose glass container with a bulb that can be broken off at the neck. A vial is a small bottle with a rubber stopper through which a needle can be inserted. A vial can contain either a single dose or multiple doses. Remember to check the vial or ampule label against the medicine card as you set up the parenteral medications.

The practice procedures at the end of this chapter will help you learn to draw up medications smoothly, accurately, and without contaminating the equipment. Be sure to observe Standard Precautions.

FROM A VIAL

To draw medication from a vial, first remove the protective cap. If the vial has been opened previously (e.g., a multiple-dose vial), wipe the rubber seal firmly in a circular motion with an alcohol wipe (Figure 19.3). This cleans the surface through which the needle will pass, thus guarding against contamination.

The air pressure inside the vial is less than the pressure outside. Therefore, some air must be injected into the vial to make the medication easier to withdraw. You should inject an amount of air equal to the volume of medication that you are withdrawing. In other words, if you plan to withdraw 1.5 cc of medication, then you should first inject 1.5 cc of air into the vial. Pull back the stopper to the point marked 1.5 on the calibrated syringe. Insert the tip of the needle, with the bevel pointing up, through the center of the rubber seal. Inject air into the vial, holding on to the plunger. You may hold the vial right side up, tilted, or inverted as you inject the air. Hold the vial securely and do not touch the rubber stopper.

Next, invert the vial and place the needle into the medication. Inverting the vial allows the fluid to accumulate in the lower half of the vial. Hold the vial between the thumb and middle fingers of your nondominant hand. Grasp the end of the syringe barrel and plunger with the thumb and forefinger of the dominant hand. Keep the needle below the surface of the liquid so as to avoid taking in air. Air pressure will fill the syringe slowly with the medication.

Before taking the needle out of the vial, check for air bubbles in the syringe. Air bubbles keep you from measuring an accurate dose. The tiny bubbles that often collect on the rubber tip of the plunger are no problem. However, if you see larger bubbles in the barrel, hold the syringe straight up at a 90° angle and tap it sharply with your finger. This will cause the bubbles to collect and join together at the tip of the syringe. Force the bubbles out by pushing in slightly on the plunger and then withdraw more medication.

When you have drawn up the medication, replace the needle cover and assemble the remaining items you need for giving the injection: a medicine card, medication record, or other appropriate record form and an antiseptic wipe. As long as the needle cover is on, you may place the needle and syringe on a tray or cart without risking contamination.

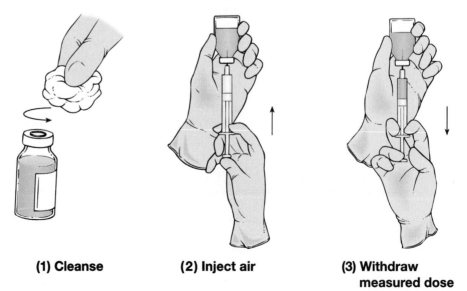

Figure 19.3
To draw medication from a vial, (1) cleanse the seal; (2) inject air; and (3) withdraw the measured dose.

(1) Cleanse   **(2) Inject air**   **(3) Withdraw measured dose**

FROM AN AMPULE

To withdraw medication from an ampule, first inspect the ampule to see if there is any medication in the top portion. If so, tap the top with your fingernail to send the medication back into the bottom portion. The scoring line of the ampule is usually marked with a colored band. Most ampules are prescored. Then, place a small gauze pad or alcohol swab around the ampule neck to protect your fingers from getting cut when you break the ampule (Figure 19.4). After covering the ampule neck, quickly snap it away from you to prevent shattering the glass toward your face or fingers.

Because the air pressure is the same on the outside and inside of the opened ampule, there is no need to inject air before withdrawing the medication. Add a filter needle to the syringe before withdrawing. Insert the needle into the ampule while holding the ampule on a flat surface in a tilted or upright position. As you pull back on the plunger, keep the needle submerged in the medication at all times. Do not allow the needle tip or shaft to touch the rim of the ampule. Some people prefer to invert the ampule while withdrawing the medication. This makes it easier to draw up all the medication without getting air bubbles.

No matter which hand position you use, be certain not to touch anything except the outside of the ampule, the outside of the syringe barrel, the flange, and the end of the plunger.

Next, check for air bubbles. If air bubbles are aspirated, do not expel air into the ampule. The air pressure may force fluid out of the ampule and medication may be lost. Remove the needle, hold the syringe upright, tap the side of the syringe to force the bubbles to rise toward the needle, draw back on the plunger, and push the plunger upward to expel air. If the syringe contains excess fluid, hold the syringe vertically with the needle tip up over a sink and slowly eject

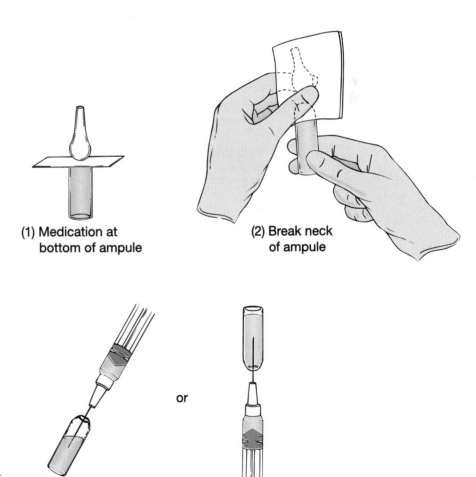

(1) Medication at bottom of ampule

(2) Break neck of ampule

or

Figure 19.4
Withdrawing medication from an ampule is similar to withdrawing from a vial, except that it is not necessary to inject air.

(3) Insert needle in ampule and withdraw medication

the excess. Replace the needle cover, and assemble the remaining items you need for giving the injection (e.g., medicine card, antiseptic wipe).

MEASURING DOSES ACCURATELY

To get an accurate dose, pay close attention to the calibrations on the particular syringe you are using. On a 2-cc syringe each mark may represent two-tenths of a cubic centimeter (0.2 cc). Count the number of marks between labeled units of measurement. If there are ten, then each mark measures off one-tenth of the unit. If there are five marks, then each mark measures two-tenths of the unit. Figure 19.5 shows how to read the calibrations when withdrawing a measured dose of medication. The bottom of the rubber plunger should be lined up with the desired dosage.

Figure 19.5
To withdraw a measured dose, line up the bottom of the plunger with the desired dose.

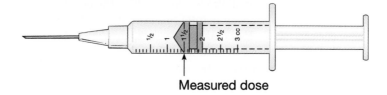

Measured dose

RECONSTITUTING POWDERED DRUGS

Certain drugs, such as antibiotics, are stored in their powdered form because they quickly lose freshness and effectiveness when in liquid form. These powders come packaged in vials and must be **reconstituted** before injection. In other words, liquid must be added to make a solution or suspension.

Drug powders are reconstituted using sterile water or saline solution for injection. To find out how much sterile water or saline solution to add, read the directions on the vial label or package insert. Then fill a syringe with the proper measured amount of fluid and inject it into the vial. If you must inject a great deal of fluid into the vial, withdraw some air as you proceed so that pressure does not build up. After adding the fluid, gently shake or roll the vial between your hands to dissolve or disperse the medication completely.

Although you may reconstitute a multidose vial, most reconstituted medications come in single dose vials. A multidose vial requires a label containing the date of mixing and concentration of drug per milliliter. Multidose vials may require refrigeration after they are reconstituted.

MIXING TWO MEDICATIONS IN A SYRINGE

When a patient is to receive more than one medication by injection, it saves discomfort for the patient if both medications can be given in the same injection. However, not all drugs can be mixed with others in the same syringe. Some drugs, when mixed together, form a **precipitate,** or granules, that cloud the liquid or settle to the bottom. Other drugs may change color when mixed. Either change can signal loss of effectiveness. Even with no visible change, the medications may still react to cancel each other's effects. Consult a pharmacist, the *PDR*®, or a drug reference book if you are unsure whether two medications may be mixed.

When premixed unit doses are not available and you wish to mix two drugs that can be mixed, use the following procedure. Inject air in both vials equal to the amount of drug to be withdrawn from the vial. Measure the first drug accurately and eliminate air bubbles in the syringe. Then withdraw the second drug. The total amount of liquid in the syringe should be the same as the two individual doses added together (Figure 19.6). If one medication must be withdrawn from a multiple-dose vial, withdraw this medication first. If both medications are in multiple-dose vials, change to a fresh needle after withdrawing the first dose to avoid getting any of the first medication in the second vial.

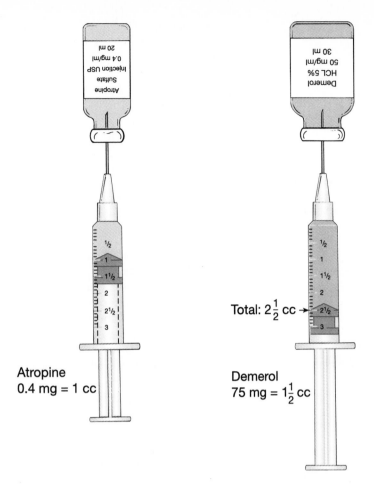

Figure 19.6
To mix two drugs in one dose, inject air into both vials, then withdraw the first medication. Change needles, and withdraw the second medication.

Atropine
0.4 mg = 1 cc

Total: $2\frac{1}{2}$ cc →

Demerol
75 mg = $1\frac{1}{2}$ cc

When mixing different types of insulin in a syringe, withdraw the fast-acting or clear insulin first and then the long-acting type.

INJECTION SITES

The exact location for an injection depends on whether it is to be subcutaneous, intramuscular, or intradermal. The doctor orders the route, but it may be up to you to decide exactly where to administer it. There are several options for each parenteral route. The specific site to choose depends on the patient's build (thin, fat, heavily muscled), age (infant, young child, average adult, elderly), and the sites of other recent injections.

INTRADERMAL SITES

Intradermal injections are usually administered into the skin on the inner surface of the lower arm (Figure 19.7 on page 346). In special cases (e.g., allergy tests), they may also be given in the upper chest area and on the upper back below the shoulder blades.

Very small amounts of medication are given by this route—usually 0.1 to 0.2 cc—so a tuberculin syringe is used with a 25–26G, $\frac{3}{8}$-inch needle. The needle, with the bevel pointing up, should be held at a 5° to 15° angle to the skin. It should pass just below the epidermis into the dermis and be inserted to a depth of $\frac{1}{16}$ to $\frac{1}{8}$ inch (you will be able to see the needle point through the skin). As the medication is injected, you should see a small bleb or blister form under the skin. If no bleb forms, withdraw the needle slightly, as you may have gone too deeply into the skin. If medication leaks out around the needle as you push the plunger, insert the needle a bit more deeply. After injecting the medicine, withdraw the needle and apply an alcohol swab. Do not massage the injection site. Massaging the site may disperse medication into underlying tissue and alter the test results.

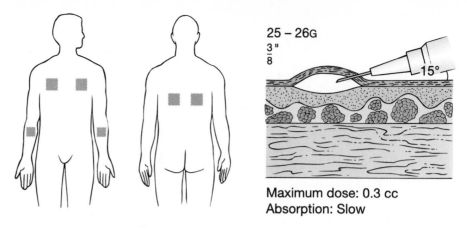

Figure 19.7
Intradermal sites
and injection
technique.

25 – 26G
$\frac{3}{8}$ "
15°

Maximum dose: 0.3 cc
Absorption: Slow

Intradermal injections are used to determine exposure to tuberculosis. About 48 to 72 hours after intradermal injection of tuberculin, the area is checked for **induration** (hardening of tissue caused by inflammation or edema) and erythema (reddening). This procedure is usually called "reading a diagnostic skin test." Induration with erythema is measured to determine exposure to tuberculosis; erythema without hardness rules out tuberculosis. An area less than 5 mm in diameter is a negative reaction. A site that is 5 to 9 mm is read as doubtful, and another test must be done. An area of 10 mm or more is a positive reaction. A similar test is used for histoplasmosis, so it is important to read the directions that come with the medication carefully.

SUBCUTANEOUS SITES

The sites for subcutaneous injection are the fatty tissues on the outer upper arm, the front of the thigh, the abdomen, and the upper back below the shoulder blades (Figure 19.8). The most common of these are the arm and the thigh with 1 inch of fatty tissue. This may be difficult to find on an elderly person, so be cautious in choosing an area. Most medication given subcutaneously is absorbed slowly because of the lesser vascularity of this tissue compared to muscle tissue.

Not more than 0.5 to 1 ml of water-soluble medication may be given subcutaneously. A 2- to 3-cc syringe may be used. The most common needle size for an average adult is 25G, ⅝ inch. The needle is inserted at a 45° to 90° angle, through the epidermis and the dermis, into the subcutaneous tissue. In an obese person, it may be desirable to use a 1-inch needle at a 90° angle. Check with your supervisor as to which angle is preferred for specific cases in your health facility. Do not massage the site after an injection of heparin or insulin. Massaging after heparin causes bleeding, and massaging after insulin may increase absorption of insulin.

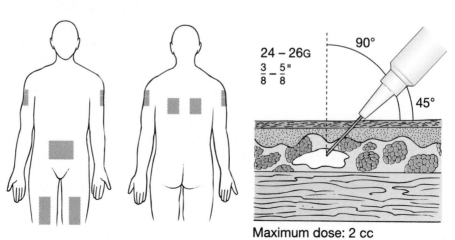

Figure 19.8
Subcutaneous
sites and injection
technique.

24 – 26G
$\frac{3}{8} - \frac{5}{8}$ "
90°
45°

Maximum dose: 2 cc
Absorption: Moderate to fast

INTRAMUSCULAR SITES

The intramuscular route places the needle deep into body tissues where there are nerve bundles, large blood vessels, and bones. Therefore, it is especially important to locate the sites properly. The danger of causing tissue damage is less when the medicine enters deep muscle, but there is a risk of inadvertently injecting medicine into a blood vessel. You should locate the sites by touch, using certain prominent bones as landmarks. Advantages of the intramuscular route are as follows:

- A larger amount of medication may be injected—up to 3 cc.
- The muscles can absorb more medication than can other tissues.
- Absorption is quite rapid because muscles are well supplied with capillaries.
- The route is appropriate for oily medications that do not come in oral form.
- It can be used with uncooperative patients, and with those who cannot swallow, to get a rapid effect from a drug and to avoid loss of drug effects.

Intramuscular injections must be made only into the thickest parts of large, healthy muscles. There are four possible sites (Figure 19.9):

- The dorsogluteal sites, both above and to the outside of the buttock area
- The ventrogluteal sites, both above and to the outside of the buttock area
- The deltoid site of the upper arm
- The vastus lateralis muscle of the thigh

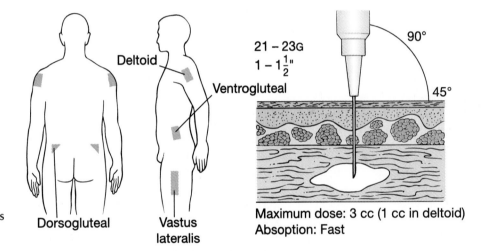

Figure 19.9
Intramuscular sites and injection technique.

In the two sites near the buttock area, the aim is to inject into large muscle masses that are as far away as possible from the **sciatic nerve,** the largest nerve in the body, and the **gluteal arteries,** which supply the muscles of the buttock area. Piercing the sciatic nerve could cause pain and possibly paralysis. The dorsogluteal or posterior gluteal site is the most commonly used intramuscular site in average-sized adults. Two ways of locating the dorsogluteal site are shown in Figure 19.10.

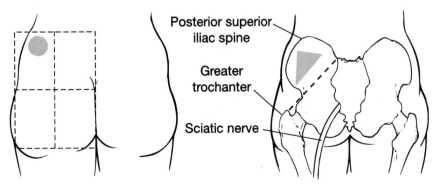

Figure 19.10
Locating the dorsogluteal site.

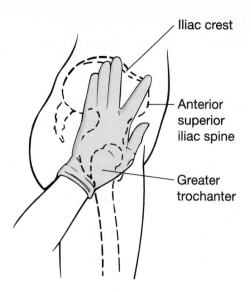

Figure 19.11
Locating the ventrogluteal site.

One method is to draw imaginary lines dividing one side of the lower back and buttock area into quarters. The injection is given in the upper outer corner of the upper outer quarter. The other method is to draw an imaginary line between the head of the femur (thigh bone) where it joins the hip (the **greater trochanter**) and the posterior superior iliac spine of the hipbone. The injection is given above and to the outside of this line. Study Figure 19.10 carefully and then practice locating the dorsogluteal site on a classmate or friend.

When you use the dorsogluteal site, the patient may lie in a prone position (on the stomach), with the toes pointed inward, or in a side lying position with the upper leg flexed at the hip and knees.

The ventrogluteal site is close to the dorsogluteal site and is usually approached from a side-lying position. The site can be located by placing the palm of your hand on the patient's greater trochanter and then feeling for two spots on the hip bone, the **iliac crest**, or highest point, and the anterior superior iliac spine. The V formed by touching these spots with your index and third fingers identifies the correct placement of the ventrogluteal injection (Figure 19.11). This site is especially useful when a large amount of medication is to be injected into a patient who must lie flat on his or her back.

The deltoid site is in the deltoid muscle of the outer upper arm, 1 to 2 inches below the spot where the arm and shoulder join (the **acromion process**). This is a small site, and it may not have much muscle even in a well-developed body. The maximum amount to inject into the deltoid is 1 cc, and a shorter needle (1 inch maximum) is used.

The vastus lateralis site is on the outer upper thigh, in the middle third of the area between the knee and the greater trochanter. This is the preferred site for infants and children, because their buttock (gluteal) muscles are not well enough developed to safely receive dorsogluteal or ventrogluteal injections.

For intramuscular injections, the needle should be long enough to pass through the subcutaneous tissue and deep into muscle tissue. A 21G to 23G, 1-inch to 1½-inch needle is usually used, with a 2- to 3-cc syringe. An 18G to 20G needle may be used for viscous medication. The needle is inserted at a 90° angle.

GENERAL PROCEDURE FOR INJECTIONS

Although the various types of injections require different sites, needle sizes, and angles of penetration, certain steps and principles (i.e., Standard Precautions) are common to all. With these general directions in mind, you will be prepared to practice the step-by-step procedures for intradermal, subcutaneous, and intramuscular injections at the end of the chapter (Practice Procedures 19.3, 19.4, and 19.5). All procedures are described for a right-handed person. If you are left-handed, simply reverse the positions.

1. **Locate and inspect the injection site.** Use the physician's ordered route and the site rotation plan, if any, to determine where to give an injection. Find the proper injection site using anatomical landmarks. Remove clothing or sheets as necessary to get a full view of the physical landmarks that enable you to locate the proper sites. If the injection is intramuscular, choose only healthy, heavy muscles that are free of tenderness. Inspect the skin carefully for signs of rash, redness, lumps, hair, or birthmarks. Rash or redness may be signs of reactions to previous injections given in that area. Do not proceed with the injection if there has been a reaction, but chart the appearance of the skin and consult the nurse in charge. Hardness in the skin or underlying muscle suggest that a previous injection was poorly absorbed or caused tissue damage. The next injection should be given at least 1 inch away or in another site.

2. **Disinfect the skin.** Use an antiseptic wipe (e.g., alcohol) to cleanse the skin so microorganisms do not enter the body at the injection site. Cleanse the skin in a circular motion. Using an antiseptic swab, start at the center and rotate outward in a circular motion for 2 inches. Allow the antiseptic to dry. This is especially important with alcohol, because it can sting if it enters body tissues. Save the antiseptic wipe and hold it between the third and fourth fingers of the nondominant hand. You will use it later when you are ready to withdraw the needle.

3. **Stretch and firm the skin.** With your left hand, hold the skin taut. Use your thumb and middle finger to stretch the skin and push it down. Alternately, when the site is on the arm, grasp the tissue from behind the arm and pull down and back. For the subcutaneous route, spread the skin tightly over the injection site, which allows the needle to penetrate more easily than through loose skin, or pinch the skin. Pinching the skin elevates the subcutaneous tissue and may desensitize the area.

4. **Insert the needle at the proper angle.** Use the correct angle of insertion for the route, site, and needle size. With your right hand, hold the needle and syringe at the correct angle in relation to the skin surface (15°, 45°, or 90°). The bevel should be facing up. Then insert the needle quickly and smoothly with a firm thrust.

5. **Release the skin and change the hand position.** Lift your left hand so that the skin is no longer stretched or pinched. Move this hand over to the lower end of the syringe barrel so that your right hand can operate the plunger. Do not release the syringe from your right hand until your left hand is holding it steady. Any sideward movement of the needle at this step could damage underlying tissues.

6. **Aspirate.** While the needle is fully inserted, pull back slightly on the plunger. This is called **aspirating.** It is a safety check to make sure that the needle has not entered a blood vessel. If it is not in a vessel, you will feel some resistance on the plunger and you will not see blood in the syringe. You may then proceed with the injection. If the needle has entered a vessel, however, blood will become visible in the syringe as you pull the plunger. If this happens, remove the needle, discard the medication and syringe, and repeat the procedure. Aspirating is important because medications ordered for subcutaneous and intramuscular injections must not be injected intravenously. If this were to happen accidentally, it could cause serious harm. There are two cases in which you should not aspirate: (1) intradermal injections, because the needle does not penetrate deep enough to contact large vessels, and (2) anticoagulant injections (e.g., heparin), because aspirating could lead to uncontrolled bleeding.

7. **Inject the medication slowly.** Still holding the syringe with your left hand, change your right hand position to push in the plunger. This forces the

medication out of the syringe and into the body tissues. It must be injected slowly to avoid overstretching and injuring the tissues. Be sure to inject all the medication by pushing in the plunger fully.

8. Firm the skin and remove the needle. The skin must once again be firmed so that the needle does not pull the skin as it is withdrawn. Hold the antiseptic wipe (which you tucked between your fingers in Step 2) near the needle and press gently on the skin. Pull the needle out quickly at the same angle at which it was inserted. This technique reduces pain and prevents tissue damage.

9. Remove and discard equipment. Do not insert the needle back into the cap. Always observe standard blood and body fluid precautions. Do not break the needle. Dispose of the contaminated syringe and needle in a puncture-resistant waste container in the working area.

If you must recap the needle, cover it and place the cap on a clean surface. With one hand, slowly insert the needle into it. The needle and syringe are now contaminated and may not be reused.

10. Chart the medication. Include the specific parenteral route (intradermal, subcutaneous, or intramuscular) and note the location of the injection (right or left arm, right or left dorsogluteal site, etc.).

11. Observe the patient for expected and adverse reactions. Try to remain with the patient for at least 1 minute, then check frequently to see how the patient is feeling. The length of time to observe depends on the drug. In certain cases, you may have to stay near the patient for a certain time (e.g., 20 minutes the first time a person is injected with penicillin). Be alert for the call button of a patient who has recently received an injection. One aim of observation is to see whether the drug is working—whether an analgesic, for example, is successfully relieving pain. The other aim is to detect unexpected side effects and adverse reactions.

Parenteral medications work very quickly compared to oral, rectal, and topical medications, so reactions can occur within minutes of the injection. Systemic adverse reactions may occur as a result of overdose or allergy. These require immediate medical treatment, so you should notify the supervisor immediately if they occur.

Local reactions result from irritation of the tissues where the drug was injected. Redness, rash, and lumpiness have already been mentioned as signs of drug sensitivity, tissue irritation, poor absorption, and extravasation. More serious local reactions can result in severe tissue damage—for example, death of tissue (**necrosis**), shedding of skin (**sloughing**), and formation of pus inside the tissues (**abscess**). These conditions require special treatment by a physician. Your duty is to chart and report any unusual signs of inflammation or irritation that appear in the injection area.

This general procedure includes specific steps required for parenteral administration. In addition to these steps, you must follow the other basic rules for administering medications, such as identifying the patient, explaining the procedure, assisting the patient into a comfortable position both before and after the injection, and observing Standard Precautions.

SPECIAL INSTRUCTIONS

SITE ROTATION

Some people must have injections several times a day—for example, penicillin for a systemic infection. Others, such as patients with insulin-controlled diabetes, must have injections daily over a long period of time. If all these injections were to be given in the same site, the tissues might be damaged and scar tissue might form, making further injections difficult. For these reasons, injection sites must be rotated according to some pattern (**site rotation**) that allows the medical staff to keep track of whether and where the last injection was given. Most health facilities adopt a rotation plan such as that shown in Figure 19.12. This method gives them a systematic way to administer regular

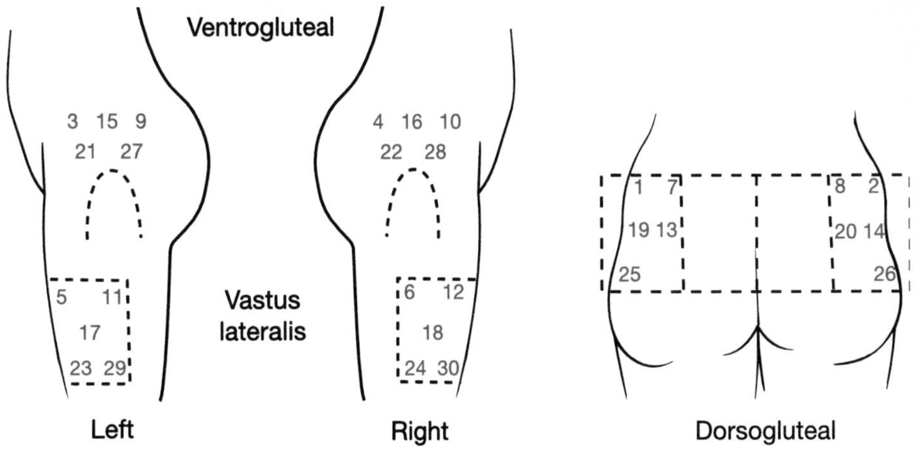

Figure 19.12 Site rotation plan for IM injections with location of injections numbered in order of administration.

Ventrogluteal

Left

3 15 9
21 27

5 11
17
23 29

Vastus
lateralis

Right

4 16 10
22 28

6 12
18
24 30

Dorsogluteal

1 7
19 13
25

8 2
20 14
26

injections without damaging body tissues. Site rotation is used with subcutaneous (except insulin) and intramuscular injections. Rotating injection sites for insulin is no longer recommended. The patient may rotate injection sites within a given area, such as the abdomen. Intradermal medications are not usually given over many days.

PREVENTION OF TRACKING

As a needle is withdrawn after an injection, it leaves a small channel or track where the needle was inserted. **Tracking** is the leaking of medication into the channel. Medication that did not clear the needle may leak into the track as the needle is pulled out. Alternately, the pressure of the medication in the tissue where it was injected may force some of the medication to back up into the track. In either case, tracking is not desirable, because the medication may irritate or stain other tissue layers. Penicillin, for example, causes a burning pain if it contacts subcutaneous tissue, and Imferon can cause stains. There are several ways to prevent tracking:

- Inject very slowly and wait at least 10 seconds before withdrawing the needle.
- Avoid massaging the injection site, which increases the pressure on the medication.
- Advise patients to wear loose-fitting clothing and to avoid heavy exercise.
- Use an air bubble or use the Z-track method.

Use of an Air Bubble. Some health facilities recommend the use of an air bubble to prevent tracking in intramuscular injections. In this method, a small amount of air (0.2 cc) is taken into the syringe after the correct dose is measured. When the medication is injected, the air bubble leaves the syringe last. It serves to clear the needle of all medication so that none can leak out as the needle is withdrawn. The air bubble also provides a space into which the medication can flow and thus lessen the pressure on surrounding tissues. Finally, the bubble seals off the needle track to block leakage. Ask your supervisor if this is the preferred procedure for intramuscular injections in your facility.

Z-track Intramuscular Injection. The **Z-track** method of injection may be used to minimize irritation by sealing the medicine in muscle tissue (Figure 19.13 on page 352). Z-track is used to give certain medications and always for intramuscular injections. A large, deeper muscle, such as the ventrogluteal, should be selected. After drawing up the medication, put a new needle on the syringe so no medication remains in the needle shaft. After cleansing the injection site with alcohol, pull the skin and subcutaneous tissues 1 to 1½ inches to the side. Hold the prepared site taut and insert the needle deep into the muscle. After aspirating for blood, slowly administer the

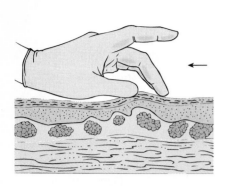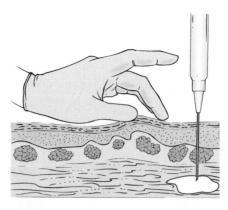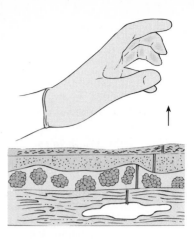

Figure 19.13
The Z-track method of injection prevents medication from backing up into other tissue layers.

medication. The needle should remain inserted for 10 seconds to promote even distribution of the medicine. Release the skin after withdrawing the needle. This technique leaves a zigzag pattern that seals the needle track, preventing the medicine from escaping into surrounding tissues. The Z-track method is primarily required when injecting Imferon.

YOUR ATTITUDE TOWARD INJECTIONS

No matter how skillful you are at giving injections, they are bound to cause fear and discomfort in some patients. This is where psychological factors come into play. You need to explain how and why you are giving the medication, as always. But more than ever, your attitude toward the procedure and the patient are crucial.

Your attitude toward the patient is important in getting the patient to cooperate in the procedure. Be a good listener and let patients know that you care about their concerns. A relaxed patient who has confidence in you will feel less discomfort than a tense, anxious patient.

Where the procedure itself is concerned, you can be only as confident as the amount of supervised practice you put into learning how to give injections. Practice must, of course, include some feedback on how well you performed the procedure. When you really understand what you are doing, your confidence will show. The key, then, is to study carefully the theoretical information about injections and then practice the injection procedures until you can perform them with 100 percent accuracy.

PRACTICE PROCEDURE 19.1
Drawing Up Medication From a Vial

■ EQUIPMENT

Medication order (e.g., regular insulin 5 U SC)

Kardex, medicine card, medication record, patient chart

Variety of syringes and needles with covers

Vial of medication (e.g., 100-U strength insulin in a multiple-dose vial); check the expiration date

Vials of sterile water for injection (for practice)

Antiseptic wipes or sponges

Sterile gauze

Continued

■ PROCEDURE

1. Read the medication order and assemble the equipment. Check for the "five rights." Read the vial label by holding it next to the medicine card (or Kardex, medication record, or physician's order if medicine cards are not used).

2. Wash your hands.

3. Select the proper size needle and syringe for the medication and the route (e.g., for subcutaneous injection of insulin, 100-U insulin syringe and 25G, ⅝-inch needle). If necessary, attach the needle to the syringe.

4. Check the vial label against the medicine card (or appropriate record) a second time.

5. Remove the metal or plastic cap from the vial of insulin. If the vial has been opened previously, clean the rubber stopper by applying an antiseptic wipe in a circular motion.

6. Remove the needle cover (pull it straight off).

7. Inject air into the vial as follows:

   • Hold the syringe pointed upward at eye level. Pull back the plunger to take in a quantity of air equal to the ordered dose of medication (5 U in our insulin example).
   • Place the vial on a flat surface. Take care not to touch the rubber stopper.
   • Insert the needle through the center of the rubber stopper of the vial. Inject the air into the vial's airspace by pushing in the plunger.

8. Invert the vial and withdraw the medication: hold the vial and the syringe steady. Pull back on the plunger to withdraw the measured dose of medication. Measure accurately. Keep the tip of the needle below the surface of the liquid; otherwise, air will enter the syringe.

9. Check the syringe for air bubbles. Remove them by tapping sharply on the syringe. If you are using an air bubble to prevent tracking, add 0.2 cc of air to the syringe after measuring the dose accurately and expelling air bubbles.

10. Remove the needle from the vial. Replace the sterile needle cover.

11. Check the vial label against the medicine card (or appropriate record) a third time.

12. Place the filled needle and syringe on a medicine tray or cart, with an antiseptic wipe and the medicine card (or appropriate record). The dose is now ready for injection.

13. Return multiple-dose vials to the proper storage area (cabinet or refrigerator). Dispose of unused medication in a single-dose vial according to your agency's procedure. (Remember, disposal of a controlled substance must be witnessed and the proper forms signed.)

Demonstrate this procedure to your instructor.

PRACTICE PROCEDURE 19.2

Drawing Up Medication From an Ampule

■ EQUIPMENT

Medication order (e.g., *Vistaril*, 25 mg IM stat)

Kardex, medicine card, medication record, patient chart

Variety of syringes and needles with covers

Continued

Ampule of medication (e.g., 1-ml ampule of *Vistaril* containing 100 mg/ml); check the expiration date

Ampules of sterile water for injection (for practice)

Sterile gauze

Antiseptic wipes or sponges

■ **PROCEDURE**

1. Read the medication order and assemble the equipment. Check for the "five rights." Read the ampule label by holding it next to the medicine card (or Kardex, medication record, or physician's order if medicine cards are not used).

2. Wash your hands.

3. Select the proper size needle and syringe for the medication and the route (e.g., a 2½–cc standard hypodermic syringe and 22G, 1½–inch needle for intramuscular injection of *Vistaril*). If necessary, attach the needle to the syringe.

4. Check the ampule label against the medicine card (or other appropriate record) a second time.

5. Tap down any medication in the top of the ampule.

6. Place a small gauze pad around the neck of the ampule to protect your fingers from broken glass.

7. Snap the neck of the ampule quickly and firmly away from you.

8. Withdraw the medication. Insert the needle into the open end of the broken ampule. Check your agency policy to see if a filter needle is to be used for drawing up the medication. Do not let the needle touch the rim of the ampule; this contaminates the needle. The needle should be kept below the fluid level to prevent drawing up air. The ampule may be tipped to allow the fluid to accumulate in one corner of the ampule to facilitate drawing up all the medicine. Pull back on the plunger and remove a measured dose of medication. The ampule may be held right side up on a flat surface or inverted. Measure accurately. (If using the sample order of *Vistaril*, draw up 1.0 ml of the drug.)

9. Check the syringe for air bubbles. Remove them by tapping sharply on the syringe. Draw back on the plunger and then slowly push the plunger upward to expel air. Be careful not to eject any of the medicine.

10. If the syringe contains too much medicine, hold the syringe vertically with the needle tip up and slanted toward the sink. Slowly eject the excess medicine into the sink. Place the syringe vertically and recheck the dose.

11. If you used a filter needle, change the needle to the appropriate size. Replace the needle cover.

12. Check the ampule label against the medicine card (or appropriate record) a third time.

13. Place the filled needle and syringe on a medicine tray or cart with an antiseptic wipe and the medicine card (or appropriate record). The dose is now ready for injection.

14. Discard the unused portion of the ampule according to your agency's procedure.

Demonstrate this procedure for the instructor.

Administering an Intradermal Injection

■ EQUIPMENT

Medication order for an intradermal preparation (e.g., Mantoux test for tuberculosis)

Kardex, medicine card, medication record, patient chart

Vial or ampule of medication for intradermal injection; check the expiration date

Sterile needle, 26G, $\frac{3}{8}$ inch with cover

Sterile tuberculin syringe

Sterile antiseptic wipes, gloves

Medicine tray

Puncture-resistant container for disposal of contaminated materials

Plastic dummy or arm for practice injections

■ PROCEDURE

1. Read the medication order and check for the "five rights."

2. Assemble equipment and prepare the injection. Use sterile technique and measure accurately.

3. Identify the patient, following agency policy. Explain what you are going to do. Wear gloves.

4. Assist the patient into a comfortable position that allows access to the injection site (lower inner arm, upper back, or upper chest).

5. Inspect the injection site. Inject only into healthy skin free of rash, redness, or lumps.

6. Cleanse the site with an antiseptic wipe and allow it to dry.

7. With nondominant hand, spread the skin over the site with forefinger or thumb.

8. With the dominant hand, hold the needle at a 5° to 15° angle to the skin surface. Insert the needle slowly until resistance is felt. Advance the needle to a depth of $\frac{1}{8}$ inch below the skin. The needle tip can be seen under the skin. Do not aspirate.

9. Inject the medication slowly and fully. It is normal to feel resistance. If you do not meet resistance, the needle is too deep, and you should remove the needle and restart the procedure. You should see a small blister or bleb, approximately 6 mm or $\frac{1}{2}$ inch, form just under the skin while injecting medication. The bleb means the medication is deposited in the dermis.

10. Withdraw the needle and apply an alcohol swab or gauze to support the tissues. There is some evidence that discomfort may arise with alcohol, and a dry gauze may be preferred. Do not massage the tissues. Massaging the tissue may cause the medicine to disperse into underlying tissues and alter the test results.

11. Dispose of the uncapped syringe into a puncture- and leak-proof container.

12. Remove gloves.

13. Stay with the patient and observe for allergic reaction. A severe allergic reaction is characterized by wheezing, shortness of breath, and circulatory collapse.

14. Chart the medication.

15. Draw a circle around the perimeter of the injection site with a pencil and return in 48 to 72 hours after the injection to evaluate the patient's response to the medication.

Demonstrate this procedure to your instructor.

■ EQUIPMENT

Medication order for a subcutaneous preparation

Kardex, medicine card, medication record, patient chart

Vial or ampule of medication prepared for subcutaneous injection; check the expiration date

Sterile needle, 25G, $\frac{5}{8}$ inch or 27G, $\frac{1}{2}$–1 inch with cover

Sterile antiseptic wipes, gloves

Medicine tray

Puncture-resistant container for disposal of contaminated materials

Plastic dummy, arm, torso for practice injections

■ PROCEDURE

1. Read the medication order and check for the "five rights."

2. Assemble equipment and prepare the injection. Use sterile technique and measure accurately.

3. Identify the patient following agency policy. Explain what you are going to do. Wear gloves.

4. Assist the patient into a comfortable position that allows access to the injection site (outer upper arm, upper back, anterior thigh).

5. Inspect the injection site. If rash or redness is present, chart and report to your supervisor and do not give the injection. If lumps are present, inject at least 1 inch away or choose another site.

6. Cleanse the site with an antiseptic wipe and allow it to dry. Secure the wipe between your third and fourth fingers for later use.

7. With your nondominant hand, spread the skin tightly or pinch the skin and subcutaneous tissue between the thumb and finger. For an obese patient, pinch the skin at the site and insert the needle at a 90° angle. Obese patients have a fatty layer of tissue above subcutaneous tissue.

8. With the dominant hand, insert the needle at a 45° angle to the skin, bevel side up. Insert the needle quickly and smoothly.

9. Use the dominant hand to stabilize the syringe. Be careful not to move the needle from side to side.

10. Aspirate by pulling back on the plunger. If no blood appears, proceed with the injection. If blood appears, prepare a new injection with fresh equipment and move to another site. *Never* aspirate with anticoagulants such as heparin.

11. Inject the medication slowly. Push the plunger all the way in to inject the full dose.

12. Withdraw the needle quickly, firming the skin with the antiseptic wipe held near the needle. Pull out the needle at the same angle (45° or 90°) at which it was inserted.

13. Do not massage the site after injecting insulin or heparin. Massaging the site after heparin causes bleeding, and after insulin, increases absorption of the insulin.

14. Dispose of the uncapped syringe in a puncture-proof container.

15. Chart the medication: name, dosage, route, site, and time.

16. Observe the patient frequently (or as ordered) to be sure the medication is working and that there are no adverse reactions. Subcutaneous injections usually take 30 minutes or more to absorb. Instruct the patient in any necessary self-care and advise the patient to rest quietly for at least a few minutes.

Demonstrate this procedure to your instructor.

Note: This procedure is geared to the average adult.

■ EQUIPMENT

Medication order for aqueous intramuscular preparation

Kardex, medicine card, medication record, patient chart

Vial or ampule of medication prepared for intramuscular injection; check the expiration date

Sterile needle, 22G, $1\frac{1}{2}$ inches with cover (1-inch size for the deltoid site)

Sterile syringe, size $2\frac{1}{2}$–3 cc

Sterile antiseptic wipes, gloves

Medicine tray

Puncture-resistant container for disposal of contaminated materials

Plastic dummy or torso for practice injections and standard injection procedure

■ PROCEDURE

1. Read the medication order and check for the "five rights."

2. Assemble equipment and prepare the injection. Add a 0.2-cc air bubble to the syringe after measuring the medication if this method is used in your agency.

3. Identify the patient following agency policy. Explain what you are going to do. Wear gloves.

4. Assist the patient into a comfortable position that allows access to the injection site (dorsogluteal, ventrogluteal, deltoid, or vastus lateralis).

5. Inspect the injection site for signs of redness, rash, or lumps. If rash or redness is present, chart and report to your supervisor and do not give the injection. If a lump is present, make the injection at least 1 inch away or choose another site.

6. Cleanse the site with an antiseptic wipe. Start cleansing at the center of the site and rotate outward in a circular motion for up to 2 inches.

7. With the nondominant hand, spread the skin taut between two fingers.

8. With the dominant hand, hold the needle at a 90° angle to the skin, bevel side up. Insert the needle quickly and smoothly, with a firm thrust.

9. Release the taut skin and use this hand to steady the inserted needle and syringe. Be careful not to move the needle from side to side.

10. Aspirate, using your free hand to pull back on the plunger. If no blood appears, proceed with the injection. If blood appears, prepare a new injection with fresh equipment and move to another site.

11. Inject the medication slowly. Push the plunger all the way in to inject the full dose.

12. Withdraw the needle quickly, firming the skin with the antiseptic wipe held near the needle. Pull out at the same 90° angle at which the needle entered.

13. Do not massage the injection site. Massaging the injection site causes underlying tissue damage.

14. Dispose of the uncapped syringe in a puncture-resistant container.

15. Remove gloves.

16. Chart the medication.

17. Return to the patient in 10 to 30 minutes to evaluate the effects of the medication.

Demonstrate this procedure to your instructor.

Define each of the terms listed below.

1. Standard Precautions _____

2. Aspirate _____

3. Viscous _____

4. Aqueous _____

Answer the following questions in the spaces provided.

5. Identify the parts of a needle and syringe on the drawing below.

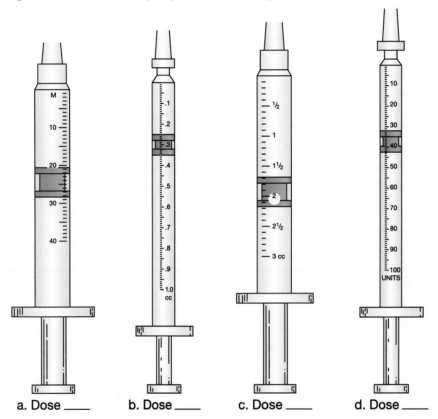

a. Dose _____   b. Dose _____   c. Dose _____   d. Dose _____

6. These syringes are filled with measured amounts of medication. Tell the exact dose in each.

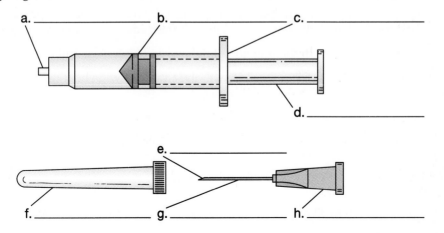

a. _____   b. _____   c. _____

d. _____

e. _____

f. _____   g. _____   h. _____

Continued

7. In item 6, name the type of syringe shown in each case.

   a. _____   c. _____

   b. _____   d. _____

8. Summarize what you have learned about parenteral routes and equipment by filling in the blanks in the table below.

	Intradermal	Subcutaneous	Intramuscular
a. Injected into (name tissue layer)	_____	_____	_____
b. Type of syringe	_____	_____ or _____	_____
c. Needle length	_____	_____	_____
d. Needle gauge	_____	_____	<u>aqueous</u> <u>viscous</u>
e. Angle of entry	_____	_____	_____

9. List at least three reasons that a physician might order a drug to be given by the parenteral route.

   _____

   _____

   _____

10. What does it mean to aspirate before injecting medication? Why is it done?

   _____

   _____

11. What should you do if you see blood in the syringe when you aspirate?

   _____

   _____

Match sites of injection to routes of injection.

_____ 12. Anterior thigh, upper outer arm, abdomen, upper back under shoulder blades

_____ 13. Vastus lateralis, deltoid, dorsogluteal, ventrogluteal

_____ 14. Inner lower arm, upper chest, upper back under shoulder blades

_____ 15. Veins of arms and legs

a. intramuscular

b. intravenous

c. intradermal

d. subcutaneous

Complete the following statements by filling in the blanks.

16. Injections in the buttock area must be placed very carefully so as to avoid the gluteal arteries and the _____ nerve.

17. When holding the needle and syringe at the proper angle to the skin, the bevel should be facing _____ (down or up).

18. Before drawing up a measured amount of medication from a vial, inject an equal amount of
_____ into the vial.

19. The neck of an ampule must be _____ before use.

20. After reconstituting a powdered drug in a multiple-dose vial, write the _____ ,
_____ , and _____ on the label.

■ CASE STUDIES FOR CRITICAL THINKING

Answer the following questions in the spaces provided.

21. Review the 12 general steps in any injection procedure. Then write them here (from memory, if possible).

_____

_____

_____

_____

_____

_____

22. List the local reactions that can occur following injections.

_____

_____

23. What should you do if the injection site you have chosen is covered with a rash?

_____

_____

24. How do practice and attitude affect your ability to give injections?

_____

_____

_____

_____

■ APPLICATIONS

Obtain a current copy of the PDR® or a drug reference book. Use it to answer the questions that follow about Fortaz, a broad-spectrum antibiotic.

25. What is the generic name of *Fortaz*? _____

26. Name two strains of bacteria that this drug can affect. _____

_____

_____

Continued

27. Give the usage and indications of this drug. _____

_____

_____

_____

_____

28. When is *Fortaz* contraindicated? _____

_____

 *Inter*NET CONNECTION

WebMD at http://shn.webmd.com is another interesting Web site with medical and health information for consumers. Here you can search for topics in many places including the Health and Medical Library. Click on Medical Encyclopedia to see thousands of entries. Click on Drug Reference to gain access to the U.S. Pharmacopeia Drug Information database.

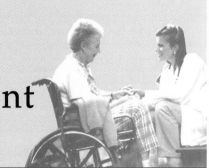

OBJECTIVES

After studying this chapter, you should be able to

- describe the major changes that take place in the various body systems during aging.
- state why treatment of elderly patients must be individualized according to each person's needs.
- describe the effects of aging on absorption, distribution, metabolism, and excretion of drugs.
- explain how medication orders are usually adjusted to account for the pharmacokinetics of an older patient.
- explain why the presence of more diseases in old age makes drug therapy more complicated.
- state what types of adverse reactions health care workers must look for in administering drugs to the aged.
- explain how elderly patients are affected by the attitudes and actions of health care workers.
- review safe medication administration practices and the principles that are specific for the elderly patient.
- list ways that patients can take an active part in their own medication therapy.

KEY TERMS

collagen: protein making up fibers in connective tissue; builds up in the lungs during aging, thus decreasing lung elasticity

geriatrics: the branch of medicine pertaining to the diseases and disorders of people 65 years of age or older

gerontology: the study of aging and problems of the aged

polypharmacy: the use of a number of different drugs by a patient who may have several different health problems

DRUGS AND THE ELDERLY

Regardless of whether you are employed in a long-term care facility or in another clinical setting, you are likely to find yourself working with an aging population. The population aged 65 years and older is the fastest growing segment of the population, increasing approximately 2 percent each year. As patients age, diminishing organ function is normal, and they become more prone to disease. Medical assistance is required to help the aged maintain the best possible health. Drugs are part of the health maintenance program; they also play a large part in disease management. The elderly are likely to be prescribed a larger number of drugs than younger adults simply because they tend to have more disorders. Also, OTC medications are primarily used by the elderly. It is estimated that 70 percent of OTC medications are used by the geriatric population. The aged are also more prone to side effects from all categories of medications.

The study of aging is called **gerontology,** and the study of diseases of the aged is called **geriatrics.** Because you will probably work with the elderly in administering medications, it is important to understand their special problems and needs. It is especially important because the elderly are often slighted in treatment. You want to be the best caregiver possible, and a thorough understanding of the elderly and their drug-related needs is an important step toward that goal.

THE AGING PROCESS

As body cells are lost through aging, the organs that they compose also slow down. Almost every organ loses some of its function, although this loss does not necessarily represent disease. These changes are normal anticipated changes in the elderly. The body also loses some of its ability to cope with stress. The body's balance-keeping systems become less finely tuned, so stress is longer-lasting and more extreme in old age. Disease and injury are forms of stress that put the body temporarily out of balance. The effect of aging is to make it harder for the elderly to "bounce back" after diseases—even minor diseases such as colds. Healing takes longer and complications are more likely to develop. That is why flu, pneumonia, and broken bones are much more serious for the elderly than for younger adults.

Aging does not occur at exactly the same rate in everyone. Body systems age at different times and at different rates. There are also wide variations among individuals in the course of aging. For some people, the first sign of aging is loss of visual sharpness—requiring reading glasses, for example. For others, it is a slowdown of the digestive system and resulting constipation. These people find they must drink prune juice or eat more bran cereals to keep regular bowel habits.

Most people react to aging by becoming less active. They take up less strenuous sports and reduce their workload. This is a normal adjustment to the changes of aging. But reducing the level of activity does not and should not mean giving up all activity. With proper health maintenance and proper attitudes in people around them, the elderly can continue to lead active and rewarding lives (Figure 20.1).

The following is a discussion of specific changes that may be expected at some time in each body system. Now that you have studied these systems, you should be able to appreciate how the changes of aging affect their functioning.

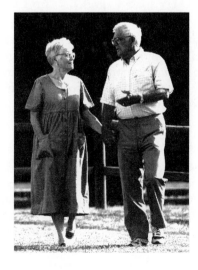

Figure 20.1
Proper health maintenance can help the elderly continue to lead active lives.

INTEGUMENTARY SYSTEM

The skin becomes thinner, drier, and loses its suppleness. The fatty layer under the skin disappears, causing wrinkles and folds and giving less protection against cold and injury. Bruising is more common. Spots of color appear on the skin, and small vessels are likely to burst, causing "spiders." Sweating decreases, and there is less blood flow to the skin. Elderly bedridden patients are at high risk of developing decubitus ulcers, or pressure sores.

CARDIOVASCULAR SYSTEM

The heart becomes less efficient, pumping less forcefully and less blood with each beat, while the number of beats per minute increases. The heart has less ability to gear up for action when the body is under stress. Various parts of the heart and the blood vessels lose elasticity, and fatty substances may be deposited on the inner layers of arteries. These deposits give more resistance to the heart's pumping action, so hypertension may develop. There is less blood flow to all parts of the body.

RESPIRATORY SYSTEM

A protein called **collagen** settles in the lungs, lessening their ability to expand. Along with reduced blood flow to the lungs, reduced expansion makes respiration less efficient, and not as much oxygen is supplied to the body. To make up for this deficiency, an older person may breathe faster than the normal 16 to 20 times per minute. Breathing is also shallower.

NERVOUS SYSTEM

Brain cells die and brain weight decreases. Less blood flow to the brain affects memory and the ability to make decisions. Confused thinking and personality changes can also result from the decreased supply of oxygen to the brain.

SENSORY SYSTEM

The ability to perceive messages received through the senses decreases. The eyes have difficulty adjusting to changes in light. The ears do not hear the higher sounds, and hearing aids may be needed. Taste and smell are dulled, so that eating becomes less pleasurable. The sense of touch is dulled. When the senses do not provide as much information as before, the elderly may become confused, especially in strange surroundings.

GASTROINTESTINAL SYSTEM

The secretions and muscular movements of the digestive tract slow down, and the elderly produce less stomach acid than normal. These changes make food harder to digest and slower to move through the system. Indigestion and constipation are common problems. If teeth are lost or inflamed, eating may be difficult or uncomfortable. Absorption of nutrients from the intestines is less efficient, so nutrition may be affected.

URINARY SYSTEM

There is less blood flow to the kidneys, and there are changes within the kidneys themselves. They do not filter the blood as efficiently, so wastes are excreted more slowly. The kidneys cannot adapt as quickly as before to changes in the fluid/electrolyte balance. Urgency and stress incontinence may occur in female patients from a decrease in perineal muscle tone. Urinary frequency may occur in males because of an enlarged prostate.

ENDOCRINE SYSTEM

All the glands secrete less of their hormones. As a result, body cell metabolism is not as well regulated and the body cannot react as quickly to stress.

REPRODUCTIVE SYSTEM

Usually between ages 45 and 52, females no longer menstruate or are able to conceive. In both men and women, sex hormone production decreases, with resulting physical changes. However, because sexual enjoyment is determined by attitudes and emotions, not just hormones, older people can still enjoy active sex lives.

MUSCULOSKELETAL SYSTEM

Muscles lose strength and flexibility. There is also an increase in the percentage of body fat, replacing muscle. The bones are more prone to demineralization and become lighter and more porous. As a result they are more apt to fracture easily and heal slowly. Ligaments and joints are subject to stiffening and thickening. Diseases of bones, joints, and ligaments are more common.

PHARMACOKINETICS IN THE AGED

Let us look at what the changes of aging do to the actions of drugs in the body. Recall that drugs entering the body undergo four processes: absorption, distribution, biotransformation (metabolism), and excretion. Naturally, the aging of the body systems has an impact on how drugs are absorbed, distributed, metabolized, and excreted. In general, absorption, metabolism, and excretion become slower, and distribution becomes unpredictable. For a person administering medications to the elderly, it is important to understand these pharmacokinetic effects of aging. This discussion will help you learn why you should be particularly watchful for side effects and unusual effects of drugs in the elderly.

SLOWER CIRCULATION, SLOWER ABSORPTION

Absorption and distribution are affected mainly by two things: slower blood circulation and slower absorption of oral medications through the intestines. Slower circulation occurs because the heart pumps less efficiently and must work against blood vessels that have lost their elasticity. The stomach and intestines have fewer of the digestive enzymes needed to help drugs break down and be absorbed through the lining. Peristalsis is weaker, so drugs do not reach the intestine as quickly. As a result, drug absorption and distribution are slower and less predictable in the elderly. Therefore, you cannot be sure that the proper dose is getting to where it is needed in the usual amount of time.

In addition, because of decreased circulation, the heart and brain compete with the rest of the body for the blood supply. They demand and get more blood, and other parts of the body get less. Distribution of drugs is affected, because more of the drugs end up in the heart and brain. This distribution can lead to abnormal drug reactions.

Biotransformation or metabolism of drugs is affected by the reduced capacity of the liver. Most drugs are biotransformed (metabolized) in the liver. In the elderly, however, the liver produces fewer enzymes to break down drugs, so they are not biotransformed as quickly or as completely. The drugs stay in effect longer and can build up in the body with repeated doses. The result may be a cumulative effect and even drug toxicity.

Excretion is affected by changes in kidney function. Reduced blood circulation and changes in kidney cells combine to make blood filtration slower. Thus drugs are not excreted as quickly. Again, they can build up in the body and show cumulative or toxic effects. Some drugs, such as urinary antiseptics, do not become active until they are excreted by the kidney. In the elderly these drugs take longer than usual to show an effect.

Finally, because of the body's lessened ability to keep a balance among all the systems, drugs are more apt to throw the body into wide imbalances. Unusual and unexpected drug reactions may occur from time to time. Also, the aged are more sensitive to the effects of certain drugs.

Because of these changes in pharmacokinetics, one must be very careful in administering medications to the elderly. As a general rule, medications for the elderly are prescribed in lower doses and less frequently to help prevent cumulation and toxicity. To aid absorption, adjustments are made in the forms of medication given and their routes.

DISEASES AND DRUG INTERACTIONS

Two other age-related factors have an impact on the effect of a drug: disease and other drugs. We have said that the elderly are more prone to disease. Adding disease factors to the age changes already mentioned, the overall picture becomes complicated. For instance, a diseased kidney or liver, a heart condition, or hypertension can further slow down the body's handling of drugs. Because the elderly tend to have more diseases, there is a greater chance for adverse drug reactions, especially cumulation.

Consider also the possible drug interactions. The elderly have more ailments, both major and minor, than do younger adults. Thus they are likely to take more drugs together. For example, they may routinely take nonprescription laxatives, antacids, or mild stimulants. Any of these can interact with drugs that a doctor may prescribe. It is extremely important for the medical staff to find out what other medications patients are taking on their own, especially OTC medications. For example, you may discover a tetracycline is prescribed for an infection for an elderly patient who may also be taking bicarbonate of soda for an upset stomach. As you know, antacids interfere with the absorption of tetracyclines.

As a situation that can be even more dangerous, consider the patient who is on corticosteroids for chronic rheumatoid arthritis, a condition common in the elderly population. Corticosteroids increase the excretion of potassium in the kidneys. Now suppose that the person develops a heart condition requiring digitalis, a cardiac stimulant. A normal dose of digitalis becomes dangerously strong (i.e., is potentiated) when there is little potassium in the body. Cardiac arrhythmias could result from the combined action of the corticosteroid and digitalis.

It is the physician's responsibility to avoid, wherever possible, prescribing drugs that could interact in a harmful way. But, as an added safety precaution, you too should be aware of possible interactions. There are times when the physician must order drugs that are known to interact because the risk of drug interaction is less than the risk of not giving two drugs the patient needs. In these circumstances, all the people who are attending the patient must be especially careful to chart any unusual signs. Examples of important drug interactions that can occur with medications for the elderly are listed in Table 20.1.

The complex pharmacokinetics in the elderly should suggest, then, that you be alert for possible adverse reactions and side effects. You must watch especially for signs of cumulation, toxicity, drug interactions, and unusual effects. All your skills of observation and communication are needed to ensure that older patients receive safe drug treatment. Talk with your patients, ask them questions, and carefully notice all their physical and psychological signs. Question the patients specifically about the use of a number of different drugs prescribed by different physicians (**polypharmacy**).

TABLE 20.1: Common Drug Interactions With Elderly Patients

DRUGS THAT INTERACT	RESULTS OF COMBINATION
Alcohol + sedatives	Both depress central nervous system and can result in toxicity
Antipsychotics + antiparkinsonian agents + antidepressants + antihistamines	All have anticholinergic effects; when combined, can cause dry mouth, blurred vision, urine retention, constipation, increased intraocular pressure
Nonsteroidal anti-inflammatory drugs + anticoagulants + acetylsalicylic acid	Increased anticoagulant effect, increased bleeding
Bisacodyl (*Dulcolax*) + antacids	Enteric coating of bisacodyl dissolves in stomach, causing gastric irritation
Tetracycline + metals (milk, antacids, and other substances containing calcium, magnesium, aluminum, or iron)	Reduced absorption of tetracycline can lessen its effect
Cholestyramine (*Questran*) or cholestipol (*Colestid*) (anticholesteremics) + acidic drugs	Poor absorption of acidic drugs may lessen their effects
Cathartics (laxatives)	Increased intestinal motility caused by carthartics can decrease absorption of any drug
Warfarin (*Coumadin*) + phenobarbital	Anticoagulant breaks down more quickly, so has less effect; increases risk of thrombus formation
Vitamin D + anticonvulsants phenytoin (*Dilantin*) and phenobarbital	Vitamin D breaks down more quickly; patient may require vitamin D supplements
Allopurinol (*Zyloprim*) + mercaptopurine (*Purinethol*) or azathioprine (*Imuran*)	Allopurinol slows breakdown of the other drugs; can lead to toxicity
Salicylates (e.g., aspirin) + acidifiers	Prolongs and possibly increases effects of salicylates; can lead to toxicity
Penicillins + probenecid (*Benemid*)	Excretion of penicillin blocked
Monoamine oxidase inhibitors + sympathomimetics (e.g., amphetamines)	Releases large amounts of norepinephrine; can cause severe headache, hypertension, or arrhythmias
Guanethidine (*Ismelin*) + tricyclic antidepressants or antipsychotics (e.g., chlorpromazine)	Decreases antihypertensive effect of guanethidine; fails to lower blood pressure
Digitalis + diuretics	Diuretics can cause potassium loss, making heart more sensitive to digitalis effects; can cause arrhythmias
Lithium carbonate + diuretics	Loss of sodium increases effects of lithium; toxicity (nausea, vomiting, weakness, sleepiness, seizures)
Digoxin + quinidine	Quinidine interferes with digoxin clearance; increases risk of digoxin toxicity (nausea, vomiting, weakness, heart rhythm changes)
Phenytoin + enteral feedings	Reduced phenytoin absorption

ADMINISTERING MEDICATIONS TO ELDERLY PATIENTS

Aging brings changes in the patterns of daily living. It also brings changes in your responsibilities as a giver of medications. Remember that you must individualize your treatment of each patient. The physician is responsible for adjusting dosages and routes, and you must adjust your care. You must be resourceful, caring, firm, patient, aware, and knowledgeable. The following suggestions may help you adjust your care to the elderly so as to achieve the best drug effect and maximize the patient's independence.

Identify the right patient. This is the first rule of the "five rights." As previously discussed, never administer medication to a patient who does not have an identification bracelet. Remember, any patient may incorrectly respond to a name. If the patient does not have an identification bracelet, have another identification bracelet made. If for some reason a patient will not leave the bracelet on, secure it to the head of the bed.

Explain what you are doing. Explaining your actions to the patient is one of the most important general rules for administering medications. Everyone likes to be told what to expect, even if they must expect some discomfort. Older people are sometimes fearful of medications. Explain cheerfully and positively why you are there, what medications you are giving, and how you will give them. Allowing elderly patients to take an active role in their own care helps them maintain their self-confidence and feeling of independence.

Be patient; do not rush. Encourage patients who are lying down to sit up before you administer medications. They will have an easier time swallowing the medication. Give one tablet at a time to swallow, and allow them time between tablets to rest. Take the time to treat each patient as an individual. A slow and easy approach on your part will encourage confidence and cooperation.

Explain what the drug is supposed to do. Explain in simple terms what the drugs are for. Encourage patients to ask questions about their medications. Questions and answers help to enhance patient compliance and drug effectiveness.

Help a patient who has trouble swallowing pills. When a patient has difficulty swallowing tablets or capsules, ask the physician to substitute a liquid medication if at all possible. Do not cut or crush a tablet or place it in applesauce or fruit juice. This practice can reduce the dose and effectiveness of some drugs. It may also cause choking or aspiration of medication particles. As a general principle, always offer a little fluid before giving a medication, to enhance swallowing. Encourage patients to drink 5 to 6 ounces of fluid after medication administration, unless a patient's condition, such as renal failure, contraindicates it. Encouraging fluid ensures that the medication leaves the esophagus and enters the stomach to speed its absorption.

When a patient appears confused, assess the reason. Confusion about identity, location, last drug taken, and so on comes from many sources. There may be a lack of oxygen in the brain. Medication that affects the nervous system may cause confusion. Or the patient may have psychological problems. Do not automatically assume that a patient has dementia or give up trying to communicate. Consider the drugs he or she is taking. Confusion and other mental status changes are frequent side effects of a number of medications. Help the patient focus on what you are saying. Encourage the patient to express his or her needs clearly and to stay in touch with reality.

Respect each patient's customs and beliefs. Be empathetic to patients' cultural and ethnic beliefs and traditions in regard to drug therapy. Be flexible and try to adapt to the patient's requests as much as the physician's orders allow.

Adapt to hearing and vision problems. The elderly may have difficulty hearing or seeing, so you need to adapt your behavior to their special problems. Speak slowly and clearly when giving instructions, and wait for signs of understanding. Stand facing the patient when you speak, so that he or she can read your lips. Write things down, if necessary, and use large letters that are easy to read. Sometimes what seems like mental confusion is merely a sign that a patient cannot hear or see what you are saying or doing. Always keep this possibility in mind so that you adjust to the patient's situation.

Blood and urine tests are important. When ordered, make sure these tests are done and the results checked. Many drugs do not have a therapeutic effect until they reach a certain level in the body. Tests are necessary to find out when this point has been reached. A patient who is fearful of tests may accept them better if you explain their importance.

Help elderly patients with eyedrops. Some patients prefer to administer their own eyedrops; others do not. Support their wish for independence. If you administer the eyedrops, take care not to contaminate the dropper by touching the eye or eyelashes. You may need to instruct the patient in self-administration. (See Practice Procedure 7.1 on page 133.)

Watch for dangers of OTC drugs. Seemingly harmless OTC drugs, which many elderly patients take, can be dangerous when they accumulate or interact with prescription drugs. Know the combined effects of OTC and prescription drugs so you can be alert to adverse reactions.

Make sure that all ordered medications are given. A good charting system and proper organization will ensure that each patient receives all ordered medications.

Explain the need for medication to asymptomatic patients. A patient who has no obvious symptoms may refuse medications. Explain to patients why they must continue to take some medications (e.g., those for hypertension and infection) even after the symptoms are under control.

Help elderly patients remember their medications and instructions. Arrange for your elderly patients to take medications at certain times each day, such as before meals. Taking medications at regularly scheduled times makes it easier for the patient to remember. If special instructions go along with the medications, explain them clearly and simply, but also write them out. If a patient has poor eyesight, label drug bottles with large letters.

Never force a patient to take medication. Explain the purpose of the medication. If your positive, encouraging attitude and your explanations of the benefits of the drugs do not get the patient to accept a drug, do not push the issue. Instead, report the problem to the nurse in charge and wait for further instructions. In some cases, medications will have to be given parenterally until the patient's cooperation can be secured for oral medication.

Keep medications secure. Never leave the medicine room unlocked. Patients may wander by and take medications that can cause them harm. Never leave the medicine cart unattended. Because you may be spending more time with elderly patients in giving their medications, you will have less time to keep an eye on the cart. On the other hand, you do not want to rush each patient. A good solution is to get an attendant to watch the cart while you help patients. When possible, lock the cart while you work with patients.

Chart medications promptly. Do your charting as soon as you finish giving medications. You will have many medications to chart, and you may be tempted to leave charting until the end of the day. This is a dangerous practice that can lead to medication errors. It can and must be avoided by properly organizing your charting procedures. The only correct time to chart medications is right after you give them. When a cart is used, the charting form for medications is usually on it for immediate charting.

Use caution with PRN medications. When a PRN order has a range of doses, try giving the smallest dose first. This dose is often enough to bring about the desired effect. Because of slow absorption and metabolism, a higher dose may produce unpleasant side effects or adverse reactions. Guard against giving a higher dose of a PRN medication just because a patient is confused. The PRN medication may actually be causing the confusion through some effect on the oxygen supply to the brain. Make sure you chart PRN medications immediately. If you put it off until later, someone else may give the patient another dose of the medication. The patient may not remember that you gave a previous dose. It is easy to overdose a patient accidentally by forgetting to chart PRN medications. You should be aware that some patients may pretend to take their medications but actually put their pills and capsules in pockets, drawers, pillow cases, plants, or anywhere. Report this to the nurse in charge and follow his or her instructions. Be aware that this can happen and try to prevent it.

ENGAGING PATIENTS IN THEIR CARE

When you give medications to the elderly, it is important to remember that they can and should take an active part in their medication therapy. They should be encouraged to take their own medications under your supervision. They can pour their own glass of water. They can apply their own ointments. They can help design a plan for remembering to take all their medications. The point is that their care includes concern for their mental health. Your treatment must leave room for independent effort. Let them do as much as they are capable of doing, even if you could do it more quickly and efficiently. Their mental health

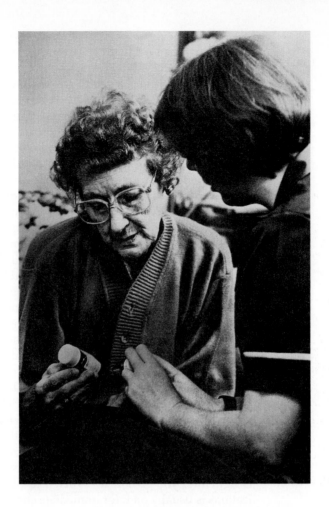

Figure 20.2
Take time to talk and listen to the patient. Encourage patients to take an active role in their medication therapy.

depends on your letting them care for themselves when they are willing and able to do so. Give medical care with the patient, not for the patient (Figure 20.2).

Finally, be prepared to meet many needs in individual elderly patients. Be supportive of their activities. Encourage them to get the most they can out of life. Show that you care about them, and help ease their physical and emotional burdens. You and your fellow workers have the power to make their lives miserable or rewarding. Do not abuse that power. The more you help them be independent and confident, the less the aged will feel like a burden, both to you and to themselves.

Define each of the terms listed below.

1. Geriatrics _____

2. Gerontology _____

3. Polypharmacy _____

4. OTC medications _____

Briefly describe the major changes that occur in the following body systems as one ages:

5. Integumentary system _____

_____

_____

_____

6. Cardiovascular system _____

_____

_____

_____

7. Respiratory system _____

_____

_____

_____

8. Nervous system _____

_____

_____

_____

9. Sensory system _____

_____

_____

_____

10. Gastrointestinal system _____

_____

_____

_____

11. Urinary system _____

_____

_____

_____

Continued

12. Endocrine system _____

_____

_____

_____

13. Reproductive system _____

_____

_____

_____

14. Musculoskeletal system _____

_____

_____

_____

Answer the following question in the space provided.

15. How and why does a doctor usually adjust the normal adult dose when ordering medications for an elderly patient?

_____

_____

_____

■ CASE STUDIES FOR CRITICAL THINKING

The following are situations or scenes that might take place in a long-term care facility or in a hospital unit that has many elderly patients. Answer the questions briefly, using the information in this chapter.

16. Mr. Jones and Mr. Smith are both 80 years old. Mr. Jones is strong and physically active and enjoys taking walks. He wears glasses to correct his failing vision. He is forgetful sometimes and tends to tell the same jokes over and over again. Mr. Smith, on the other hand, is frail and walks with a cane, but his watchful eyes take in everything that goes on. His mind is sharp, and he entertains the nursing home staff with his views of current political and social events. Why are these men so different in their physical ability and mental alertness, even though they are the same age? What does this mean for their medication therapy?

_____

_____

17. Ms. Peach is taking life easier than she used to, because she finds that her energy runs out more quickly now that she is 72. Her breathing has become slightly faster and shallower than before, which the doctor says is normal for a person her age. What changes has her respiratory system probably undergone as a result of aging?

_____

_____

_____

Continued

18. Doc Webster is a grand old man who is full of stories about the days when he practiced surgery in a big city hospital. He is taking a number of medications for heart disease and a nervous condition. Today, when you go to his room, he does not answer to his name and has forgotten where he is. It's hard for you to give him his medication instructions, because he can't seem to concentrate on what you are saying. What possible reasons might explain why he appears confused?

_____

_____

_____

19. In giving elderly Mrs. Nimitz her medications, you want to be sure to treat her as an independent, intelligent adult. How can you help her be responsible for taking her medications?

_____

_____

_____

20. Mr. Redbone is under medication for an infection and several other minor disorders. Because of his advanced age, you know that his liver and kidneys are not working as well as they once did. What effect does a weakened kidney or liver have on how the body handles drugs? What adverse reaction should you be on the lookout for?

_____

_____

_____

21. Mrs. Mendoza is suffering from phlebitis and must take an anticoagulant to keep blood clots from forming. She keeps a bottle of aspirin in her purse for occasional arthritic pain. She also has an old bottle of tranquilizers her sister gave her. She hasn't mentioned the aspirin and tranquilizers to her doctor, but she asks if you think it would be all right to take them when necessary. What should you say?

_____

_____

_____

22. Your facility has recently admitted a number of new patients, so the staff's workload is heavier than usual. You are busy giving medications and carrying out your other duties. You would like to put off your charting until the end of the day, but you're not sure you should. How will your decision affect the welfare of your patients?

_____

_____

_____

23. A new elderly patient, Mr. Minassian, is getting his first dose of medicine. You are instructing him on the usual side effects of the drug. He is smiling and nodding, but he does not seem to understand what you are saying. What can you do to make sure he gets the information he needs?

_____

_____

_____

24. Ms. Brill sweetly declines any medications you offer her, saying that she doesn't need them. You are worried because you know that her blood pressure could become dangerously high if she fails to take the antihypertensive, and she needs *Diabinese* to control a tendency toward high blood sugar. What should you do?

_____

_____

_____

 Inter*NET* CONNECTION

An Internet Web site that focuses on aging is the National Institute on Aging at http://www.nih.gov/nia. Click on What's New. Listed are a variety of topics related to aging; explore some of these to observe the type of information abailable. Click on Health Information and select the heading of Alzheimer's Disease. Click on the heading to get a better understanding of the disease, including information on the most recent drug clinical trials.

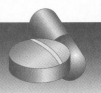

INDEX

Hyponatremia, 239
Hypotension, 163
 orthostatic, 170
Hypothalamus, 270
Hypothyroidism, 268–269
Hypovitaminosis, 96
Hypoxia, 192
Hytone (hydrocortisone), 147, 153, 279
Hytrin (terazosin), 257

IBS (irritable bowel syndrome), 213
Ibuprofen *(Advil; Haltran; Medipren; Midol 2000; Motrin; Motrin IB; Nuprin; Pamprin; Rufen)*, 294, 308
IDDM (insulin-dependent diabetes mellitus), 274
Idiosyncrasies, 23t, 24
Ileocecal valve, 209
Ileum, 209
Iliac crest, 348, 348f
Imferon (ferrous sulfate), 25, 102, 173
Imipramine *(Tofranil)*, 317, 321
Immune system, 108, 329
Immunity, 108
Immunization, 109
Immunomodulating agents, 333
Imodium (loperamide), 217
Impotence, 254
Impulses, nerve, 301
Imuran (azathioprine), 292, 304
Incident reports, 80, 81f
 filling out, 85
Incontinence, 236
Inderal (propranolol hydrochloride), 162, 170, 175, 245
Indian tobacco *(Lobelia inflata)*, 101t
Indications, 5
Indigestion, 210
Indocin (indomethacin), 294
Indomethacin *(Indocin)*, 294
Induration, 346
Indwelling catheter, 243, 245–246
Infants, drug action in, 19
Infections, 107–110. *See also specific types of infections*
 bacterial, 117t
 of bones, 289
 of brain, 306
 chlamydial, 117t
 drugs for. *See* Antibiotics; Anti-infectives
 of gastrointestinal system, 212
 immune system and, 108
 immunization against, 109
 nosocomial, 108
 parasitic, 117t
 patients at risk for, 109–110
 protozoan, 117t
 respiratory, 187
 rickettsial, 117t
 sexually transmitted, 256–257
 of skin, 146
 spirochetal, 117t

staphylococcal, 110
superinfections, 112
of urinary tract, 236–237
vaginal, 255–256
viral, 117t
Infectious diseases, 107, 117t
Infertility, 258
Inflammation, 142–143
 of brain, 306
 drugs for. *See* Anti-inflammatory drugs
 gastrointestinal, 213
 respiratory, 187
 vaginal, 255
Infusions, intravenous, 59–60
INH (isoniazid), 187, 195
Inhalation, 58
Inhalers, metered-dose, 198
Injections. *See* Injection sites; Parenteral administration route
Injection sites, 345–348
 intradermal, 345–346, 346f
 intramuscular, 347f, 347–348, 348f
 locating and inspecting, 349
 rotating, 350–351, 351f
 subcutaneous, 346, 346f
Inoculation, 109
Inorganic substances, 99
Insect bites and stings, 149t
Insertion, of topical medications, 58
Insomnia, 303, 316
Instillation, 58
Insulin, 3, 273, 275t, 275–276, 276f
 administration of, 280–281
 drugs interacting with, 278, 279t
 produced by body, 210
Insulin *(Humulin N; Humulin R)*, 275
Insulin-dependent diabetes mellitus (IDDM), 274
Intal (cromolyn sodium), 189
Integumentary system, 141. *See also* Skin
 aging of, 364
Interferon alfa-2a *(Roferon A)*, 322
Interferon alfa-2b *(Intron A)*, 322
Interstitial fluid, 164
Intestinal motility, 211
Intestine. *See also* Gastrointestinal system
 inflammation of, 213
 large, 209
 parasites in, 213
 small, 209
Intra-arterial injections, 60
Intracardiac injections, 60
Intracutaneous administration route. *See* Intradermal (intracutaneous) administration route
Intradermal (intracutaneous) administration route, 59
 administration procedure for, 355
 sites for, 345–346, 346f
Intramuscular administration route, 59, 60f
 administration procedure for, 357
 sites for, 347f, 347–348, 348f
 Z-track method for, 351–352, 352f

Intraspinal injections, 60
Intrathecal injections, 60
Intravenous administration route, 59–60
Intravenous infusions, 59–60
Intron A (interferon alfa-2b), 322
Intropin (dopamine), 168
Iodine, 3, 4, 100t
 radioactive isotopes of, 273
 thyroid function and, 269
 tincture of, 54
Ions, 101
Ipecac syrup, 215, 219t
Ipratropium *(Atrovent)*, 189
Iron, 3, 100t. *See also* Ferrous sulfate *(Feosol; Fer-In-Sol; FeSol; Imferon)*
Iron deficiency anemia, 168
Irrigation, 58
 of bladder, 243
Irritable bowel syndrome (IBS), 213
Islets of Langerhans, 270
Isocarboxazid *(Marplan)*, 317
Isolation, 110, 117–120, 118t
 medication administration to patients in, 119, 119f, 122–123
Isoniazid (INH), 187, 195
Isoproterenol *(Isuprel)*, 189
Isopto Atropine (atropine sulfate), 133
Isopto Carpine (pilocarpine hydrochloride), 132
Isordil (isosorbide), 169
Isosorbide *(Isordil)*, 169
Isotretinoin *(Accutane)*, 144
Isradipine *(DynaCirc)*, 170
Isuprel (isoproterenol), 189
Itching, 143
Ivy Dry Cream, 149t

Jaundice, 212
Jejunum, 209
Johnson's Medicated Powder, 149t
Joints, 288f, 288–289. *See also* Musculoskeletal system

Kaolin, 217
Kaolin + pectin *(Kaopectate)*, 217, 219t
Kaon (potassium supplement), 102, 170, 241, 245
Kaopectate (kaolin + pectin), 217, 219t
Kardex file, 69
Kato Powder (potassium chloride), 55
K-Dur (potassium supplement), 102, 170, 241, 245
Keflex (cephalexin), 114
Keflin (cephalothin), 114
Kemadrin (procyclidine), 309
Kenalog (triamcinolone), 147, 153, 189, 279
Keratin, 141
Keratolytic agents, 144, 147, 152
Keratosis, 143
Keri, 149t
Ketoacidosis, 275
Kidney(s), 234–235
 disorders of, 235–237

Kidney failure, 237
Kidney stones, 236
Kilogram, 34t
Kilometer, 33
K-Lor (potassium supplement), 102, 170, 241, 245
K-lyte (potassium supplement), 102, 170, 241, 245
KNOWN/UNKNOWN formula, 39
Kwell (lindane), 146, 148
Kytril (granisetron), 333

Labeling instructions, 63
Labia, 252
Lacrimal glands, 128
Lactinex, 217
Lanoxin (digoxin), 161, 171, 175
Large intestine, 209
Larodopa (levodopa), 309
Larynx, 183, 183f
Lasix (furosemide), 170, 171, 240–241, 244
Laws. *See* Legislation
Laxatives, 211, 217–218, 223
LD (learning disability), 316
Learning disability (LD), 316
Legislation, 7–10, 8t, 9t
  health team responsibilities and, 10
Lesions, 143
Leukemia, 168
Leukeran (chlorambucil), 332
Leukine (GM-CSF), 333
Leukocytes, 108, 164, 309
Leukopenia, 333
Levodopa *(Dopar; Larodopa)*, 309
Levodopa + carbidopa *(Sinemet)*, 309, 311
Levonorgestrel *(Norplant)* implants, 260
Levophed (norepinephrine), 168
Levothroid (levothyroxine sodium), 270, 281
Levothyroxine sodium *(Levothroid; Synthroid)*, 270, 281
LH (luteinizing hormone), 272
Libritabs (chlordiazepoxide hydrochloride), 9t, 318, 322
Librium (chlordiazepoxide hydrochloride), 9t, 318, 322
Lidex (fluocinonide), 147
Ligaments, 289
Lindane (gamma-benzene hexachloride; *Kwell*), 146, 148
Liniments, 55
Lioresal (baclofen), 293, 295
Liothyronine sodium *(Cytomel)*, 280
Liotrix *(Euthroid)*, 280
Liquids, 53t, 54. *See also* Fluid(s); Solutions
  aqueous and viscous, 341
  pouring, 73
Liter, 33, 34t
Lithane (lithium carbonate), 318–319, 323
Lithium carbonate *(Eskalith; Lithane)*, 318–319, 323

Liver, 209
  disorders of, 211
Lobelia inflata (asthma weed), 101t
Local effects, 22
Lomotil (atropine sulfate + diphenoxylate hydrochloride), 9t, 223
Loop diuretics, 169–170
Loperamide *(Imodium)*, 217
Lopid (gemfibrozil), 171
Lopressor (metoprolol tartrate), 170, 175
Lorazepam *(Ativan)*, 9t, 317, 322, 333
Lorelco (probucol), 171
Lotions, 55
Lovastatin *(Mevacor)*, 171
Lovenox (anoxaparin sodium), 172, 306
Loxapine *(Loxitane)*, 318
Loxitane (loxapine), 318
Lozenges, 56
LSD (lysergic acid diethylamide), 9t
Lubricants, laxative, 218
Ludiomil (maprotiline), 317
Lumen, of needle, 341
Lung(s). *See* Respiratory system
Lupron Depot, 256
Luteinizing hormone (LH), 272
Lymph, 164
Lymphatic system, 164
Lymphokines, 333
Lysergic acid diethylamide (LSD), 9t
Lytren, 243

Maalox (aluminum hydroxide + magnesium salts), 25, 67, 214, 215, 219t
Maalox Plus (aluminum hydroxide + magnesium salts), 25, 67, 214, 215, 219t
Maceration, 149
Macrodantin (nitrofurantoin), 244
Macrolides, 114–115
Macrominerals, 99, 99t
Madderwort *(Artemisia absinthium)*, 101t
Mafenide acetate *(Sulfamylon)*, 144, 153
Magmas, 55
Magnesium, 99t
Magnesium hydrochloride (milk of magnesia), 3, 55, 67, 214, 219t
Magnesium salts, 217
Magnesium salts + aluminum hydroxide *(Gelusil; Maalox; Maalox Plus; Mylanta)*, 25, 67, 214, 215, 219t
Magnesium sulfate (Epsom salts), 3, 217
Major tranquilizers, 318–319
Male reproductive system, 253f, 253–254
Malignant tumors, 330. *See also* Antineoplastic drugs; Cancer
Mammary glands. *See* Breasts
Mandelamine (methenamine), 240
Manic-depressive illness, 318–319
MAOIs (monoamine oxidase inhibitors), 25
Maprotiline *(Ludiomil)*, 317

MAR (medication administration record), 70, 70f
Marezine (cyclizine), 215, 219t
Marijuana, 9t
Marinol (dronabinol), 216, 333
Marplan (isocarboxazid), 317
Mask, oxygen therapy administered by, 199f, 199–200
Master gland, 268
Maxair (pirbuterol), 189
Maxzide (hydrochlorothiazide + triamterene), 170, 240
Mazicon (flumazenil), 318
Measurement, of hard to measure drugs, 34
Measurement systems, 32–34
  converting among, 34–36, 35t, 36f, 36t
Mechlorethamine hydrochloride *(Mustargen)*, 332, 334
Meclizine *(Antivert; Bonine)*, 215, 219t, 222
Medical abbreviations, 64t, 64–65
Medicated baths, 151
Medication(s). *See* Drug(s); *specific drugs and drug types*
Medication administration record (MAR), 70, 70f
Medication error(s)
  avoiding, 74
  reporting, 80, 81f
Medication error form, 80, 81f
Medication forms, abbreviations for, 53t
Medication orders, 60, 61f, 62f, 62–63. *See also* Physician's order sheet
  basic parts of, 62–63
  keeping track of, 69–72
  PRN, 63. *See also* PRN drugs
  questioning, 64
  routine, 66
  self-terminating, 70–71, 71f
  standing, 63
  stat, 63
  transcribing, 81–82
  verbal, 62
Medicine cards, 69
Medicine cart, 67–68, 68f
  dispensing unit-dose medications from, 84–85
Medicine room, 67
Medicine tray, 68, 69f
Medipren (ibuprofen), 294, 308
Mediquell (dextromethorphan), 188, 189, 193
Medi-Quick, 149t
Medrol (methylprednisolone), 217, 279
Medroxyprogesterone acetate *(Depo-Provera; Provera)*, 259–260
Megace (megestrol), 259
Megadoses, of vitamins, 98–99
Megestrol *(Megace)*, 259
Melleril (thioridazine), 318
Menopause, 254
Menorrhea, 254